ADVANCED ADJUSTING TECHNIQUES

CHIROPRACTIC CARE FOR PHYSICALLY COMPROMISED PATIENTS

William J. Ruch, D.C

Table of Contents

ACKNOWLEDGEMENTS

I would like to thank those folks that were helpful in getting this book published. My reviewers were very helpful with their suggestions and comments. They are Dr.'s Rebekah Connors, Kerri Duggins, Roger Coleman, Eric Fredrickson, Christophe Mulinghaus and Victoria Nelson, also Margaret Kelly. Susan Hesse was our final editor and we owe her a lot because, as a layperson, this is a difficult text to evaluate.

This book makes use of patients as models to demonstrate adjusting or examination procedures. They were all very patient with us as we set up various shots. They are Susan Paulson, Mynor Ohlinger, Zora Katz, Zoe Tamano-Hill, Victoria Nelson, Rachel Ruch, Sonia Escobar, Yarka Cleary, Shayestah Talai, Margaret Kelly, Michael Delcollo and Dr. Samantha Ma.

The "Z's", Zoe and Zora have become quite efficient at set lighting for photo shoots.

Paul Marcus has done his usual excellent work with typesetting, and Kim Lemoine has provided final formatting and graphic elements..

INTRODUCTION

The need to modify my technique was made clear to me with my first patient in my new office in 1987. She was 36-years-old, walked with a cane, had persistent swollen legs and ankles, had not liked the "cracking" type of manipulation and was now giving up on the Activator Technique as ineffective.

Before I went to the chiropractic college, I was in the residential remodeling business. I was a superintendent of construction for a large firm. I knew all the trades, having worked my way up the ladder, so although I no longer had my tool belt on, I was telling people what to do. I had critical thinking skills, and it was now time to apply them.

Going into an older home to do renovation and upgrading is quite different from new construction; a different approach is required with different tools and skills. Delicate work is needed to work on older homes. Not that 36 is old, but having had 20 years of instability and dysfunction made her a complex case. Everyone in her past had ascribed her problems to the spine, but they hadn't even evaluated her knees and ankles.

I was trained in Chiropractic Biophysics, which does not offer extremity protocols. I had taken a series of Extremity Adjusting classes in the College curriculum in addition to attending a number of weekend seminars on the subject. I felt none of them had prepared me for someone with chronically swollen lower legs and an obvious joint dysfunction of the ankles and feet. Big yanking and distraction-type manipulations were not an option for her, since she was too sensitive.

I could see her lower limbs were deformed and inflamed and in need of intervention. I knew there was a building code to the body and my goal became to reduce the building code violations (reduce the subluxations). So that is what I did. She taught me a lot, as did all the patients that have followed. Many of my patients have terrible stories: hip replacements gone bad, failed back surgeries, genetic disorders, you name it, they have come through my doors.. Yet they've shared the will and drive to keep working and get better. I am forever honored and grateful for their willingness to let me help them achieve better functioning bodies and improved quality of life. That first patient was off the cane in three weeks, but she needed it again, 23 years later, in her final days when she was in chemotherapy, to keep herself steady as she walked with terrible weakness.

So began my journey toward the development of these gentle yet effective adjusting techniques to address the needs of the injured, impaired and suffering patients with multiple injuries and other health problems.

May this book help you with that task.

CHAPTER ONE

Protocols of Care: General Concepts for Evaluating, Treating and Managing Patients with Special Needs

Some of the joint limitations we may find above and beyond the chief trauma would include fusion from surgery, natural degenerative changes, or prostheses. The adjustive approaches described in this text involve multiple low-force impulses with instruments, by hand or drop table, according to the extent of injury to the joints and injury to the surrounding joints.

For example, the knee and hip adjustments that follow were designed for patients with knee/hip replacements, bony fusions (with cadaver bone) and/or with spinal rods, wires and screws. These adjustments involve the use of a drop table, the Thuli speeder board and a spring-loaded adjusting instrument (Activator type). These procedures are also effective on patients with less severe injuries.

All musculoskeletal evaluative procedures include an assessment via static palpation, some motion palpation (it is amazing how many patients have normal Range of Motion with subluxations), mechanism of injury (patient history) and X-ray and/or Advanced Imaging analysis. Some of these displacements can be clearly viewed on radiographs. Some, not so clearly.

Projection error obscures pubic symphysis subluxation on anterior-posterior (AP) lumbopelvic views. The signs of rib cage subluxation at the spine on X-ray or MRI are not recognized by the radiographic community. This can complicate arriving at a correct diagnosis.

The resolution of symptoms is mostly dependent on the effectiveness of the intervention, but also the age of the patient, their conditioning, the type of injury, length of time since the trauma and the individual's unique body type and ligamentous integrity. Careful patient management and the patient's ability to follow instructions will be essential for progress. The patient must be instructed how to modify their daily activities to maximize healing and function. Sharing the goals with the patients allows them to be co-managers in their recovery.

Patients with advanced arthritis and spinal surgeries or joint replacements have had some kind of traumatic event – in most cases, years earlier. I find most of these patients are victims of modern injuries, the type currently being treated in the United States and other industrialized countries in the 21st century. Most of the patients that I've evaluated and treated have a history of traumatic events that their grandparents or great grandparents could never have suffered.

Ligament injury and the accompanying joint instability equal the etiology of osteoarthritis. So in evaluating a patient with osteoarthritis, I'm looking for joint dysfunction and ligament injury throughout their whole body. Treating these individuals requires an understanding of the full extent of their injuries.

In chiropractic education, many techniques approach a single issue that needs to be addressed and assumes joint integrity of the rest of the structures in the region. Patients that have suffered moderate injuries frequently have no uninjured limbs and no stable joints. This creates challenges for not just the treatment, but the management of the multiply-injured patient. It has been my experience that managing the injuries is more difficult than adjusting them.

Ligament injuries are tough to manage and take a long time to recover, if ever. Most patients with advanced arthritis and surgical replacements are past the age of 40, and healing time is greatly increased. The older you get, the longer your repair time – and this can be very frustrating for quite a few patients. Along with their gray hair and grizzled appearance, they are experiencing a new feature of their lives – being old and injured. They resent it and their frustrations can make managing their cases difficult. But patients with multiple health problems who regain some of their mobility as well as more understanding, and therefore get more control of their condition can be forever grateful. Someone who is frail with advanced arthritis, hip replacement and cardiac problems will be helped significantly when their pelvis and lower extremities are restored to normal alignment. The increased mobility not only improves their quality of life but also their prognoses for cardiac problems and arthritis.

MODERN INJURIES

"Modern injuries" is my term for the results of an event or events that disrupt the integrity of the spine, pelvis, and rib cage, including the anterior joints of the chest and extremities. There is a global, or complete effect on the body. In my experience, most of the injuries will become arthritic if enough time passes. Most of these "modern injuries" occur in incidents that involve a high rate of speed and rapid deceleration. The way we get hurt in these accidents is something that's of recent origin. A hundred years ago, what kind of car accidents were we having? Cars didn't travel very fast and there weren't many of them. Now, most people I encounter as patients and students have been in at least one, but often multiple motor vehicle accidents. Most people are still suffering from the effects of those accidents despite chiropractic care.

The advent of motor vehicle accidents is a major factor in patients' lives and is something that we as chiropractors are having to deal with often. There were 10,000,000 motor vehicle accidents in the U.S. per year from 1990 to 2009, according to the National Safety Council – which means there were as many as 200 million accidents over that entire period of time. Most of these accidents were multiple vehicle and multiple occupant events. So the incidence of spinal trauma and other joint injuries, including the anterior joints, could be in the 15,000,000 to 20,000,000 range per year. A lot of these injuries will never have full recovery. By these numbers, we can easily see that two-thirds of the U.S. population has been exposed to spinal trauma and other joint injuries – and therefore, future osteoarthritis.

A typical high-speed, rapid-deceleration crash involves a lot of instantaneous overstretching of the spine, shoulder and extremities. In my opinion, the therapy to recover from these events should not reproduce the event. A lot of traditional chiropractic manipulation involves instantaneous overstretching. For joints and ligaments to recover from an injury involving instantaneous overstretching, it does not seem sensible to perform instantaneous overstretching as a therapeutic intervention.

With regard to chiropractic care, the traditional manipulative procedures sometimes called the "Flying Seven" can cause further injury and harm to motor vehicle accident injuries. I feel this approach does not analyze, or take into account the possibility of anterior joint injuries. In my experience, a lot of the population has a negative impression of chiropractic care because of the rough nature of the procedures on the type of injuries commonly suffered by the population. A common story I hear is that a forceful cervical manipulation has caused a feeling of injury to the neck. When evaluating a patient with that complaint I find costosternal and sternoclavicular joint injuries, which cause rigid scalene muscles and sternocleidomastoid muscles. These relax when the affected joints are brought back into alignment. In my opinion, a forceful manipulative chiropractic treatment with rigid musculature from unresolved subluxations only complicates an injury that is already difficult to treat.

The type of injuries patients are sustaining are different from the type of injuries they were being treated for decades ago. The traditional manipulative procedures were developed, in some cases, more than a century ago. According to our own studies (JMPT 2010), chiropractors are treating approximately five percent of the population. The same statistic was used at the 1974 Palmer graduation ceremony, which means that nothing has changed in the profession in over 40 years.

My contact with various groups from the community would indicate at least 80 percent of the population is somewhat wary or frankly afraid of us. I feel this has a lot to do with our profession not responding appropriately to these new types of injuries. Injuries to the sternal joints and pubic symphysis will not respond to side posture manipulation, anterior dorsal or posterior dorsal procedures.

The Rotary Break for cervical spine manipulation has caused a lot of people to be terrified of chiropractic care. Most of my patients can describe injuries from manipulative procedures. I personally have been hurt by chiropractic care. In retrospect, in analyzing my particular experience, assumptions were made that I had an intact, healthy chest wall, (I do not). Also, there was an assumption that my leg pain was radiating leg pain, when in fact I have injured legs, (no one ever examined my legs). The decompression therapy I did for a number of years on an inversion table added to the destabilizing of my lower leg and ankle ligaments and contributed to the chronic nature of my problems. So this illustrates another one of the principles of this work: when evaluating somebody's injuries from a motor vehicle accident or other rapid deceleration event, assume all components of the patient's body have been injured and look to the areas of pain to find the injury. Do not assume that leg pain is coming from the spine, it's likely to be an injured leg; for shoulder and arm pain, it is likely that the arm and shoulder are injured.

There is a study in *Spine* magazine from 1996, involving 96 people, who claim to have had no back injury or back pain and yet, 46 of them had herniating or bulging discs – all of them asymptomatic. Of course, from a clinical point of view, these are 46 people with damaged spines who deny trauma – which should be of interest in and of itself. Understating or omitting previous trauma is common and should be anticipated when interviewing a new patient with multiple health challenges or injuries.

In dissecting more than 250 spines, I discovered most had signs of having been in traumatic events, like motor vehicle accidents. There was osteoarthritis of the sternal joints in a lot of the bodies. Some of the osteophytes on the inside of the chest wall impinged on the great vessels. In my opinion, this was a complex protective mechanism. The body felt it was more important to keep the chest wall intact, even if it meant some intra-thoracic space was sacrificed to accomplish the task. Additionally, I found the pubic symphysis was injured and misaligned on most of the spines. These discoveries led me to start to evaluate these joints in my patients. I rarely had a patient tell me they had chest wall pain or pubic symphysis pain, but the vast majority of them had a +2 or +3 flinch response on palpation of those joints. This meant that the posterior joints connected to these anterior structures could not be aligned. The vast majority of these same patients complained of back pain, not anterior pain.

This is one of the cornerstones of my method – **if you do not look for it, you will not find it.** The same thing can be said of leg pain and arm pain: if you don't evaluate the extremities and instead assume everything is coming from the spine, you will have marginal, if not ineffective outcomes.

I do feel very strongly that realigning the joints and stabilizing ligaments is an essential, if not the only rational approach to treating and managing moderate injuries. Therefore, I am proposing gentle adjusting that is repetitive in nature to carefully realign the joints and appropriate use of soft braces to help stabilize ligaments.

My construction analogy could continue, describing the motor vehicle accident as a seismic event for the human body. If your house suffered an earthquake, what part of your house would you want your contractor to ignore concerning its repair? Every component of the house suffered some seismic force, deforming it. From the foundation to the roof rafters, everything should be inspected and assessed for structural integrity. I feel our patients deserve the same comprehensive approach.

GENTLE ADJUSTING USING REPETITIVE MOVEMENTS WITH THE SLI OR DROP TABLE/DROP PIECES

Gentle adjusting of the spine, rib cage, pelvis and extremities with the use of a spring-loaded adjusting instrument and drop table or drop piece is my preferred way to realign the joints and treat these types of injuries. When doing these adjustments, we want to avoid reproducing the way the injury occurred, so we use a careful application of force. I can't stress this truth too often. The spring-loaded adjusting instrument, the drop table and a small drop piece allow me to do gentle adjusting at the site of injury by using controlled, isolated force and does not involve other parts of the body, which have also probably been injured.

Defining manipulation and adjusting as different approaches in manual medicine is not a unique statement. There has been a long history of discussion on this topic. Most manipulation techniques assume an intact and stable core, rib cage and pelvis. This is not the case with a lot of my patients, including their limbs. I am defining "manipulation" as long axis motions taking articular structures into a para-physiological position, (not achievable with normal movement). "Adjusting" is the application of a small controlled force to realign articular components. The spring-loaded adjusting instrument and the drop table and the drop piece all allow low-force, repetitive yet gentle adjusting to the specific joint complex that's being targeted.

We also have patients that have advanced arthritis. They are not only living longer, but the injuries that generate the arthritis are occurring at a younger age. So I treat a number of patients in their 30s that have advanced arthritis. They were involved in motor vehicle accidents in their childhood or teenage years. Twenty years later, they have advanced arthritis and degenerative discs and other arthritic joints affecting their quality of life. We also have patients that have surgical joint replacement and spinal implants in their 20s and 30s. Cancer is occurring in younger people, so we have cancer survivors in their 30s and 40s with a history of surgery – in some cases, multiple surgeries. These previous procedures can make standard prone adjusting impractical and painful.

There is a prevalence of motor vehicle accidents at all ages, especially among young children and teens. I have patients in their 50s and 60s that were in serious accidents as children, and they still suffer from the effects of the accident. These injuries include damage to the spine, rib cage, pelvis, shoulders, arms and legs, including the knees and ankles. I have a patient that was 12 years old when I first examined her, with arthritis in her thoracic spine, from an accident at age six, she's now 34 and a mother. She still needs regular care to manage the pain.

For some, obesity and heart disease are part of the situation, making these very tough cases to manage. Some obese patients are only in their 20s or 30s, and many are deconditioned. Conditioning can be especially difficult for patients with injuries to the pelvic girdle and lower extremities. Injuries to the knees and ankles in childhood or young adulthood will influence the pattern of activity or lack of activity, building influence throughout their lives. All the conditions being discussed here can affect functional capacity greatly, sometimes to a debilitating extent.

Getting people moving, increasing their activity levels by lessening the joint dysfunction of their knees and feet can drastically change their lives. I have severely arthritic patients that were headed towards lives in wheelchairs that are out and about, maintaining their independent lives. Many studies show the benefits of increased activity and conditioning for cardiovascular problems, depression, obesity, arthritis and osteoporosis. Chiropractic care can be very helpful to these patients. Additionally, the cancer patients I have treated resent the limitations of their affliction and welcome any improvement in their functional capacity and reduction of pain without further medication.

SOME CONTRAINDICATIONS FOR MANIPULATION:

- *Advanced arthritis*
- *Advanced osteoporosis*
- *Spinal surgeries including hardware and fusions*
- *Hip replacements*
- *Knee replacements*
- *Apprehension and fear of manipulation*
- *Certain types of cancer*

THE BODY HAS A BUILDING CODE

As I said earlier, I have a construction background in residential remodeling. I often view the human form as analogous to a structure and its framework. Most of my patients have suffered seismic events and a disruption of the major components of their structural residence.

Because of this background, I use construction analogies: I feel that rough framing, where I am driving 3 1/2 inch nails with a 24 ounce framing hammer with full force, is my example of the big manipulation techniques I was taught in school. However, the gentle isolated repetitive thrusts that I advocate for the arthritic, terrified or frail patients, I compare to cabinet work.

In cabinet work, there are no forceful hammering activities, no big nails to drive. Everything is done with care and precision, so as not to challenge the integrity of the frame or its parts. You don't want to mar the finish or damage the milling. Everything is handled with great care. It takes longer to build the kitchen cabinets and install them than it does to build the walls and roof of the kitchen. So there is a time-consuming aspect to treating these types of patients, but there is the priceless payoff of taking a completely disabled patient with multiple injuries and giving their lives back to them via chiropractic care.

THE BODY HAS VITAL CAVITIES

I've treated a number of patients with spinal injuries, and they have taught me a lot. One of the main principles I've learned is how much the spinal cord controls things, even below the cord break. A quadriplegic will still have Patellar and Achilles tendon reflexes. A reflex is defined as a spinal cord mediated response to stimuli, such as tapping a tendon. What also is intact below the cord break are guarding reflexes that protect the vital cavities and extremities.

The vital cavities are: the spinal canal, the rib cage and the pelvic girdle. The vital cavities are labeled as such because the disruption of the cavities would be fatal. Luxation is complete disarticulation. Subluxation is less than a complete luxation. The body will resist any changes to the shape of the vital cavities by developing muscular rigidity. Frequently, rigid tight muscles are misread as "misbehaving" or in need of stretching. Instead, they are involved with a spinal cord mediated response to joint distress of a vital cavity.

In my view, when a subluxation occurs to a component of a vital cavity, the body's response is as to an "impending luxation," an impending fatal event. In my opinion, this programmed response of the central nervous system is a valid protective mechanism that should be given all due respect and accommodated fully. This is a hardwired response of the spinal cord, and there are only three ways to get this response to stop: adjusting the joints, general anesthesia and death. When assessing patients, look for what is being protected. A lot of pain patterns are related to a joint that's injured and biomechanically distressed at the opposite end of where the pain is. I term this "remote, but related pain."

In my experience, the diagnosis of fibromyalgia and other similar conditions are manifestations of the body's spinal cord reflex guarding mechanisms that are chronically engaged. If the guarding mechanism stays in place and becomes chronic, then trigger points, contractures and lymphatic drainage problems will all become part of the permanent condition.

Giving this chronic state a name and prescribing medications is the standard of care in allopathic medicine. But I've seen a number of chiropractors and other alternative health care providers suffering from fibromyalgia and unfortunately, they feel they are doomed to just take their medication, and then consider that the only form of treatment available to them. This is not true, I have had patients whose "Fibromyalgia" disappeared with regular appropriate care.

GENERAL PRINCIPLES OF ADJUSTING MULTIPLE ISSUE PATIENTS

Basic principle number one is to just be gentle and gentle and gentle!

In my experience, repetitive gentle force can replace a large force. Most of the population, in my opinion, are afraid of chiropractic care because of the big forceful manipulations that have been traditionally employed to treat patients. Most people, especially, do not want to have their neck manipulated.

Another principle is the application of force should be isolated to the area of interest at the moment. For instance, if I'm going to adjust an elbow, usually it is connected to an injured shoulder. So I want to be careful that I do not provoke or irritate the injured shoulder while I am adjusting the elbow.

Another principle is the development of different approaches or techniques for various patients and their problems. For example, with some patients, I will never do prone adjusting on them because their unstable anterior joints make it necessary for me to avoid putting them on their stomachs. Sometimes the sternal joints are so unstable that they cannot be helped in that position. Patients with facial lacerations, or recent surgeries present other reasons to avoid prone adjusting.

ADVANTAGES TO GENTLE ADJUSTING

Some of the advantages of the gentle adjusting approach is that, as a doctor, this technique choice is easier on my body. I am now in my 30th year of practice and I am a victim of motor vehicle accidents from decades ago and suffer severe osteoarthritis of my spine. I have unstable ligaments and joint injuries in all my extremities. This gentle approach is keeping me in practice. Additionally, I feel I have suffered fewer injuries in my office than some of my colleagues who use more aggressive approaches. Some of these have already retired.

I've had numerous patients tell me in the exam room they will not tolerate manipulation. Also, I have had many patients tell me that they appreciate this gentle approach and had suspended care with another chiropractor because they felt the adjusting was too rough. One patient recently said her last chiropractor's office was like a torture chamber. "You are not doing any of those big manipulations that hurt so much, I will be bringing my children to see you," – and she did!

Also, by focusing on the anterior joints as the basis for neck, shoulder and low back pain, the patients can learn to self-assess their subluxation patterns and become better managers of their injuries.

ADJUSTING WITH A SPRING-LOADED ADJUSTING INSTRUMENT

When adjusting with a spring-loaded adjusting instrument (SLI), I use my fingers to direct the force by using the instrument on my fingers. There are a number of reasons why this should be done. When dealing with the multiply-injured, multiply health-challenged patient, the issue of safety becomes paramount. With multiple injuries, you need to restrict your application of force to very specific areas, not involving nearby areas that have also suffered injury. Also, using the SLI helps me accomplish adjustments with patients that have positional limitations. Another concern is regarding the issue of anxiety about manipulations, which is very common for most patients in chronic pain – the

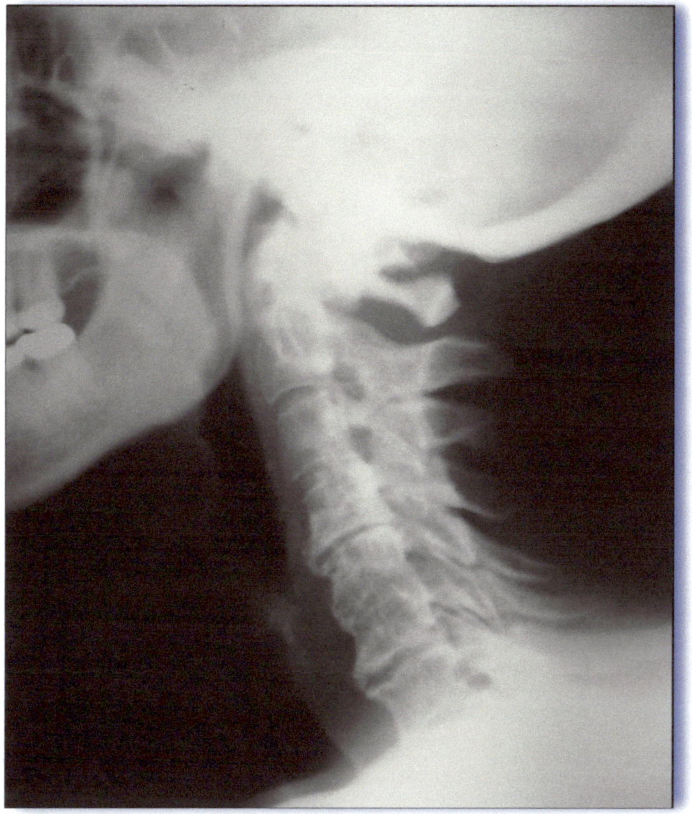

FIGURE I-1. ADVANCED DENEGERATION OF THE CERVICAL SPINE

This patient was thrown through a windshield 50 years earlier as a child. Her chief complaint was neck stiffness. There was no pain on the spine, but adjusting her rib cage improved her range of motion by 70 percent

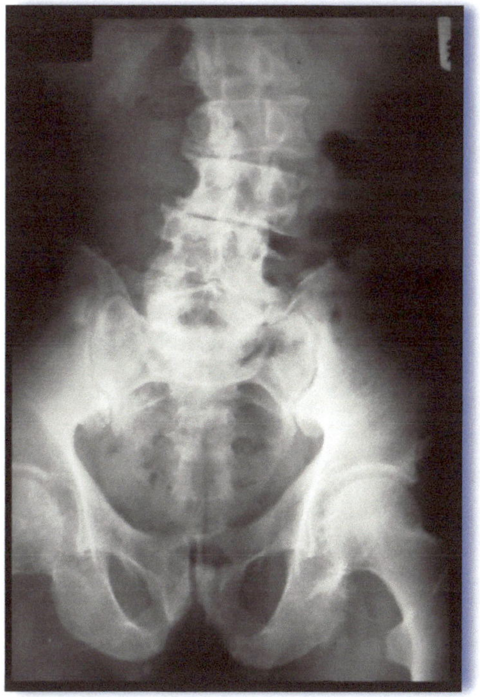

FIGURE I-2. ADVANCED ARTHRITIS OF THE LUMBAR SPINE

This patient, age 72, was playing tennis daily at tournament level,. (men's national champion in his age group), at the time of a lifting injury. Adjusting his pelvic joints returned him to the court.

gentle, controlled force of the SLI eliminates the need for manipulations and thus the anxiety the patient may have.

Additionally, when dealing with acute trauma, we have the need to be extremely careful, as the patient might still be in a state of shock. So we want to be very gentle, but highly effective in realigning joints, and using the SLI accomplishes this task very well.

DROP TABLE ADJUSTING

When adjusting with the drop table, gentle repetitive drops are key. If I want to make them more gentle, then I use my thigh or my hip up against the drop piece to initiate the drop when I thrust on the patient. I will coordinate my thrust with the motion of my thigh. This is done so that the thrust and the drop are simultaneous. The use of the drop table lets me also have broad contacts with the patient, which is almost invariably more comfortable for the patient. Again, I find the drop table reduces anxiety for the patients that have fear and anxiety about chiropractic care. Sometimes I will have a new patient who is very fearful watch me adjust another patient – with, of course, that patient's permission.

CHIROPRACTIC CARE FOR PATIENTS WITH ADVANCED ARTHRITIS

Advanced arthritis or osteoarthritis is caused by subluxation, which is caused by physical trauma. As I've pointed out previously, the amount of physical trauma that the US population is suffering is massive. There are 26 different types of arthritis, but 96 percent of the arthritis that occurs is osteoarthritis. (Rheumatoid arthritis has a two percent occurrence rate and that leaves a total of two percent for the other 24 types of arthritis.) According to testimony before Congress, 85 percent of Medicare claims are due to arthritis. So the amount of trauma suffered by our population presents a huge financial burden as well.

Disability claims are at an all-time high, with back pain and arthritis being the leading causes of the claims for early disability. The motor vehicle accident insurance companies know the outcomes of their liabilities and do their best to close the cases before arthritic changes take place – leaving Medicare and Social Security Disability to cover the disability and medical claims.

This approach to dealing with the chronic effects of motor vehicle accidents should be rethought. In my opinion, some of the many disability claims should be assessed by Medicare and Social Security Disability for sharing the chronic injury claims with the private insurance companies. As long as insurance companies have stockholders to pay dividends to, there will never be any changes to the current system – if you'd like to call it a system.

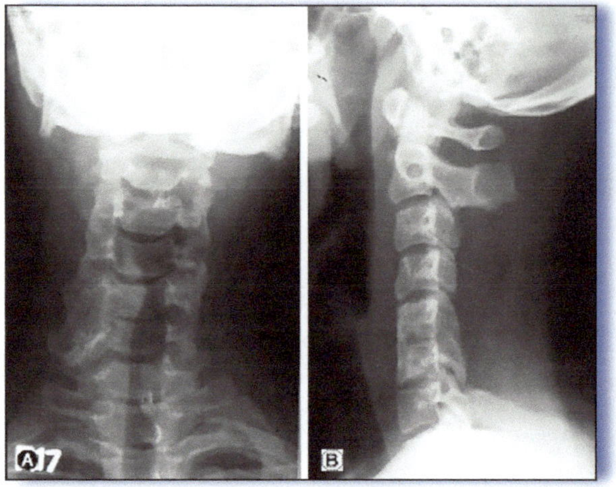

FIGURE 1-3. AP AND LATERAL X-RAYS OF A CERVICAL SPINE WITH A LAMINECTOMY HAVING BEEN PERFORMED.

Notice the lack of spinous process on the lateral and the missing lamina on the AP.

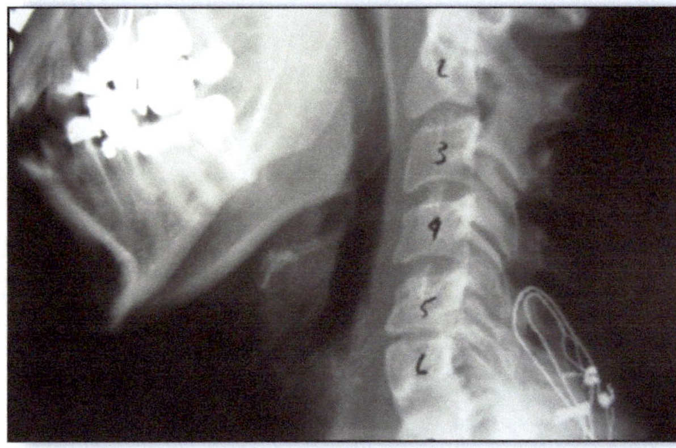

FIGURE 1-4. LATERAL X-RAY OF CERVICAL FUSION FROM MVA

This patient has two types of stabilization: wire fixation (posteriorly) and fusion with cadaver bone (anteriorly at C6-7). Note the lack of a cervical lordosis by surgical procedure. Upper extremity paralysis was almost enirely caused by rib cage injury.

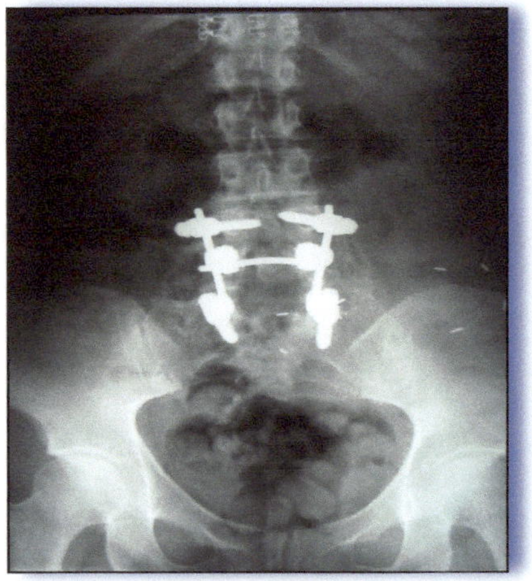

FIGURE 1-5. LUMBAR FUSION OF L-4, 5 TO THE SACRUM

This patient had surgery (18 years before this film was taken) for relief of severe back pain and left leg pain. At age 48 she was on disability and could barely walk. Adjusting her pelvic joints and left fibula and talus restored her ability to walk with ease and grace. The last contact I had with her she was walking five miles a day.

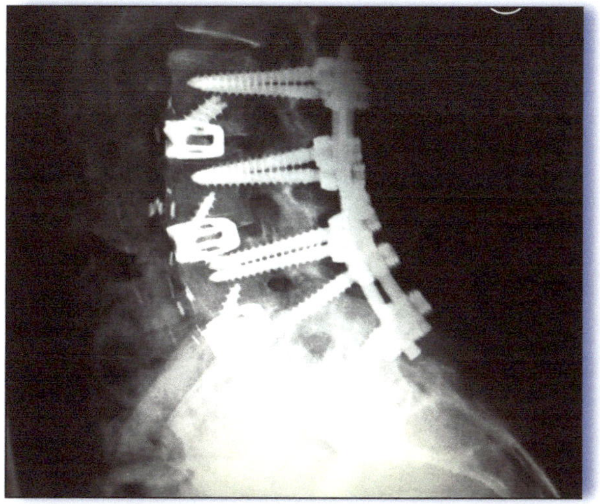

FIGURE 1-6. ROD AND SCREW STABILIZATION OF L3-SACRUM.

Anterior fixation was used as well as posterior appliances. Outcome was poor, altered gait and lots of medications persisted post surgery.

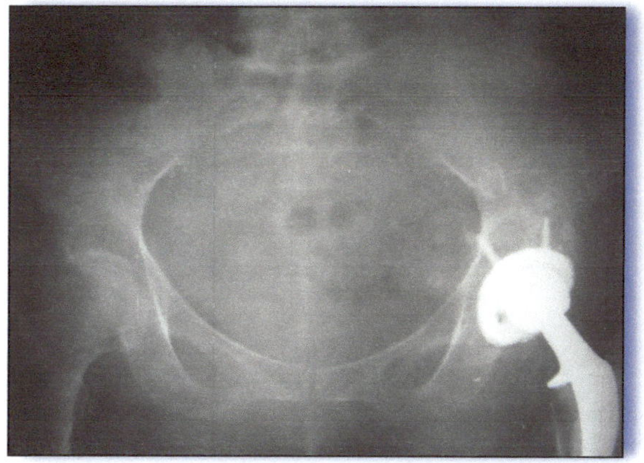

FIGURE 1-7. X-RAY OF A LEFT HIP REPLACEMENT

This patient had suffered left hip pain and an altered gait for many years. We restored her pelvic alignment and improved her conditioning and normal gait with chiropractic adjustments. .

CHIROPRACTIC CARE FOR PATIENTS WITH PRIOR SURGERIES

Most patients with advanced arthritis will present with some contraindications for manipulation. That doesn't mean they will not benefit from being adjusted. My experience with many seniors is that gently restoring any misaligned joints will help mobility and reduce pain. *(See Figures 1-1 and 1-2.)*

There are multiple types of spinal surgeries. For older folks who have canal stenosis, the laminectomy or decompression surgery is performed. The lamina and spinous processes are removed because of the osteophytes and disk bulging has caused narriowing or stenosis of the canal *(see Figure 1-3).* By removing the back of the spinal canal, the spinal cord will not be compressed.

Fusion surgery uses the patient's bone or cadaver bone to replace the damaged disc and fuse the vertebra. These can be done in the cervical, thoracic and lumbar spines.

Stabilization surgery *(see Figures 1-4, 1-5 and 1-6)* uses wire or rods and screws that cover multiple segments.

The newer approaches of Disc Herniation surgery involve smaller incisions approaching arthroscopic type of procedure. Microdiscectomy is such a protocol. It removes disc material that is in the spinal canal and is minimally invasive.

Spinal surgeries are much more common than they used to be, and younger people are getting them done after years of chronic pain and dysfunction. With a patient who has a prior spinal surgery, you should assume that there are multiple subluxations left unaddressed, or even created, by the altered biomechanics of the surgical procedure. Every patient that I've treated with a history of spinal surgery has had a traumatic event that affected the whole body. A lot of the soft tissue structures like discs and other ligamentous structures have been removed at the time of surgery. These are no longer causing pain. The pain patterns are being generated by the guarding mechanisms of the structures that haven't been fused but are still misaligned or subluxated. (*See Figures 1-3 and 1-4.*)

I have assisted a number of patients who have had hip replacement procedures, and every single one of them had injured, unstable pelvic joints which were adding to their pain pattern and affecting the hip joint. I have had more than 20 patients who came to me for care before the hip replacement, and all walked into the hospital to have the surgery done. This was in part due to our care and the patient's desire to stay fit and conditioned prior to the surgery. My stated goal when we undertake this preparation process, is that I want the physical therapist standing over the patient two weeks after the surgery to tell them they are making more progress than any patient they've ever seen in their age group. So far we are batting 1000 on this goal. *(See Figure 1-7)*

I have one patient who was in a severe car accident at age 17 that shattered her left hip. The hip was replaced at age 22. When she arrived in my office at age 56, she was on her third hip replacement on her left side. Her left leg was three and a half inches shorter than the right and she walked with a terrible "rock and roll," as she called it. This added to her mobility problems. Realigning her pelvis dramatically changed the way she walked. She started accidentally leaving her cane in public places. She had her first hip replacement on her right side at age 70. I might add that she did not have one stable or aligned joint in her body. The chiropractic care, improved ergonomics and focused exercise have given her a mobility and quality of life she could not have imagined. She calls me her "miracle worker," but I tell her that I am not licensed to do that. She has to remain mindful and follow her regimen. She is currently pain free and doing daily pilates and hydrotherapy and says she is "feeling just fine."

There are more than 600,000 knee replacements a year in the U.S. In every case I've treated, I've found a subluxated joint involved. Most of the replaced knees that I have worked with, whether partial or complete, were found to be subluxated. Most patients have additional joint dysfunction in the region of the surgery that has been ignored. For instance, with a hip or knee replacement, the sacroiliac joints and pubic symphysis are often subluxated, affecting pain levels, gait and overall quality of life.

Of course, as chiropractors, we would like to do all we can with chiropractic care and avoid a surgical intervention entirely. One issue to be aware of with some of the younger patients is the limited lifespan of the replaced parts – only 15 to 20 years before another replacement has to be done. A patient in his 50s facing a joint replacement who lives into his 80s, will need another replacement along the way. Sometimes the second surgeries can be more difficult to recover from. A t Duke University Medical Center, a study of 354 patients with orthopedic surgeries between the ages of 60 and 94 were evaluated for cognitive impairment. Fifty nine percent showed some levels of cognitive decline post surgery. Discussions of surgery procedures should consider the recommendation that titrated anesthesia be administered with a brain wave monitor to keep the brain activity just below consciousness to lower the risk of cognitive impairment post surgery.

By the mid 1980's, advanced imaging became available to most hospitals. I also feel that the use of advanced imaging, particularly magnetic resonance imaging, is leading to more failed surgical outcomes. This is due to the replacement of thorough examinations involving palpation with advanced imaging instead. Indeed, failed back surgery syndrome is a diagnosis with its own ICD code number since 1989, because of the prevalence of failed outcomes. The definition of this new condition is that the patient is "frankly worse" after the surgery.

I have three patients I see regularly. They have injured legs and they have had surgeries (multiple) on their spines. No one examined their legs before surgery. But an MRI study showed damaged discs. They still have injured legs after surgery but now they have more damage to their spines.

Open-heart surgeries disturb the integrity and alignment of the rib cage. Pain patterns post surgery can occur throughout the torso, shoulder, neck and head due to the subluxation of the costosternal joints and the costotransverse and costovertebral joints that occurred during the surgical procedure. If there was a history of motor vehicle accident or other rib cage trauma, the post-surgery pain pattern can be severe. Neck pain, headaches and a significant loss of shoulder range of motion can be the result of an unresolved rib cage injury.

Cancer surgeries, especially breast cancer surgeries, can cause multiple problems post surgery. This is especially true if there's been any history of a motor vehicle accident or other trauma to the chest. The procedure in breast cancer surgery is to have the patient under general anesthesia with the arm on the surgery side dropped off the table. The weight of the arm, under general anesthesia, can pull the rib joints apart leaving the patient with tingling and numbness of the upper extremity, severe neck pain and headaches post surgery from the neglected subluxated costosternal and sternoclavicular joint subluxations.

FUNCTIONAL CAPACITY

Functional capacity for disabled people is a huge issue. Independent living is a status that more and more people are having to give up because of their health. Maintaining independent living is absolutely imperative for most people. It takes a conditioned person to run a household and participate in all these daily activities. By the time most people are in their mid-70s, they are having problems.

The 20 year study by the state of Oregon showed that within 10 years of the person developing a slow, cautious gait for any reason will have measurable cognitive decline. The source of the gait problem could vary from stroke to a bad ankle to an arthritic hip, it didn't matter. A key to remaining active is remaining ambulatory. This means that care should be delivered to the pelvis and lower extremities to maintain the ability to walk. I have seen a number of elderly patients whose independence is threatened by an arthritic knee. With a little bit of chiropractic care, their whole challenge to remaining ambulatory can be resolved.

BASIC PRINCIPLES:

- *Evaluate everything, especially the anterior joints. The only assumption is that everything has had an opportunity to be injured. If you do not look for it, you will not find it.*
- *All joints have a building code or a "normal" alignment with their component parts. Even if motion is normal, it doesn't mean the joints are aligned.*
- *All joint injury involves the ligaments.*
- *After providing a thorough evaluation, stabilizing ligaments can be the most important intervention — after the joints have been realigned.*
- *The muscles of the body do not randomly misbehave. (If you look at most of the explanations of injury, the main focus is the "misbehaving" tight muscles, i.e., Iliotibial Band Syndrome). Chronic muscle rigidity is a manifestation of a reflex guarding mechanism initiated by the nervous system when subluxation occurs, to prevent "impending luxation".*
- *Isolate the thrust to just the area of interest: the elbow is subluxated, but so is the wrist and shoulder. You have to be mindful of all the injuries as you adjust each component.*
- *Gentleness is absolutely required when adjusting; hardly anyone likes to be handled roughly. Repeated gentle thrusts are also easier and less stressful for both the chiropractor and the patient.*

DECONDITIONING

The deconditioning of our elderly population, and even of some much younger people, is a growing problem. Getting someone through a disabled period in their lives and returning them to full functioning can involve reversing a number of personal habits. It takes time on the part of the doctor to assess, usually remotely, the effects of poor ergonomics or diet, and to reverse a disability status. Sometimes this is not possible. But I've had a number of cases where something like changing the type of motor vehicle someone is driving can change their health status. For the elderly or the chronically injured, pain is a main factor in reducing activities. If all of a patient's injuries are addressed, then increased activity becomes possible.

CONDITIONING

Independent living requires a minimum level of conditioning. If you get winded walking from the bedroom to the bathroom, you will not be able to go grocery shopping. There is a minimum level of physical energy required to run a household with all of the duties required. Full-time employment requires a much higher level of conditioning. If a patient has lost the ability to work, this in of itself can result in deconditioning. Loss of work for any reason should be resisted by maintaining an activity level through exercise or other activities to avoid deconditioning. In a study I read many years ago, it stated that there is a loss of one to two percent of aerobic capacity for every day in bed. Recovering from cancer or other surgery can leave a person without the ability to run their household, let alone go back to work.

When reconditioning an elderly patient, or someone who has been sick or disabled for a long time, the first thing to do is to find a base level of activity, even if it's just five minutes of walking. They need to do that activity every day for seven days. Then on the eighth day, they need to increase the activity to seven minutes, and then do that for seven days. Then on that second round of eight days, increase the walking by two minutes, so now the patient is active for nine minutes per day for seven days. Repeat. The goal is to walk one hour daily with a strong purposeful gait. The U.S. long-term studies show that after one year of walking one hour a day, there will be a lower cholesterol level, lower body mass, and lower blood pressure. This constitutes a sizeable improvement in the patient's health – just from daily walking.

If a patient is recovering from a disability and needs to return to work, the task is a bit more difficult. You again establish a baseline of activity, whatever it is – say, 5 minutes of walking. The walking is incrementally increased for two weeks. At the start of the second week, the patient starts a second daily session of activity – in this case, 20 minutes of walking. Then, that second daily session increases incrementally. After four to six weeks of maintaining two daily sessions of walking or other activity, then you start a third daily session. So morning, midday, and afternoon sessions are being done with incremental increases every week. When a patient has reached three to four hours a day on their feet, walking or exercising, they are ready to discuss a return to work. This takes motivation, patience and persistence by both the patient and the doctor. The doctor should keep in mind one of the basic chiropractic principles: **the body wants to heal.** Never waver from this.

Look for links throughout this book for related online content

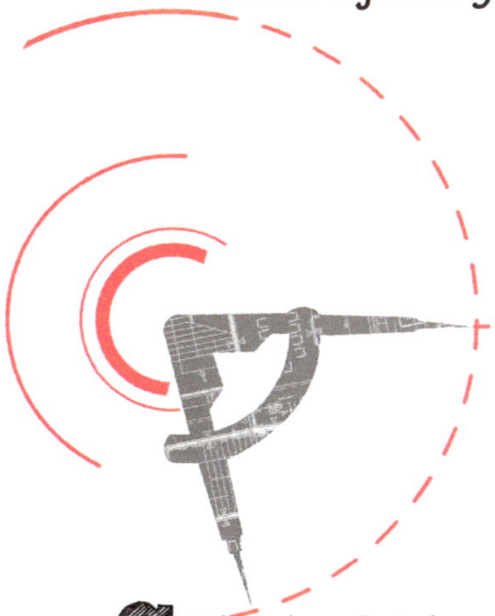

CHAPTER TWO

Evaluating, Adjusting and Managing the Pelvis

Studies show that almost half the population is walking around with damaged intervertebral discs that are asymptomatic. The focus on the disc as the only source of pain pervades the orthopedic and chiropractic professions. I feel from my observations in treating patients with advanced arthritis, spinal surgeries and hip replacements that the alignment of the pelvic bones and distress of the pelvic joints is the major factor in pain, immobility and disability. In my method, the three joints of the pelvic girdle have to be evaluated in a three-dimensional approach.

I have treated 16 patients that needed hip replacement surgery. Our treatment goal was to keep the pelvis level and functional, leaving the patient able to be conditioned and fully ambulatory by the time the surgery was performed. As I said earlier, another treatment goal was to have the physical therapist standing over the patient two weeks after the surgery saying, "I've never seen anyone making as much progress as you in your age group." We are batting 1000 on this set of treatment goals. These patients post surgery need little additional care, as long as their pelvis stays level. They invariably know, even years after the procedures, when to come in and get adjusted.

Complete evaluation of the physical injuries is critical. In the case of the pelvis, this includes evaluating the pubic symphysis. I find the pubic symphysis to be subluxated in almost every patient with complaints of pain in the lower back. In speaking at chiropractic conferences or seminars, I will ask for a show of hands of doctors experiencing unresolved low back pain, despite chiropractic care. It seems incredible to believe, but in the times I've done this, 100 percent of the doctors with chronic lower back pain had a subluxated pubic symphysis that was unknown to them. In almost every case, the pain at the pubic symphysis was greater on palpation than any of the posterior structures or areas that were giving them conscious pain. In every case, the pubic symphysis was not a source of conscious pain. Very few patients will draw a doctor to evaluate their groin, anterior or abdominal regions with complaints of pain – but I find +2 and +3 flinch response to be common during an initial physical examination.

I intend to show that the displacement or subluxation pattern of the hip bones or innominates is a significant source of low back pain and lack of mobility. This would be consistent with the prevalence of motor vehicle accidents in our patient population. The motor vehicle accident scenario for most patients is that they are seated at the moment of impact, and their sacroiliac joints are in a flexed and loaded position when the impact occurs. Studies show that with every impact, regardless of the direction, the occupants of the vehicle lift out of their seats and slam down hard, back onto the seat.

Persistent sitting post-accident can be a source of constant inflammation and continued pain. Also, the axial direction of forces of vehicle crashes shear the intervertebral discs and set off the chronic degenerative processes of degenerative joint disease and osteoarthritis. This will manifest itself years after the event, so we are left mystified as to why we have such advanced arthritis in so much of our young and middle-aged population. The earliest literature I can find about this is Schmorl and Junghanns *The Human Spine in Health and Disease*. In 1932, he stated that motor vehicle accidents are a primary source of osteoarthritis of the spine. So this has been known for a long time.

As with the other parts of this book, I will be demonstrating and advocating gentle, repetitive adjusting of the injured and arthritic spine and pelvis. In part two of this chapter, I will be talking about and demonstrating how to adjust the acute low back patient with limited positions. This is usually a patient who cannot be put into the prone position for various reasons.

I start by adjusting the pelvic girdle when possible, because 70 percent of the body's muscle mass attaches to the three pelvic bones. The patient is usually much more comfortable when their pelvis has been adjusted. It is easier to work on the cervical and upper body injuries and certainly it is easier to assess the lower body injuries if the guarding patterns of the pelvis are abating. The muscles of the back, the erector spinae, all key off the pelvic joints. Subluxation in the sacroiliac (SI) joints can mean constant burning pain in the shoulder region or terrible knee pain with walking. A retired Osteopath said he was taught that the SI Joint is the strongest joint in the body until it's injured. Then it becomes the weakest.

All the injuries that are discussed here are ligament injuries to a vital cavity. The muscular guarding pattern to protect the integrity of the pelvic girdle is mediated by the spinal cord. It is truly a reflex generated by joint distress that we as chiropractors call subluxation. So muscles at rest that are on guard mode are doing so for valid protective reasons. They are *not* misbehaving and in need of stretching and exercise. Our goal is to properly assess the injury and bring relief to the system.

Part one of this chapter is for the patient who can be in a prone position.

Let's review the anatomy that's relevant to our discussion. In dissecting over 250 spines, I have assessed that approximately 70 percent of the body's muscle mass is attached to the three pelvic bones. I believe the pelvic girdle, like the spinal canal and rib cage, is a vital cavity. I mean the central nervous system and in particular, the spinal cord, views the integrity of the three pelvic joints as vital to survival. The disruption of the integrity of any or all of the pelvic joints is viewed by the central nervous system as a threat to survival. This threat will cause a response that I regard as a spinal cord guarding reflex pattern. And, as mentioned earlier, there are only three ways to get a guarding reflex pattern to stop: adjusting the joints, general anesthesia and death.

RELEVANT ANATOMY IN THIS CHAPTER

- *Three bones, three joints and three planes in space*
- *Different morphology of sacroiliac joints*
- *Anatomy and importance of the pubic symphysis*
- *The musculature that attaches to the three pelvic bones*

THREE BONES, THREE JOINTS AND THREE PLANES IN SPACE

In my simplest explanation of the pelvic girdle, I state that there are three bones, three joints and three planes in space. So I use the Cartesian coordinate system that is used by other health care professionals to evaluate pelvic bone misalignment or subluxation patterns. (*See Figure 2-1*).

This system is new for most chiropractors. I am stating that the pelvis can be injured in such a fashion that traditional methods of manipulation are contraindicated. In traditional chiropractic teachings, the sacroiliac joints rotate or nutate around the sacrum in an AS (anterior-superior) or PI (posterior-inferior) pattern. We will call these types of injuries "physiological injuries", because they are subluxation patterns in the normal range of motion for the sacroiliac joint. There should be minimal ligament injury with this type of injury. I am adding the displacement of the innominate in a superior and or posterior subluxation pattern relative to the sacrum and the other innominate.

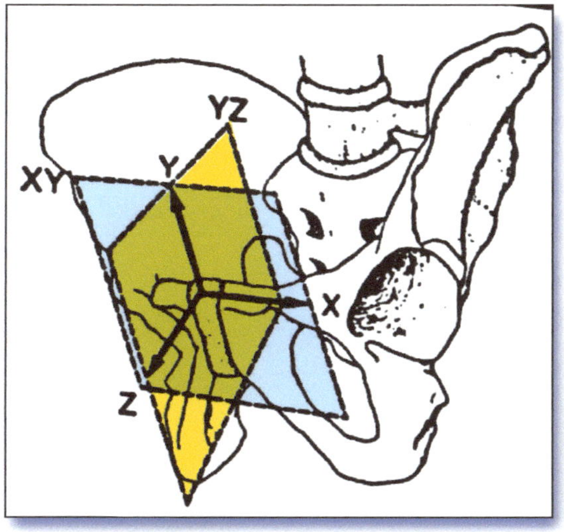

FIGURE 2-1 A DEPICTION OF THE THREE BONES, THREE JOINTS AND THREE PLANES IN SPACE.

These should be considered three sets of facts. Which aspect should be neglected in the evaluation of a patient's pelvic injury?

Online lesson at: https://youtu.be/B_rIn0x36RI

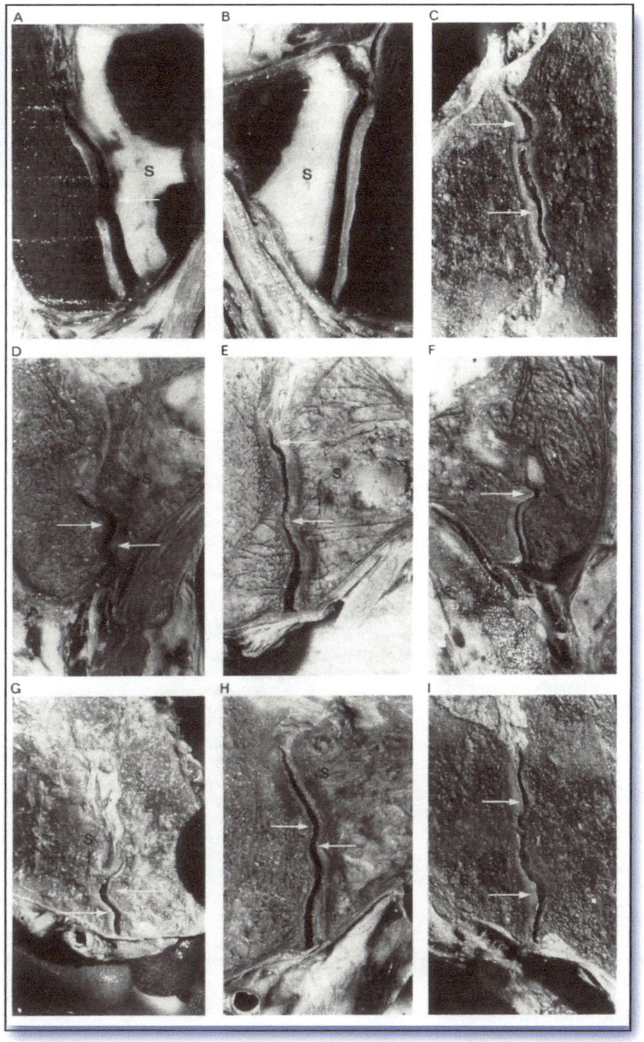

FIGURE 2-2 FRONTAL SECTIONS OF THE SI JOINTS OF EMBALMED MALE SPECIMENS.

S indicates the sacral side of the SI joint. A and B concern a 12-year-old boy. C to I concern male specimens older than 60 years. Arrows are directed at ridges and depressions. The ridges and depressions shown are covered by intact cartilage, which was checked by opening the joints afterwards.

With permission of Dr. A. Vleeming. Originally published in SPINE (European Ed.), 1990, 2: 130-132

These are "non-physiological injuries" because these are motion patterns of displacement that are not in the normal motion pattern and constitute ligament injury.

DIFFERENT MORPHOLOGY OF THE SACROILIAC JOINT

An interesting and complicating feature to the pelvic girdle is the different morphology, or shape that individuals have of their sacroiliac joints. Figure 2-2 shows the different contours among a few individuals of the joint between the sacrum and ilium. In my studies in the anatomy lab, they can be profoundly different among individuals. I believe this can explain the findings most chiropractors will have that patients with the same diagnosis and the same manipulative or adjusting protocols get different results among different patients. It stands to reason that these individual differences are a possible explanation for the variation in various patients' responses. (*See Figure 2-2.)*

I cannot find any studies or even any interest in the variation in the population of the shape of the joint and its components. The SI joint has two components: the auricular portion and the fibrous portion. Each can be different in shape and size. Some individuals have small auricular portions and large fibrous portions and some have just the opposite. (*See Figure 2-3.)* I don't know which type responds and recovers from injury better than the other, but I believe this a factor that we have to know is present even though we can't control or determine what influence it has.

ANATOMY AND IMPORTANCE OF THE PUBIC SYMPHYSIS

The pubic symphysis is regarded by some as an immovable joint that has no clinical significance or need to be evaluated. This fibrocartilage disc has annular rings and a pulpy center. (*See Figure 2-4.*) It is avascular. The physiology and structure would imply that imbibition is the only mechanism for nutrient supply and waste elimination. This assumption has led to the notion that the pubic bones have articular motion with normal activity.

Evaluating the pubic symphysis requires direct palpation. If you are uncomfortable with this, start by taking the patient's hand and putting it on the front of the pubic bones. Press their hand gently into the pubic bones and ask if there is any tenderness there. There usually is with low back pain complaints, and I ask if I can evaluate that myself. I have had no one refuse. With the prevalence of modern injuries in our population, I can easily say that more than 90 percent of your patients will have a positive flinch response and signs of subluxation.

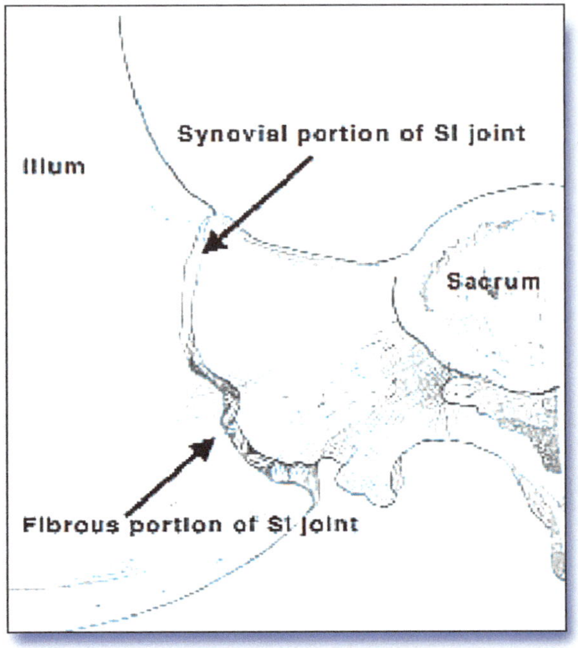

FIGURE 2-3. THE SACROILIAC JOINT FROM THE SUPERIOR VIEW.

The synovial joint is adjacent to the pelvic rim, the fibrous joint is more posterior.

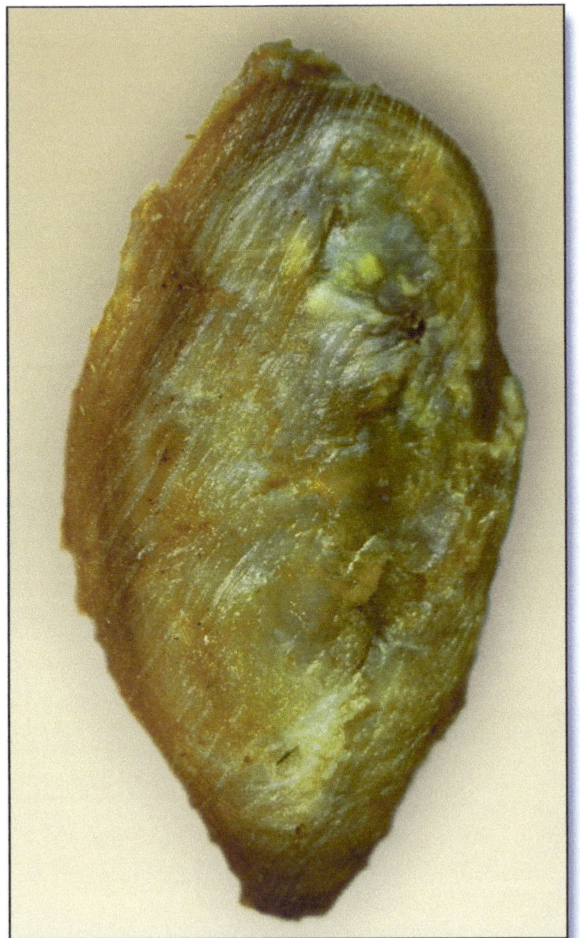

FIGURE 2-4. THE PUBIC SYMPHYSIS DISC

Note that is an avascular fibrocartilage structure that implies motion and flexibility.

THE MUSCULATURE ATTACHED TO THE THREE PELVIC BONES

The musculature that attaches to the three pelvic bones, as I mentioned, is extensive. In Figure 2-5, "A" shows the abdominal wall muscles, "B" equals the hip flexors, "C" shows parts of the erector spinae (they are attached to the cervical spine and, in some people, the underside of the occiput), and "D" is the deeper hip extensors. Not shown are parts of the medial tract of the thigh that arises off the innominate and attaches to the tibia in the pes anserinus area below the knee.

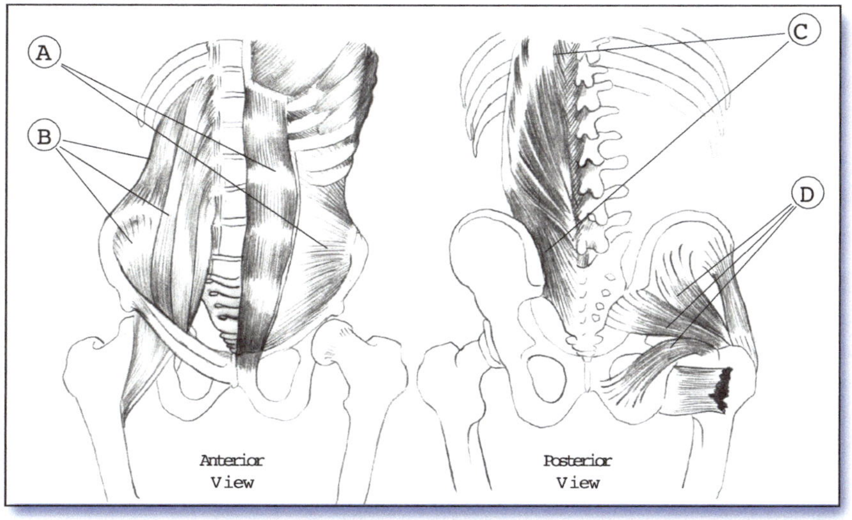

FIGURE 2-5. PELVIC MUSCULATURE

The anterior and posterior upper body musculature that attaches to the three pelvic bones, not shown are the thigh muscles.

(A) The abdominal wall which include rectus and transverse abdominus, internal and external oblique muscles.

(B) The major hip flexors: psoas, iliacus and quadratus lumborum.

(C) The erector spinae muscles.

(D) The deep hip muscles include gluteus minimus and medius, piriformis, gemellus inferior and superior, obturator internus and quadratus femoris. (Note: the gluteus maximus is not shown in this illustration.)

FIGURE 2-6 NORMAL MOTION OF INNOMINATES AND SACRUM

The "tilt" of the pelvis varies between individuals, so there is a "range" of normal tilts. Anterior tilts (left) tend to be more common in females, while posterior tilts (right) tend to be more common in males.

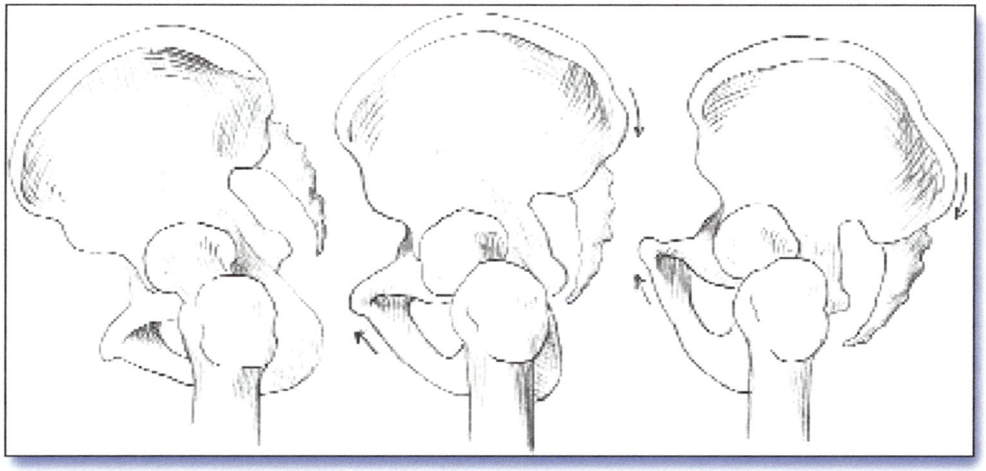

I've had patients complaining of headaches that turned out to be from sacral subluxations and patients complaining of knee pain that turned out to be pelvic subluxation causing medial tract pain at the pes anserinus. A frequent complaint besides low back pain is shoulder pain. Upon evaluation, a common cause of the shoulder pain is the erector spinae in the upper dorsal region responding to a subluxated pelvis.

I have a different view of muscular activity than most of our professional colleagues. Muscles at rest should be soft and relaxed. If they are not, I assume the spinal cord reflex guarding patterns are at play. I do not believe muscles randomly misbehave, and I will refer you to the basic physiology textbooks on muscle physiology to support this notion. Muscles respond to their neurological input. If the joints that a muscle operates are in distress, the nerves will direct the muscles to protect the joints. It is a highly developed protective system, as the body is an exquisitely designed piece of equipment.

THE EVALUATION AND PALPATION OF THE PELVIC GIRDLE

To evaluate the physiological subluxation, contact all five bony landmarks to compare the relative positions. If everything is normal, all landmarks are level. Each posterior superior iliac spine (PSIS) can be uneven and all else level.

Quadratus lumborum on the posterior inferior (PI) side shows increased rigidity and distress. One PSIS is inferior if compared to the other side. If stressing the ilium into the anterior position gives relief, then that direction of thrust is indicated.

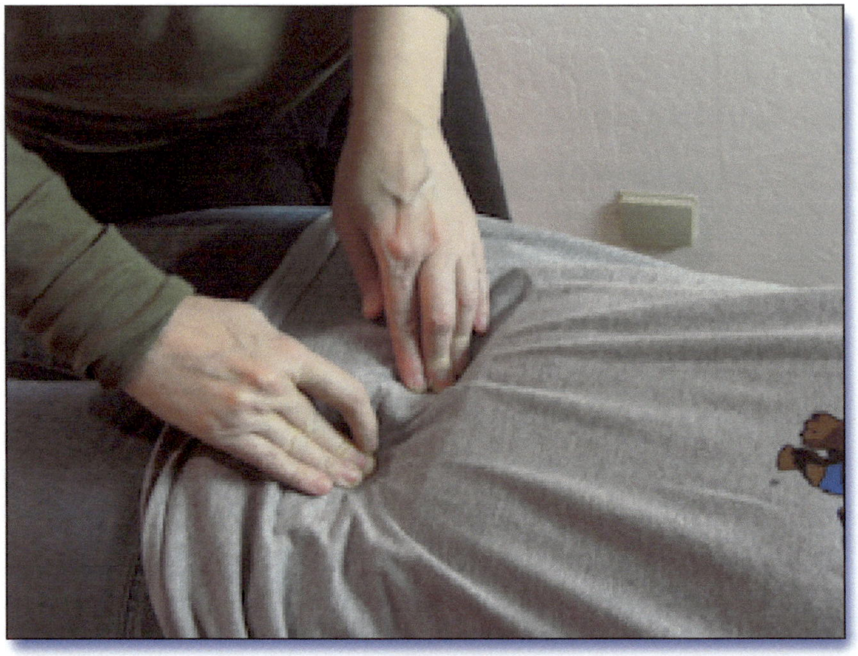

FIGURE 2-7. EVALUATION OF THE PUBIC SYMPHYSIS

Initial palpation of the pubic symphysis should be done with the patient's hands first.

THE BONY LANDMARKS OF THE PELVIC GIRDLE

- *Pubic Symphysis (both the superior and anterior surface)*
- *Anterior Superior Iliac Spine (ASIS) In the prone position:*
- *Iliac Crest*
- *Posterior Superior Iliac Spine (PSIS)*
- *Ischial Tuberosities*
- *Leg length evaluation is done, usually the superiorly displaced side has the short leg.*

POSTERIOR INFERIOR/ANTERIOR SUPERIOR (PI/AS) (PHYSIOLOGICAL SUBLUXATION)

A physiological subluxation is the fixation of the innominate or sacrum in the flexed or PI position or the extended or AS position. For example, the patient is standing up and the innominate is still in a flexed or PI position – normal motion is impaired. This subluxation is within the normal motion pattern of the joint, and ligament damage is minimal to moderate depending on the forces involved and the health of the joints. *(See Figure 2-6.)*

ADJUSTING THE PHYSIOLOGICAL SUBLUXATION

PI Ilium: The patient lies prone. The doctor raises the involved leg with the inferior hand contacting superior to the patella. The superior hand contacts the inferior border of the PSIS and thrusts posterior to anterior.

AS Ilium: The patient is prone and a wedge is put underneath the ASIS. The doctor contacts the ischial tuberosity on the same side and performs a drop table thrust that is posterior to anterior.

PELVIC SHEARING (NON-PHYSIOLOGICAL SUBLUXATION)

Due to the unnatural forces (e.g. motor vehicle accidents and other high impact events) occurring in our environment, the injury to the ligaments of the pelvis can exceed the limits of the tissues. The result is a ligament injury that leaves the innominates and sacrum in non-physiological positions. By that, I mean the normal positions available are exceeded and the ligaments involved are significantly injured. One innominate subluxates superior and/or anterior compared to the other. *(See Figure 2-8, A and B.)*
To get a 3-D picture of the displacements, you need to palpate all five bony landmarks.

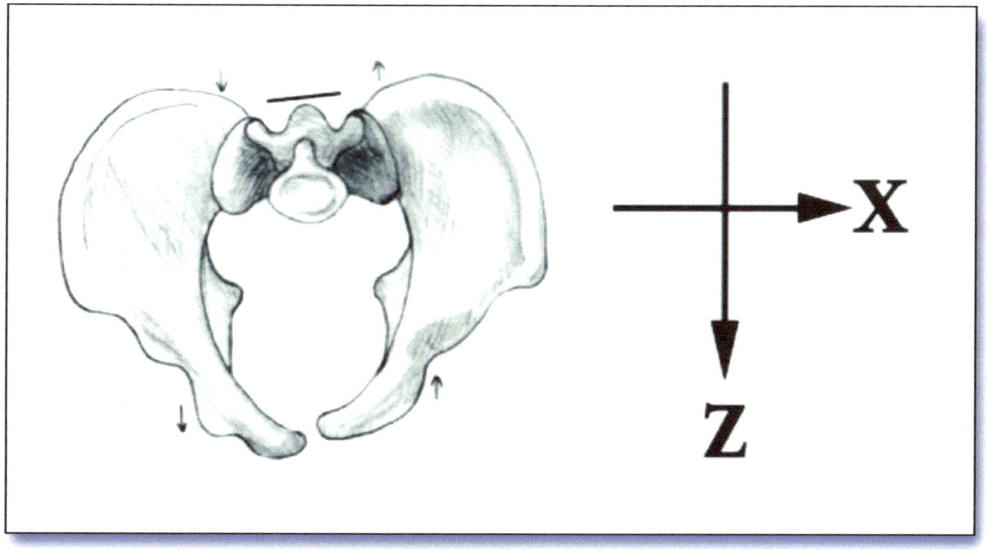

FIGURE 2-8A ANTERIOR OR Z PLANE SUBLUXATION

The pubic bones as well as the whole innominate shifts forward (in the Z Plane) or backwards relative to the other. This type of injury involves the pubic symphysis as well as both Sacroiliac Joints. Sacral rotation is implicit in this deformation.

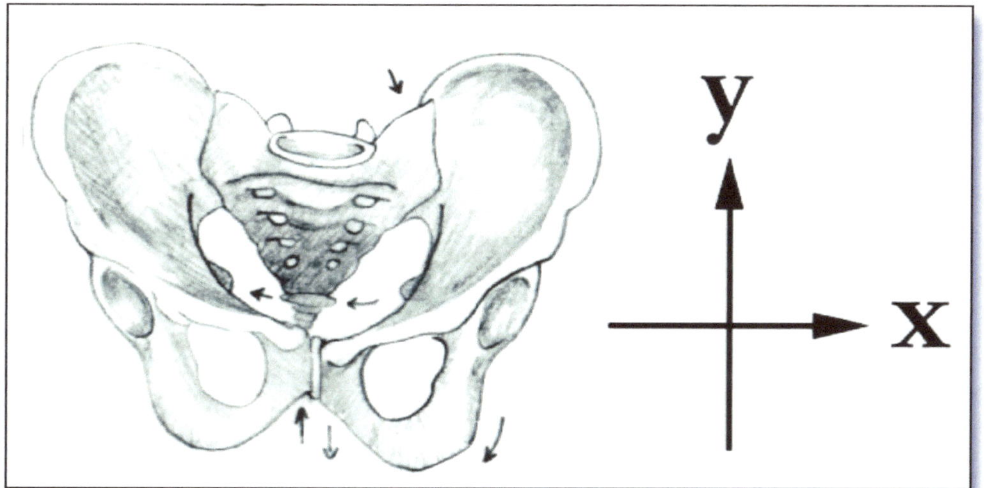

FIGURE 2-8 B. SUPERIOR OR Y PLANE SUBLUXATION

This type of injury causes the most pain and altered motion. Severe antalgia occurs when both innominates have been subluxated superiorly. This involves the pubic symphysis and both Sacroiliac Joints and Sacral tilting is implicit, commonly to the more superior side.

THE EVALUATION AND PALPATION OF THE NON-PHYSIOLOGICAL PELVIC SUBLUXATION WITH NO POSITION LIMITATIONS

One innominate's position is compared to the other one. Start the patient in a supine position and palpate the ASIS on each side. Compare the relative height as well as anterior to posterior positions of the innominates. Often, there is a difference in height between the two sides and a difference in their anterior to posterior positions.

To find the pubic symphysis, palpate the ASIS and move toward the medial and inferior along the inguinal ligament. (*See Figure 2-7*) The anterior surface of the pubic symphysis is the most useful landmark for evaluating the anterior displacement pattern (Z component). The superior surface of the pubic bones are the best indications if one of the pubic bones is superior to the other. If the abdominal wall is ridged and too hard to palpate the pubic bones, then the positions of the ASIS is the best guide. To confirm the pubic symphysis findings, go back and check the ASIS positions. Next, with the patient prone, palpate the alignment of the iliac crest, PSIS, ischial tuberosities and the leg length. The most reliable landmark for the superior displacement (Y component) is the ischial tuberosities. All the findings should be compared with each other to give the mental image of a 3-D subluxation pattern.

Pubic symphysis involvement is characterized by tenderness to palpation, or the inability to palpate it, and by rigid abdominal wall musculature. *(See*

Figure 2-7.) When the pubic symphysis is subluxated, the sacroiliac joints are involved as well. Further, the iliopsoas muscles may be so tight the patient cannot lie supine, the quadratus lumborum is rigid, and guarding of the erector spinae from the iliac crest up to the mid-thoracic area may be present.

THE X-RAY ANALYSIS OF THE PELVIS

An X-ray analysis of the subluxated pelvis is unreliable. An experiment with models of the pubic bones (the simplest part of the innominate) has shown that projection error is part of the X-ray appearance. We must physically evaluate the patient's joints; imaging, whether advanced or X-ray, does not give the full picture of pelvic subluxation.

THE EVALUATION AND PALPATION OF THE SACRUM

If the sacrum is subluxated, it is not aligned with the gluteal crease. The sacral apex is off to one side, indicating a sacral subluxation. Find the gluteal crease. Then compare the distance of the sacral borders to the gluteal crease bilaterally. The wider distance indicates a sacral apex deviation to that side. Upon palpation, gluteus minimus usually feels very tight in this pattern. *(See Figures 2-9, 2-10 and 2-11.)*

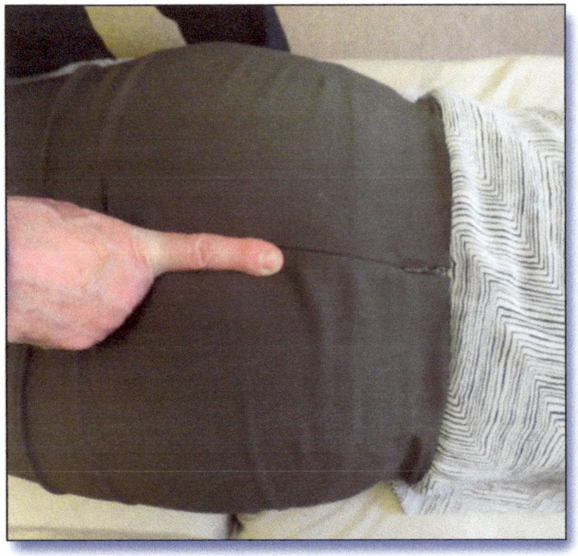

FIGURE 2-9 STEP ONE, FINDING THE GLUTEAL CREASE.

The Doctor's index finger is on the gluteal crease of the patient.

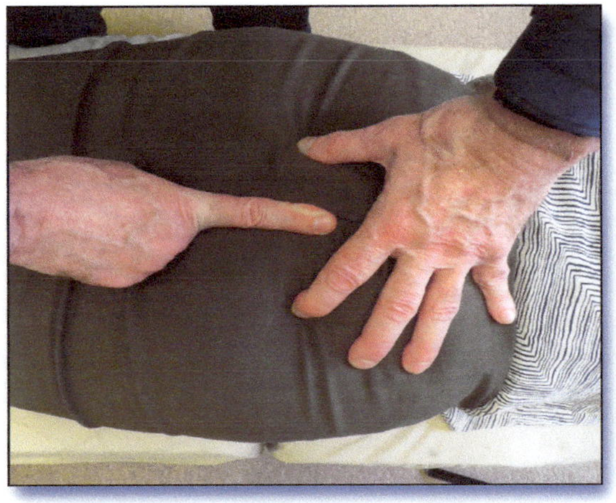

FIGURE 2-10 STEP TWO, FINDING THE SACRAL BORDERS.

The Doctor's left thumb and index fingers are on the sacral borders. The right hand still has contact with the gluteal crease. Note there is more sacrum on the patient's left side.

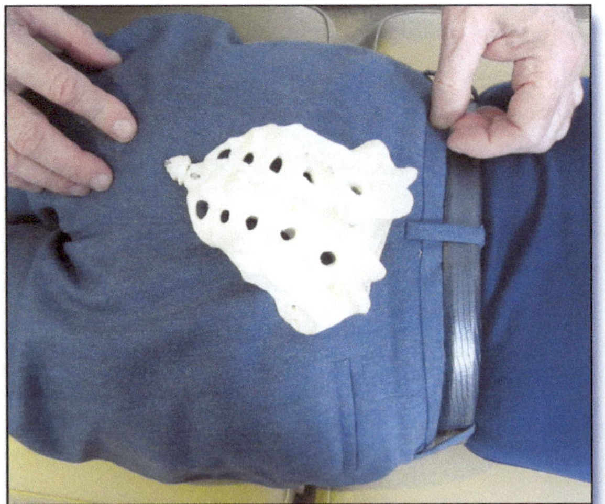

FIGURE 2-11 PICTURE DEPICTING SACRAL SUBLUXATION.

The bony sacrum is positioned on the patient in the same manner as the palpation revealed.

ADJUSTING THE SACRUM

Adjusting the Sacral Apex: The doctor will stand ipsilateral to the side of deviation to use the superior hand's fleshy pisiform to contact the lateral border of the sacrum. The correction with this hand is posterior-anterior (PA). The inferior hand pushes the sacral apex to the other side. *(See Figures 2-12 and 2-13.)*

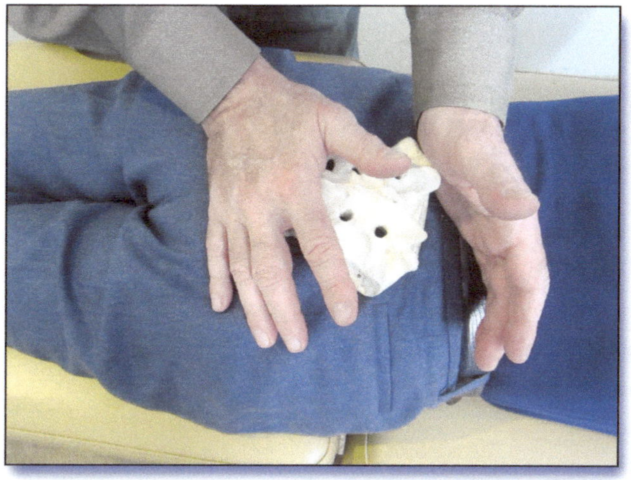

FIGURE 2-12 THIS IS THE SETUP FOR ADJUSTING A SACRAL APEX LEFT.

The Doctor's hands are, above, on the high side of the sacral base and the lower or right hand is on the sacral apex.

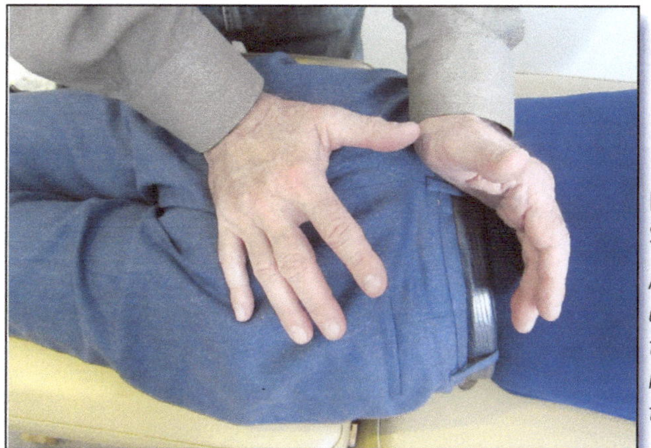

FIGURE 2-13 ADJUSTING THE APEX LEFT SACRUM SUBLUXATION.

Adjusting Sacral Apex: Stand ipsilateral to the side of deviation using the superior hand fleshy pisiform contacting the lateral border of the sacrum. The correction with this hand is PA and S-I. The inferior hand pushes the sacral apex to the other side. See Figure 2-14

ADJUSTING THE NON-PHYSIOLOGICAL PELVIC SUBLUXATIONS

The adjustment for the Superior or the +Y component: For a +Y on the right, contact the right iliac crest with a broad contact. The doctor can even use the greater trochanter as well if there is no hip replacement. An assistant might stabilize the opposite ischial tuberosity while the adjusting thrust on the right iliac crest is directed in an inferior direction. *(See Figure 2-14.)*

The adjustment for the Anterior or the +Z component: The contact for a posterior innominate is on the +Z (or posterior) side, (a broad contact on the whole side of the hip region.) *(See Figure 2-15.)* Note that the plane line of the sacroiliac joints is oblique from medial to lateral because of the shape and orientation of the sacrum. The sacrum is wider in the front than it is in the back, so the thrust should be through that plane line, posterior to anterior.

ADJUSTING THE SACRUM IN THE NON-PHYSIOLOGICAL SUBLUXATION

Sacral Subluxation: First, find the sacrum. Start by locating the gluteal crease. *(See Figure 2-9)* Second, find the sacral borders and compare the distance of the sacral borders to the gluteal crease bilaterally; the wider distance indicates a sacral apex deviation to that side. Upon palpation, the gluteus muscle can be tight in this pattern. *(See Figures 2-10 and 2-11.)*

Adjusting Sacral Apex: Stand ipsilateral to the side

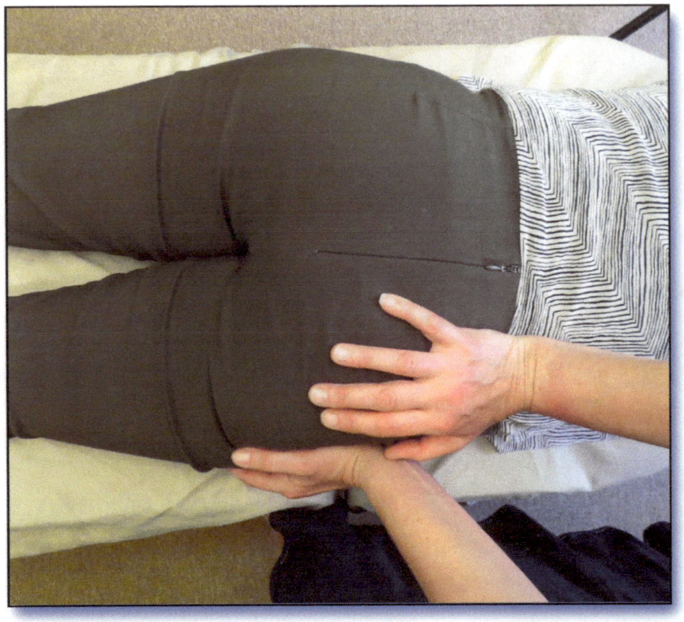

FIGURE 2-14. THE PRONE ADJUSTING FOR THE SUPERIOR OR +Y INNOMINATE

Adjustment for the Superior, or +Y component: Use a broad contact on the iliac crest on the superior side. The greater trochanter can be used as well if there is no hip replacement. The adjusting thrust is directed in an inferior direction.

of deviation and use the superior hand's fleshy pisiform to contact the lateral border of the sacrum. The correction with this hand is PA and SI. The inferior hand pushes the sacral apex to the other side. (*See Figures 2-12 and 2-13.)*

FIGURE 2-15. THE PRONE ADJUSTING OF THE ANTERIOR OR +Z INNOMINATE.

+Z Correction: The correction of the right anterior innominate will require using a wide angled block under anterior or +Z side. It should be placed under the whole innominate. The contact is broadly on the –Z side from behind and the thrust is directed in the posterior to anterior direction with noting the oblique angle of the SI joint. (The Sacrum is wider in the front than the back so the SI Joint is angled from medial to lateral, from back to front). (See Figure 2-8.) The adjusting is done gently and repetitively. (See Figure 2-7.)

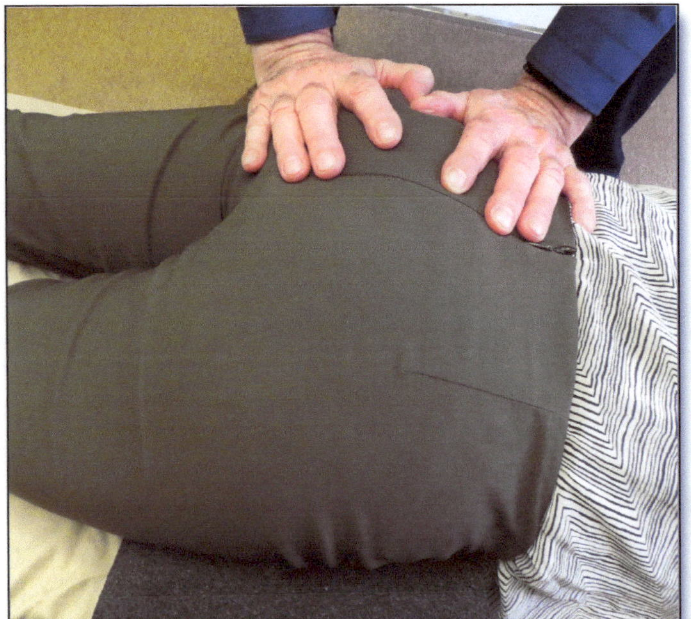

Online lessons at:
https://youtu.be/Fflsdqkzlng
https://youtu.be/orphOolwVag
https://youtu.be/HRyvjNA2C5o
https://youtu.be/ebgYtH2ShLU

PART TWO: PATIENTS WITH ACUTE INJURIES OR LIMITED POSITIONS.

Patients With Positional Limitations Include:

> *An acute injury to the back and pelvis with severe antalgia*

> *Facial lacerations or other injuries to the head or face (dental work)*

> *A severe shoulder or rib cage injury*

> *A late stage pregnancy*

> *Hospital care*

> *A port for chemotherapy in chest*

> *Surgical procedures*

These protocols are for patients who cannot assume a prone position. This would include the acute lower back injury and pelvic girdle injury that is usually characterized by severe antalgia. Also, this group can include patients with lacerations on the face, chest or knees, or patients with recent dental work. In addition, patients that have suffered a stroke are initially too infirm to lay on their stomachs.

For patients that have shoulder separations or rib cage injuries including a broken sternum, I prefer to keep them in the supine position. What I mean by supine is that they are in a reclined position on a table that's tilted up to the head and shoulders, and above the hips. This is also appropriate for patients in late stage pregnancy, especially if they are overdue. I also use this position for patients that have just been in a car accident, especially if I have not seen them prior to the accident.

These protocols can be especially useful in the hospital. Hospital beds generally will have the patient tilted up or reclined. Hospital beds pose their own challenges to providing chiropractic care, but it can be done. I've also had a number of patients in chemotherapy and who have a port in the chest, so prone work is not appropriate for them. Patients with cancer and chemotherapy have subluxations that can produce pain that alters significantly their quality of life. The adjusting is for the relief of musculoskeletal pain and to improve nerve function, not to eliminate the cancer.

Also, I would like to note that some of these patients have quite a bit of pain medication in their system for the cancer and surgery and often the musculoskeletal pain from subluxation is not affected by the pain medication given. These are different types of nerve endings that are in wounds from surgeries, compared to those that are involved with ligament injury, inflammation and muscle spasms.

I've attended a patient in the hospital with a pulverized calcaneus, shattered talus and patella, multiple broken ribs and a surgery to remove his spleen. He was on the maximum IV morphine allowed but he was in excruciating back pain from the subluxation patterns of his pelvis and ribs. When the subluxations were reduced, he dropped his hands off the rails of the hospital bed, which he had been gripping with white knuckles. I asked him how his pain level was and he said he was out of pain. I asked him how the leg felt, (he had a full length cast on it), and he said it was throbbing. The morphine was not touching the musculoskeletal pain.

There are also the patients who are in chemotherapy with ports in their chest, and surgery sites that are still considered wounds. Just like when patients have the flu and are in bed for the week, low back pain can be a real problem. The bed rest required for chemotherapy or cancer surgery can exacerbate a low back injury and produce worse pain than the port and the surgeries – this is not relieved by medication. So being able to adjust the pelvis and release the lumbar spine in the supine position can be very helpful for these patients.

The patient that cannot be put in a prone position can still have the pelvis adjusted. The evaluation is limited to the ASIS and the pubic bones. *(See Figure 2-7.)* The adjusting of the anterior innominate is shown in Figure 2-16; see that the doctor has a broad contact on the anterior upper thigh and ASIS, with a large wedge under the posterior or Z side. Gentle, repetitive thrusting is done until the pubic bones are level. This approach is needed with an advanced pregnancy and other patients that cannot be prone, i.e., a patient in a hospital bed.

The adjusting for the +Y or superior innominate with limited positions is performed by contacting the iliac crest and the trochanter (if there is no hip replacement), and gentle repetitive thrusts are made in the superior to inferior direction. *(See Figure 2-17.)*

In the case of advanced pregnancy, the +Y or superior side can be adjusted by taking hold of the affected side's leg, above the knee and above the ankle. Then, a gentle inferior pull is made with the unaffected leg placed against the doctor's leg to stabilize the patient's body. *(See Figure 2-18.)*

ADJUSTING THE POSTERIOR-INFERIOR INNOMINATE IN THE SUPINE POSITION

Place a small sacral wedge under the PSIS, while the doctor's hand goes in between the wedge and the PSIS. The patient then raises their leg and the doctor pulls up on the PSIS while pushing down on the leg. Stay off the patella when doing this maneuver. This adjusting is generally needed by a patient involved in a motor vehicle accident. (*See Figure 2-19.*)

Note: After these patterns are adjusted, repalpate, because an underlying pattern will often become obvious after the initial adjustment is performed. For example: the +Y component can switch sides due to the fact, that in actuality, the subluxation is a bilateral displacement, but one side is more severe than the other. Repeat, gently, until the pubic bones are level and the musculature has responded.

The whole series of supine pelvic adjusting (+Y, +Z and PI) on the patient with limited positions is very likely needed.

ADJUSTING THE ANTERIOR SACRUM

Subluxation of the anterior sacrum can occur from violent falls or accidents. Both inominates are pushed posteriorly relative to the sacrum. One indication that this has happened is the patient has severe pain when forward pressure is applied on the back of the sacrum. Also hurting to sit can be an indication that this has occurred.

The patient is placed in the supine position. Figure 2-20 shows the doctor's hand position on a plastic model. The hands of the doctor go right over the top of the pubic bones and as deep as possible. This should put the doctor's fingers at the top of the base of the sacrum. The pelvis is held up from the table top by a pair of foam wedges placed under each PSIS. (*See Figure 2-21.*) This allows the sacrum to move posteriorly. The drop table is then used repeatedly. The patient will experience a range of reactions from being very uncomfortable to being in pain with this procedure. It is common that the first drop gives a sharp pain followed by relief. Each subsequent drop is not so distressing. After being adjusted, the sacrum should not be as painful to palpate. The patient should avoid sitting as much as possible. When sitting is required, either a donut or a wedge cushion with a space open for the sacrum should be used.

MANAGING THE INJURED PELVIS

Important Points:

> *Review the ergonomics of the ligament injury.*

> *Review the sleeping positions.*

> *Keep the legs together, either side or back; decide what side of the bed to get into.*

> *Reduce sitting as much as possible.*

> *Avoid sitting in low chairs or couches — the higher the hips the better.*

> *Review all car behavior.*

> *Avoid climbing into or out of a car that's either too high or too low.*

Managing the injured pelvis is a challenge regarding cars and chairs. I usually start by having the patient walk after the first adjustment. I call this a "ligament stability test." Can the patient hold the corrections just applied to the pelvic girdle with weight bearing? If the patient cannot hold a correction after three to five

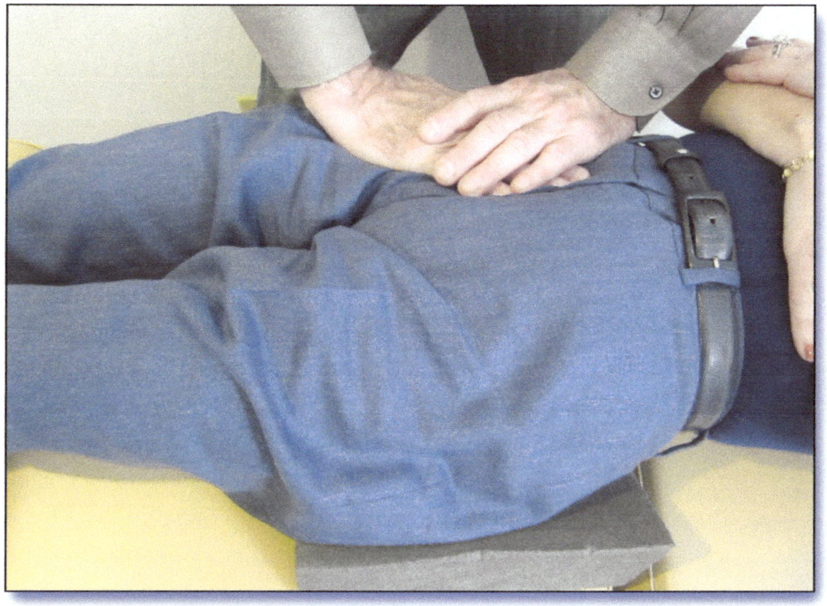

FIGURE 2-16. SUPINE ADJUSTING OF THE ANTERIOR OR +Z INNOMINATE.

Note the large wedge is under the patient's left side, while the contact is on the right side which is anterior to the left.

The contact is on the posterior side or – Z side, with the large wedge under the anterior side or + Z side. Note the broad contact of the doctor's hands.

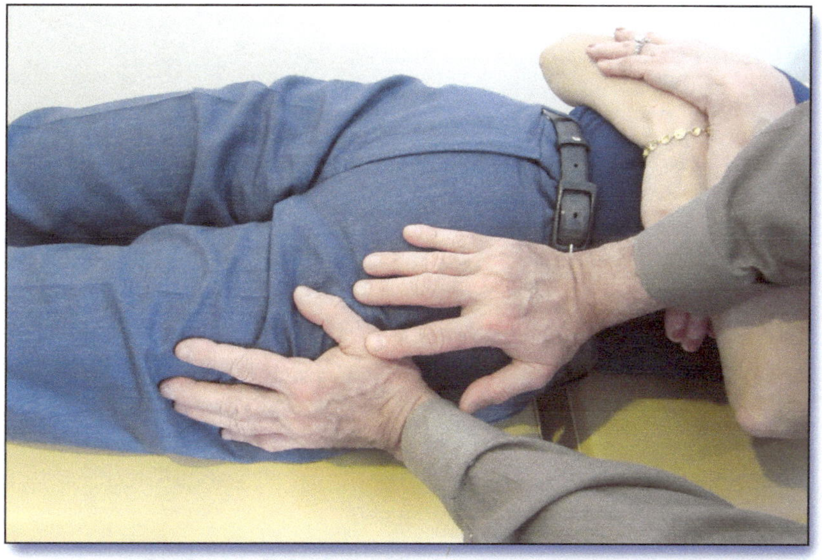

FIGURE 2-17. SUPINE ADJUSTING OF THE SUPERIOR OR +Y INNOMINATE.

Notice the doctor is contacting the iliac crest while facing the feet to facilitate the direction of the thrusting.

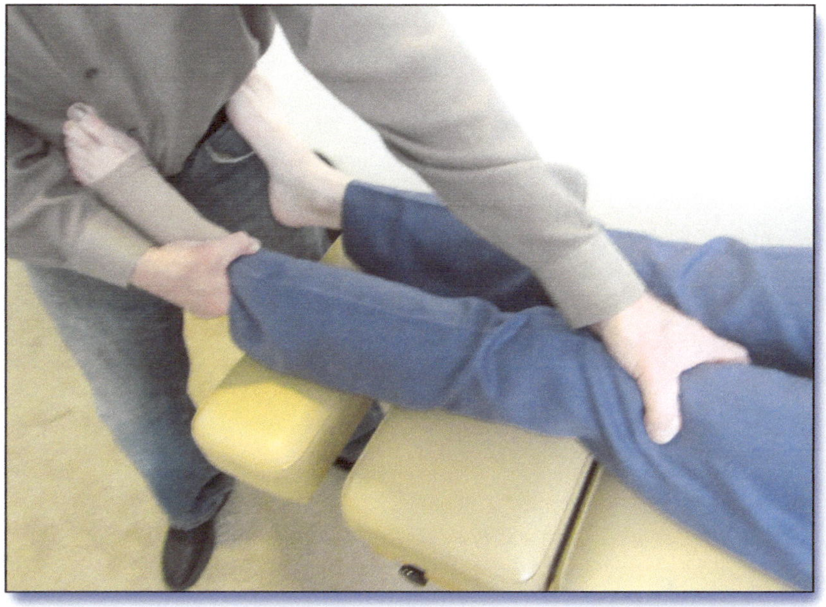

FIGURE 2-18. SUPINE ADJUSTING WITH THE LEG PULL TECHNIQUE.

Notice the patient's foot is against the doctor's thigh to stabilize the patient so they are not pulled off the table or bed.

minutes of walking, then a supportive brace should be used to help hold the injured joints in place. This is a sign of ligament failure. This is a shift in thinking for most practitioners. The muscles are not misbehaving, they are responding to the ligament failure.

In managing the injured pelvis, discovering the ligament injury that has to be at the root of the diagnosis is very difficult and important. When the sacroiliac ligaments and pubic symphysis are unstable, the guarding reflexes will make the muscles in the region tight, restrict motion and be the source of pain. Most patients want to exercise and think that some repetitive activity will restore the lost ligament integrity. That's not how it works. As with any other part of the body, a diagnosis of ligament injury is not something you want to hear. Bones heal faster than ligaments. Some ligament injuries will only heal incompletely, leaving permanent limitations on activity and motion. Modern injuries occur with such speed and force that ligament injury is very common.

Ligament injury leads to arthritic degeneration. In discussing the ergonomics of ligament injury, we start by going into the details of the things not to do. We don't want anything that pulls the pelvis apart with motions of the legs, which are huge levers. For instance, this means no lunging (this would include unilateral hamstring stretching), yoga and Pilates. When it comes time to stretch the hamstrings, we have to do it bilaterally. Remember the tightening of the back, thigh, hip and hamstring muscles are part of the guarding reflex initiated by the spinal cord to protect the injured unstable joints.

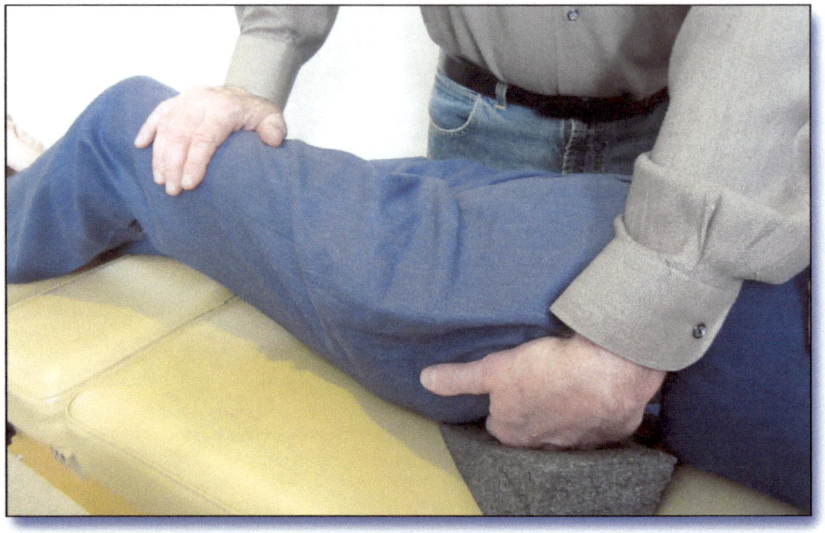

FIGURE 2-19 SUPINE ADJUSTING OF THE PI INNOMINATE.

Place a small sacral wedge under the PSIS, while the Doctor's hand goes in between the wedge and the PSIS. The patient then raises the leg and the Doctor pulls up on the PSIS as (s)he pushes down on the leg while using the drop table. Stay off the patella when doing this maneuver. This adjusting is needed by anyone involved in a MVA.

Habits that are well established, some from childhood, can now keep a new injury inflamed and unresolved, turning into a chronic debilitating condition. You must review the sleeping habits and positions, the type of bed the patient uses and its condition. Any one of these factors or all of them in combination can keep a low back and pelvic girdle injury from healing.

Once the pelvic girdle is unstable, sitting exacerbates the condition. Avoiding sitting becomes necessary. At the very least, reducing the amount of daily sitting is recommended. I can't stress this too often. Sitting when optional should be eliminated. At home, recliners are best. Sitting on soft couches or soft armchairs where the hips sink lower than the knees, is to be avoided at all costs. It is better to take the cushions off the couch and put them on a dining room chair and boost the seat height so that the hips are higher than the knees. This reduces the struggle to get up from the seated position.

Cars are an integral part of our lives, yet they are responsible for many of our injuries and the chronic arthritis that plagues the nation. Discussing with your patient the type of vehicle they have is necessary to manage the injured pelvis. I've had a 6-foot tall, 285-lb lawyer in a Miata with a clutch, whose chief complaint was left leg pain and hip pain. When he had to travel back east for family reasons, he drove a rented SUV with the automatic transmission that

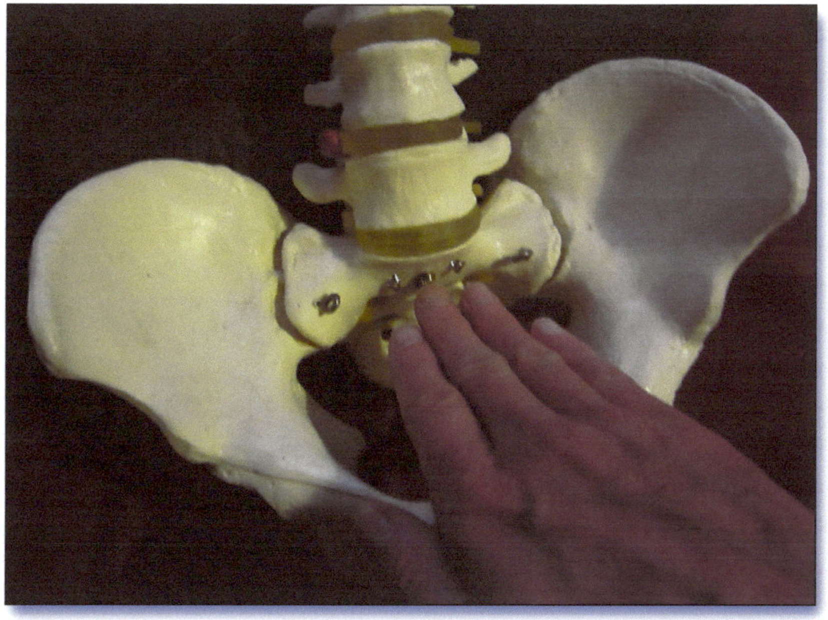

FIGURE 2-20. CONTACT FOR ADJUSTING THE ANTERIOR SACRUM

The doctors fingers go over the top of the pubic bones and into the abdomen, as deep as possible.

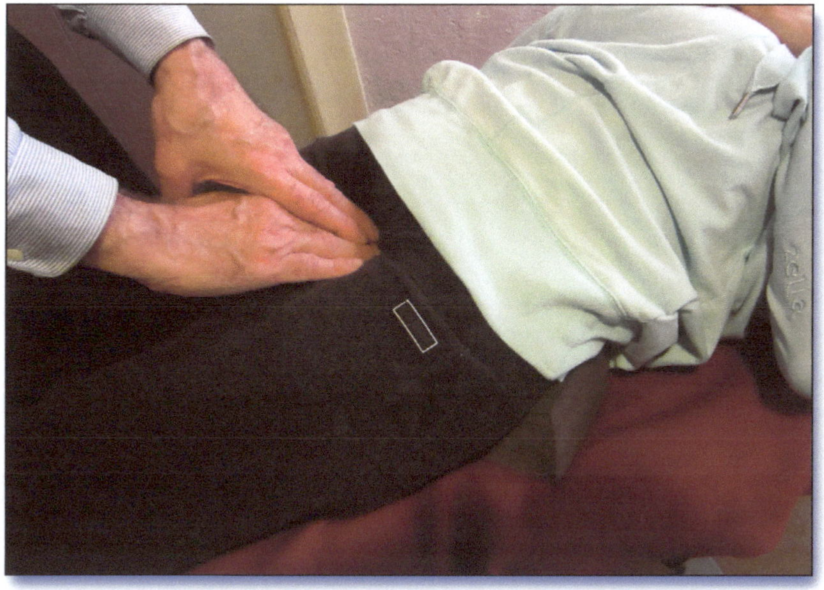

FIGURE 2-21. ADJUSTING THE ANTERIOR SACRUM

The patient is supine with the doctors fingers placed over the top of the pubic bones pressing deep into abdomen. Both PSIS's are raised off the table top. Foam wedge under the patient on both sides, left side visible.

seemed to lead to improved pain levels and ability to walk. He didn't think there was a connection (I think I mentioned he was a lawyer). So climbing out of a bucket seat for a large person is contraindicated for managing an unstable pelvic girdle. Also a small person, 5-feet tall, getting into a Cadillac Escalade, involves climbing. If you have an unstable pelvic girdle, should climbing be a daily activity? If we are writing work limitations, don't we routinely eliminate bending, twisting and climbing from the patient's activities at work? Why should they do this in their personal lives? This ergonomic evaluation must be done with all of our patients who are diagnosed with pelvic girdle injuries.

I want to review with patients what they are doing to manage their condition, especially if they've had contact with an orthopedist or physical therapist. Most exercises given by PT's for low back pain will continue to keep the unstable pelvic ligaments unstable. They have a different paradigm: they think tight muscles and pain are from lack of exercise and the major cause of the pain the patient is suffering. There are no studies to prove this, also they imply that everyone who does not exercise should be in pain. Since most people don't exercise, they should all be in pain, and we don't find that to be true. So it's necessary to review and modify the stretches and exercises the patient has been doing. In managing the injured pelvic girdle, there should be no seated exercises, no leg presses, leg extensions or upper body exercises. Being seated overloads the lumbar spine and pelvis, and this is not how to treat injured and unstable ligaments.

I'm a big believer in using anything I can to get the patient moving again. I use a lumbosacral brace every day at work to protect myself from my activities of working with severely injured patients. I have chronic shin splints and I do use braces and lace-up boots to keep my lower leg bones in place while I perform manual medical procedures on patients. I would be in a lot of pain and unable to perform as a chiropractic doctor without my braces to manage my chronic joint and ligament instability. I recommend the lumbosacral brace or something similar to everyone who comes in our office with these types of problems.

Walking is the best prescription for the recovery of an unstable pelvic girdle. In the gym, the treadmill should be the most effective piece of equipment. Some people have problems walking on the treadmill, so it should be approached with caution. If the patient has an unsteady gait, the treadmill can be a hazard. If the foot, or part of the foot, misses the tread, it can send them to the floor. So initial walking exercise for an unsteady person should be done with a walker, or possibly in the pool. This reduces the chances for falling.

Later, an elliptical machine can be brought in to increase fitness and vary the routine. The common complaint of rehabilitation activities is that they are boring. I preach boring until we can get up to five miles of walking without the pelvis coming apart. At that point, we are able to advance to more complex exercises and activities. Absence of pain is not a sign of joint stability. As I tell my patients: goal number one is to get you out of pain, goal number two is to get the injured joints to stabilize. Sometimes when we accomplish goal number one, we screw up goal number two. This is especially true of anyone under the age of 35.

PREGNANCY AND THE INJURED PELVIS

(If Mommy isn't happy, no one is happy.)

THE EVALUATION

Pregnancy and the pelvis require special attention if there has been a previous history of injury to the pelvic joints. Most pregnant patients will tolerate normal pelvic adjusting procedures that have been covered in the previous part of this chapter. Once the third trimester has started, we generally stop prone adjusting. This is something that is a judgment call on the part of the doctor and the patient. Once it becomes precarious to get the patient on and off the table, I opt for the supine procedures we will cover here. This protocol is appropriate for late stage pregnancy, and when distress patterns can be significant. The significant displacement of the pubic bones relative to each other is a major producer of pain and debilitation. *(See Figures 2-8a and b.)* Evaluating the pattern of subluxation is critical.

Place the patient in a supine tilted up posture. (*See Figure 2-22.*) Have the patient find her ASIS on each side. (*See Figure 2-23.)* Note any asymmetry and tenderness. The doctor should verify the findings. (*See Figure 2-24.*) Then have the patient find her pubic synthesis, if she can. If she can't reach it, the doctor should palpate the pubic synthesis by starting at the ASIS on each side and sweeping the palpating fingers underneath the abdomen until they reach the midline. If there is any sensitivity or pain, then the pubic symphysis is likely misaligned, especially if asymmetry at the ASIS is noted. (*See Figure 2-25a and b.*) If there is tenderness and pain you need to note the anterior or forward side of the two bones and then a higher or more superior ASIS of the pair. The doctor might have to verify the subluxation pattern. (*See Figure 2-26 a and b.*)

THE TREATMENT

1. The high or superior side will be the side for the leg pull, similar to the Limited Positions earlier in this chapter. (*See Figure 2-18.)* The patient will have the opposite side's leg straight against the doctor's thigh. (*See Figure 2-27.*) This process is done slowly, repetitively and firmly while noting the patient's response. The doctor does this until there is no pain at the top or superior part of the pubic bones.

2. The forward side will have a small firm pillow or wedge placed underneath the opposite side. (*See Figure 2-29.*) The doctor's hands are placed on the thigh and hip of the forward side and gently push towards the table or posteriorly at an angle in the direction of the midline of the patient. (*See figure 2-30.)*

Both the leg pulling and the backward pushing are done until the evaluation of the pubic symphysis is painless. (*See Figures 2-31a and b.)* Please compare Figure 2-23 to Figure 2-32. I admit this can be pretty subtle, especially as care proceeds. Tenderness and limited motion are indications of guarding patterns from joint distress.

The patient can be taught how to evaluate and monitor her movements and resulting subluxation patterns. The patient depicted has two small children

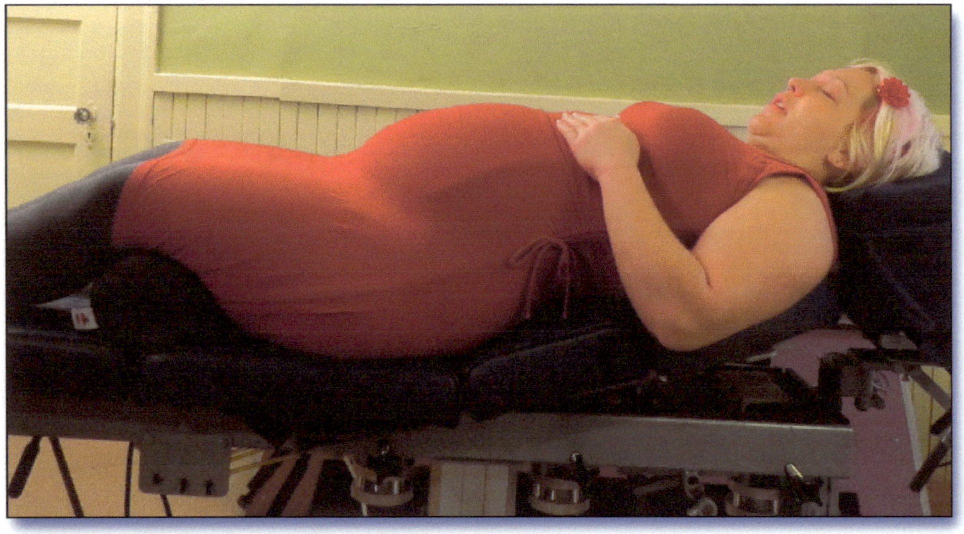

FIGURE 2-22 SUPINE POSITION OF PREGNANT PATIENT

Patient is supine on a table that is "tilted" up at the head and shoulders. This is usually the most comfortable position for the patient instead of flat on her back.

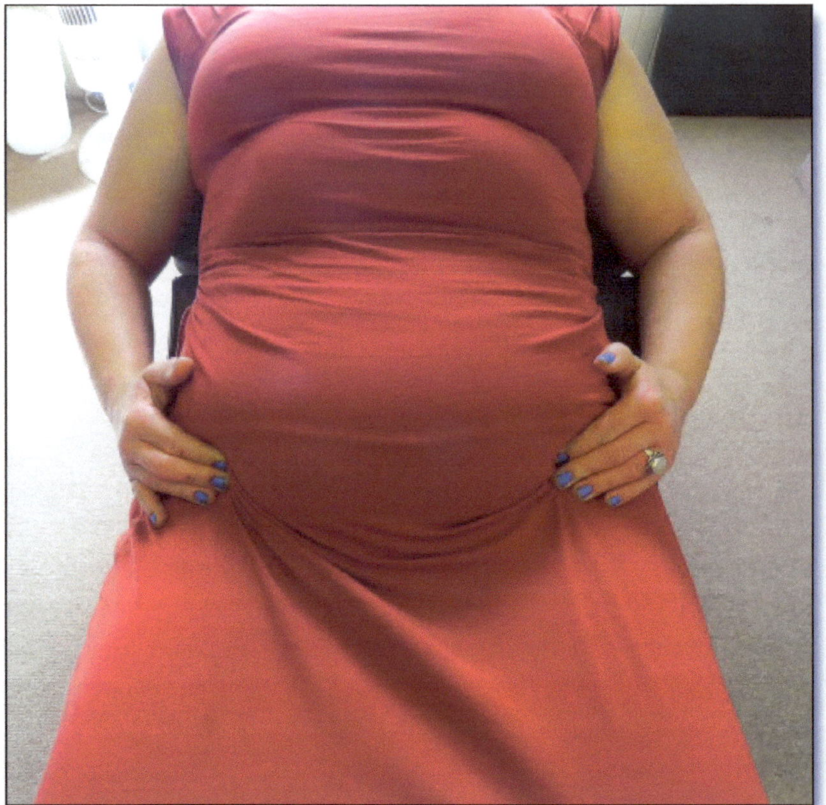

FIGURE 2-23 THE PATIENT FINDS HER ASIS ON EACH SIDE

Have the patient put her fingers on her ASIS on each side and note any asymmetry in height and posteriority. This patient's left ASIS is superior and posterior relative to the right side.

and is pregnant with her third. There are lots of ways for her to get hurt. We have taught her husband how to keep her adjusted and mobile. (*See Figures 2-32a and b – Self-evaluation*).

THE MANAGEMENT OF THE PREGNANT PELVIS

The pattern for a majority of women with pain and mobility problems during pregnancy is that the high side, as determined by supine evaluation, will have the uterus – and therefore the baby shifts to that side. Depending on pelvic tilt, the shift could put the fetus into contact with the Psoas. This muscle lifts the leg. Some women will have a hard time walking and standing. The goals we have with these protocols is multiple.

1. We want the partner, or whoever is helping, to be doing the leg pulling and the backwards pushing to keep the pelvis level. One main reason is to benefit the mother. She needs to have her usual ability to walk around with minimal pain. There is a universal rule that **if mommy isn't happy, no one's happy**.

2. The second reason is that we want the baby to be comfortable and experiencing the needed movement of the mother walking around and being active. The baby thrives when this is happening, but when the mother is distressed, the baby is distressed.

3. The third reason that we want this routine to happen is we need the partner to know how to keep the mom's pelvis level, not only through the remainder of her

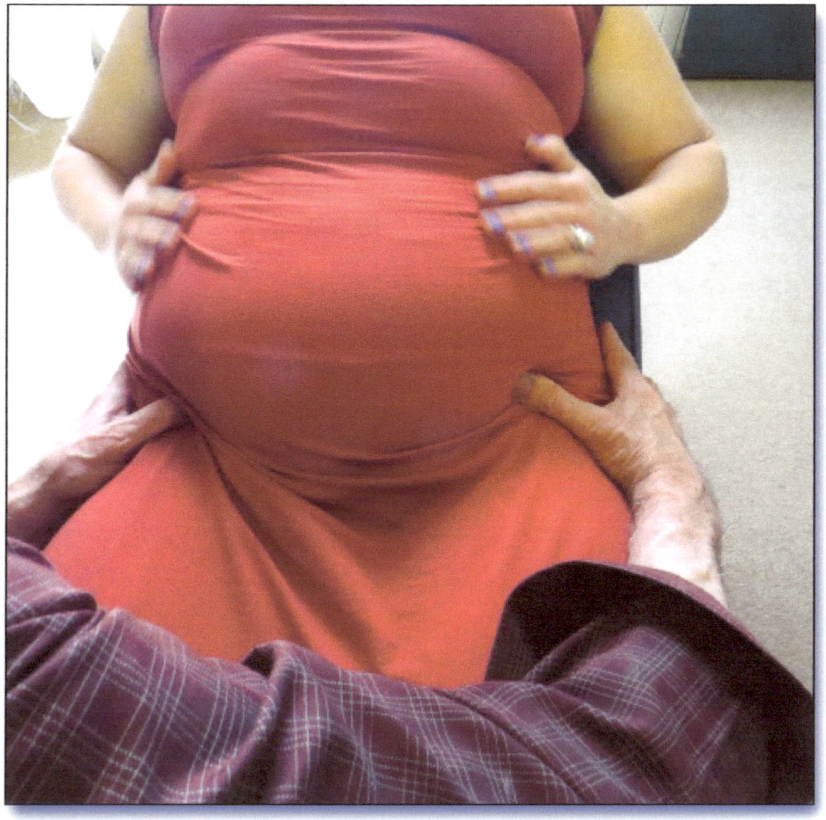

FIGURE 2- 24 THE DOCTOR VERIFIES THE POSITIONS OF THE ASIS ON EACH SIDE.

The doctors hands are on the ASIS on each side to verify that the left ASIS is superior and posterior relative to the right side.

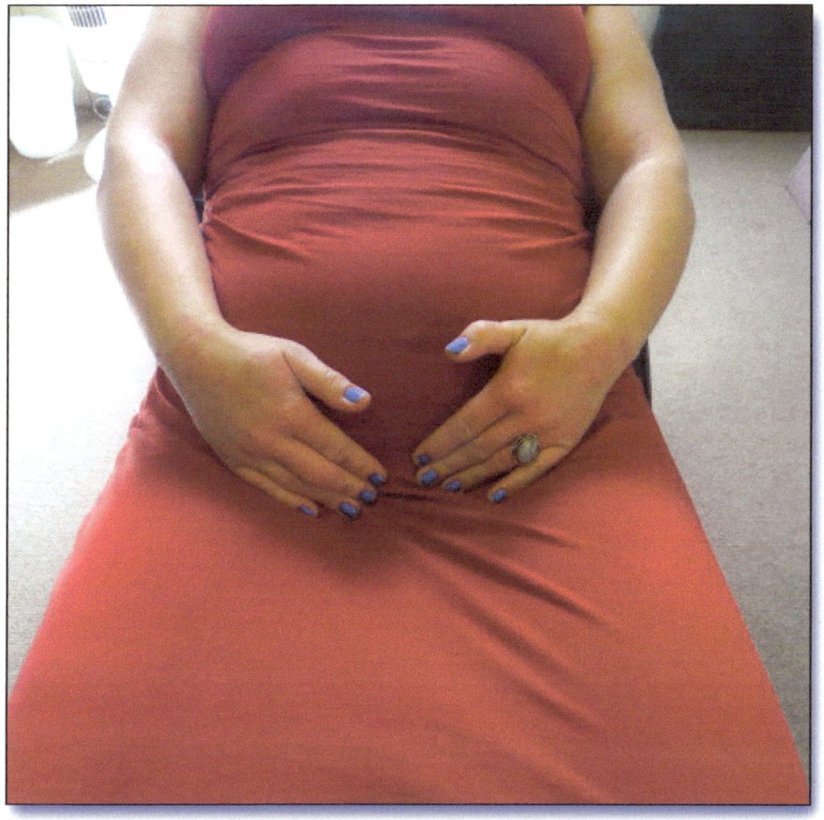

FIGURE 2-25A THE PATIENT CONTACTS HER PUBIC SYMPHYSIS, ANTERIOR SURFACE

Pain at this joint is very common when it is subluxated. Treatment is focused on reducing or eliminating pain at the pubic symphysis. This patient has significant pain at the pubic symphysis. Note the posterior position of her left hand.

pregnancy, but, through the labor and delivery as well.

I feel most of the difficulties in labor and delivery are due to uneven or subluxated pelvis. We know that the uneven pelvis and its relationship to labor and delivery is not understood by the midwives and the OB/GYN's. Our experience is that for a lot of our patients, when the pelvis is level at delivery, things go pretty smoothly and quickly.

We recommend that the pelvic leveling take place three times a day if possible: First thing in the morning, midday or as early in the evening as possible and then at bedtime. As a general rule, in the third trimester, I recommend not sitting on soft couches or the floor, or anywhere where you sink into something or have to twist and climb to get on your feet. This could mean the bathtub has to be given up.Managing an unstable pelvis requires changing personal behavior. It's much better for the patient to perch on a stool or take the cushions off the couch and put them on the kitchen chair so her hips are raised above her knees. This is especially important if the

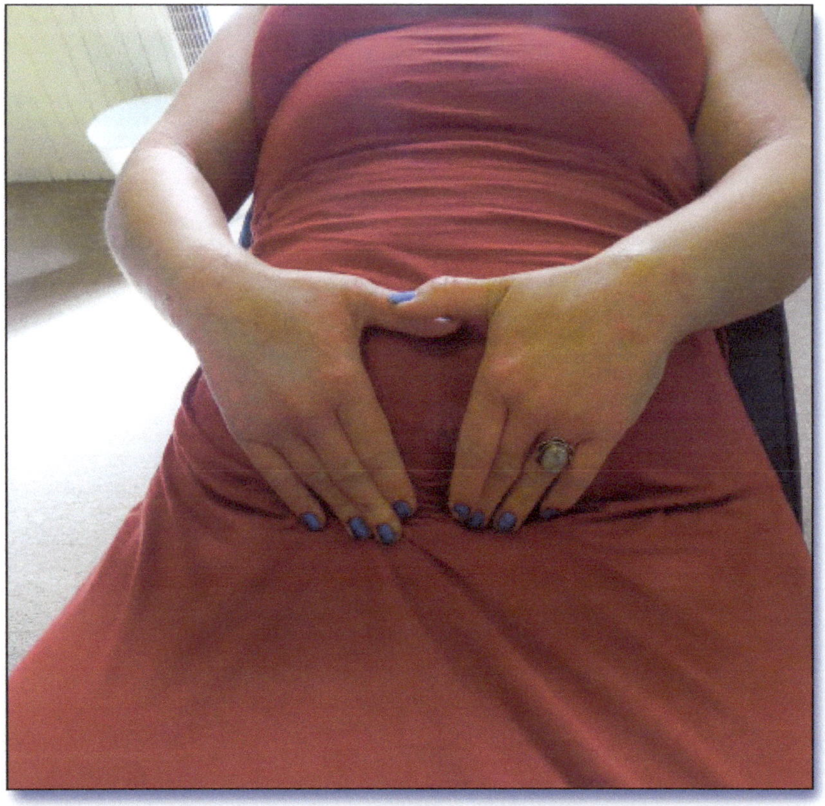

FIGURE 2-25B THE PATIENT CONTACTS HER PUBIC SYMPHYSIS ON THE SUPERIOR SURFACE

The patient, sometimes can't get into the top of the pubic symphysis, the superior displacement of the innominate is the most pain-full and debilitating of the subluxation patterns.

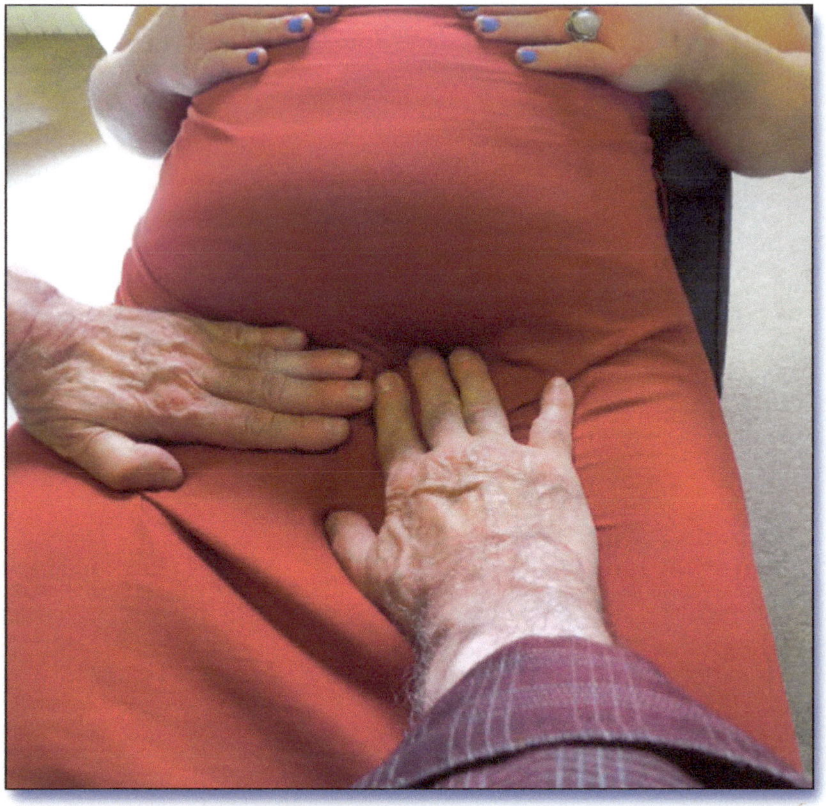

FIGURE 2-26A THE DOCTOR'S HANDS ON THE ANTERIOR PUBIC SYMPHSIS

The doctor's hands are on the anterior surface of the pubic bones. Sometime the patient is so big they cannot feel their own pubic bones. Note misalignment and pain. Reduction of subluxation and pain are the treatment goals.

patient is also suffering from wrist hand and shoulder injuries. Pushing and managing her position changes in advanced pregnancy is a factor in managing those additional injuries. (*See chapters 5, 6 and 7.*)

Pelvic instability, if pre-pregnancy, could be a lifetime problem. The presence of the relaxin hormone will be influencing the pelvic stability for weeks or months after the delivery. This period of time gets longer with each pregnancy. The additional work of baby care followed by childcare can set the patient up for chronic pain.

A STORY

A few years ago, my daughter Rachel arrived at the house we rent at the beach and she could not get out of the car without help. She was due in four days. She could barely stand or walk. As she started for the front door with a staircase to follow I directed her to

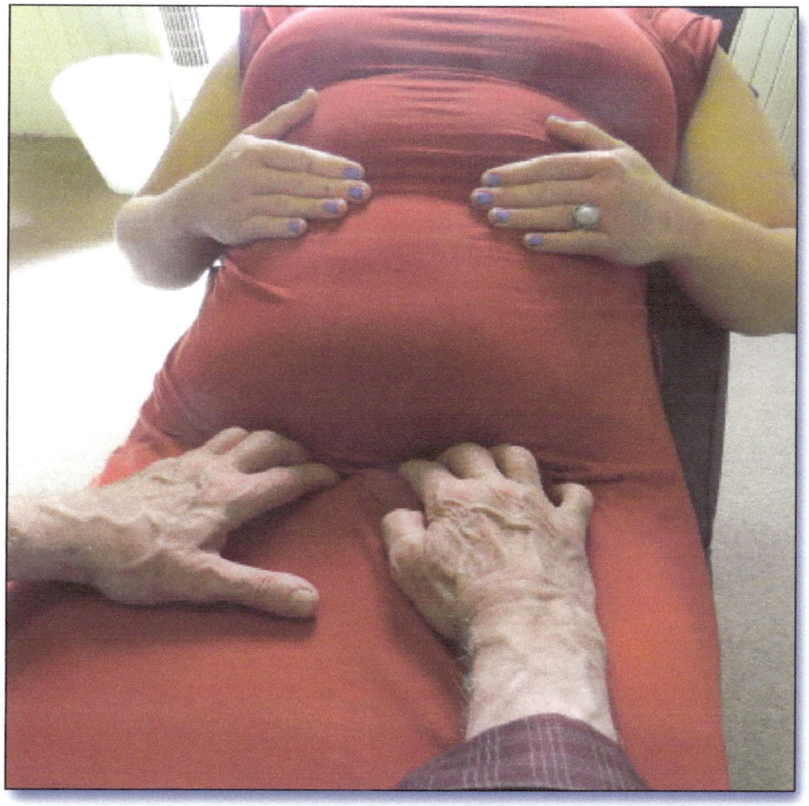

FIGURE 2-26B THE DOCTOR'S HANDS ON THE SUPERIOR PUBIC BONES

The doctor's fingers are on top of the pubic bones evaluating the subluxation pattern. Note the hand on the patients left side is more superior.

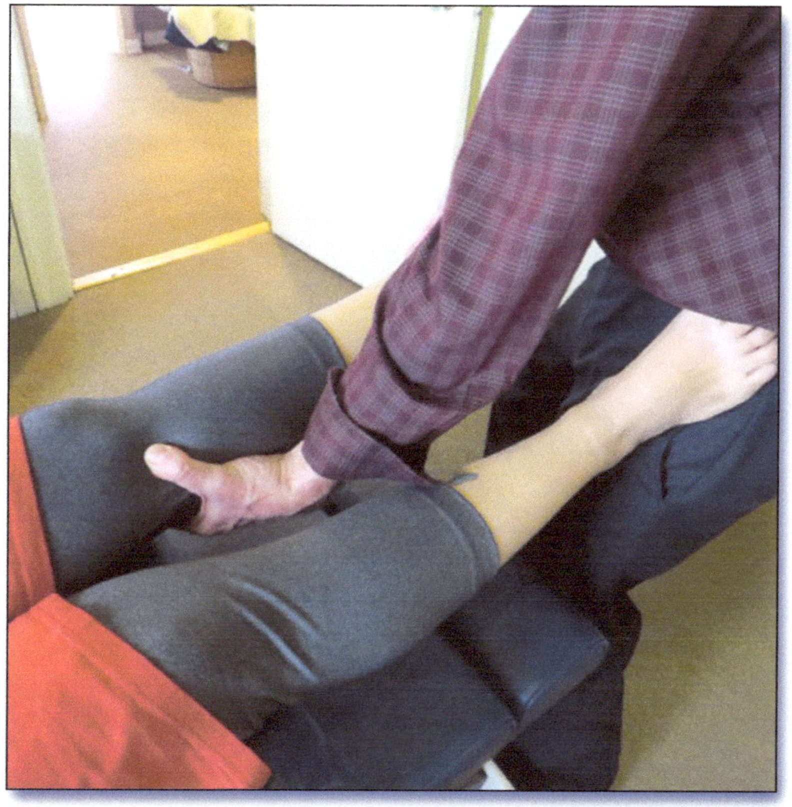

FIGURE 2-27 PERFORMING THE LEG PULL

The patient's foot is up against the doctor's thigh, the doctor has a hold of the leg of the high side of the patient. The pulling is firm but gentle. It is done many times rather than all at once and this allows reduced forces. This procedure is done until the top of the pubic bones are level or aligned across the top of the pubic bones and the pain is gone.

the sidewalk alongside the side of the house and to the deck in the back where a chiropractic table was ready for her. She needed help to get onto the table. We placed her in the supine tilted position. (*See figure 2-22.*) I evaluated her and then had her partner, Randall, reconfirm my evaluation. He confirmed my findings, Rachel was in severe distress and the pubic symphysis was significantly subluxated. Palpation of the ASIS's showed that she was high on the left side and palpation of the pubic symphysis showed that she was anterior on the right side. I then showed Randall how to do the leg pull on her left side and the backwards push to her right side. We repeated each maneuver five to six times, then rechecked the pubic symphysis until there was no tenderness and the bones were aligned anteriorly and superiorly. The ASIS's were level. We then had her roll onto her right side to sit up. Note that she was high on the left side and we do not want her loading that left side with changing positions or lifting things. *This is a major management issue.* At that moment, Rachel was able

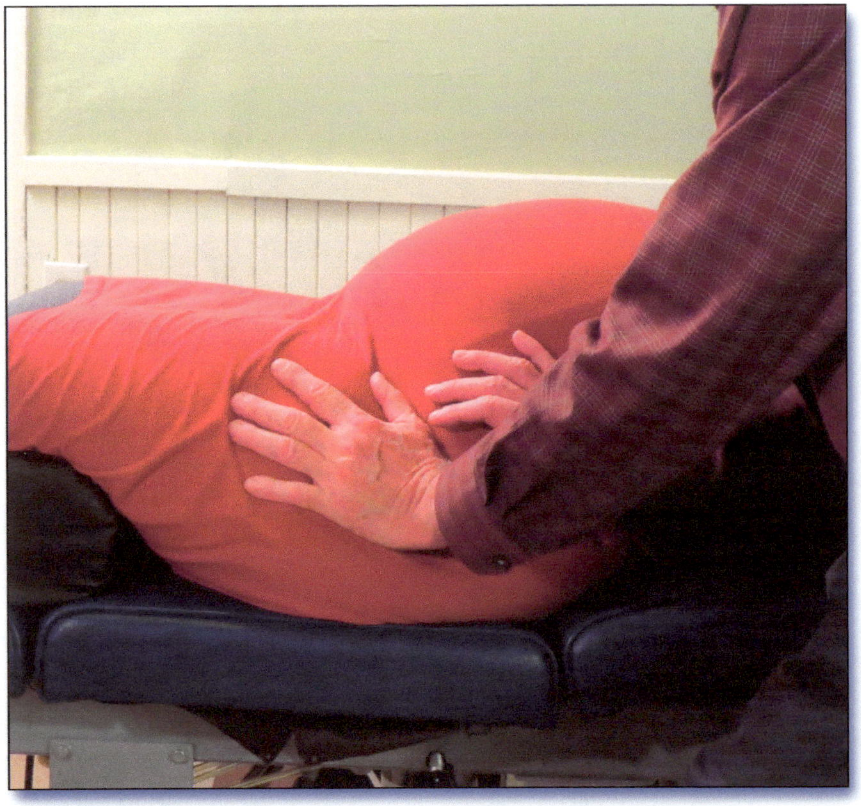

FIG. 2-28 HIP BONE PUSH

An alternative to the leg pull is the hip bone pushing. The helper contacts the iliac crest and the top of the leg bone. The pushing is towards to the feet. This might have to be done during active labor if the leg pulling is not working.

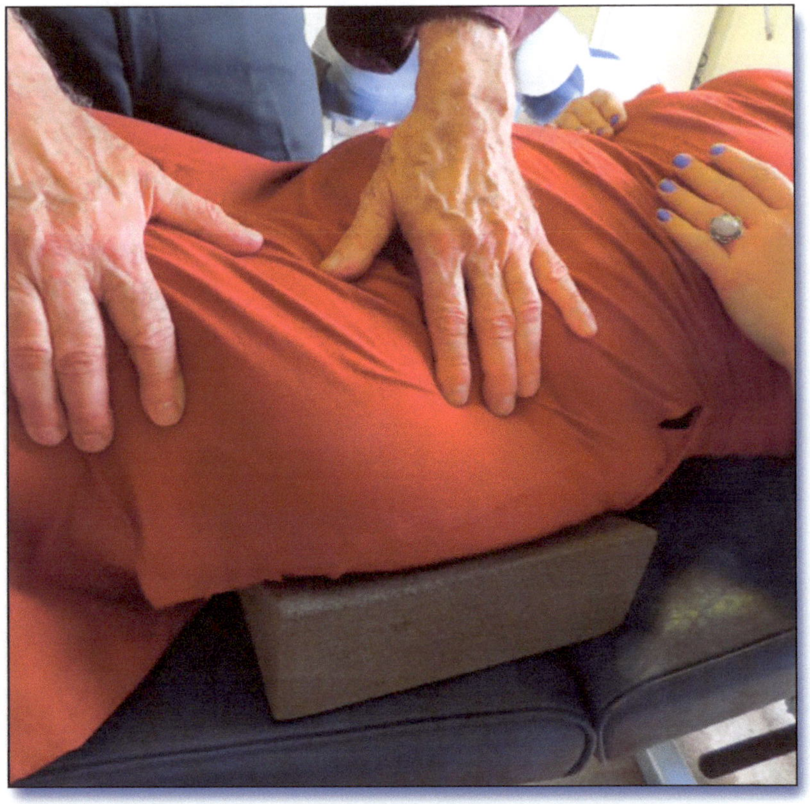

FIGURE 2-29 SETTING UP THE BACWARDS PUSH

The patient will have a cushion or support under the opposite Posterior side.

to stand up and walk around without distress. She did a few deep knee bends, declared herself fine and then went for a walk with Randall on the beach. I had Randall practice a few more times through the weekend. They went for long walks on the beach. Early Monday morning, they disappeared because she started labor, but it was a false labor. Tuesday morning she went into labor and delivered in eight hours. She had a natural childbirth without complications. When I arrived shortly after, I was told by an inside source that Randall was a great help to Rachel.

In just a few short minutes Rachel's partner was able to learn a simple adjusting technique and use it to turn a potentially painful and traumatic experience into a happy, healthy delivery.

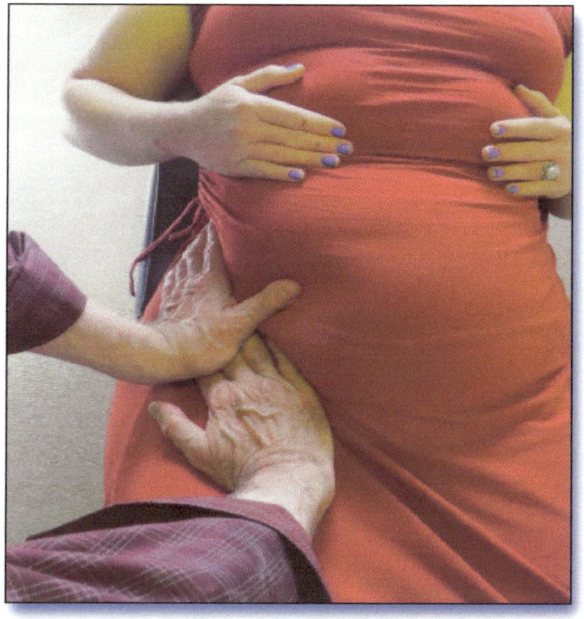

FIGURE 2-30 PERFORMING THE BACKWARD PUSH

The doctor's hand is on the thigh of the anterior or forward side of the patient. Gentle, repetitive thrusts are done towards the patients back at an angle towards the midline. This done until the pubic bones are aligned in the front or anterior surface and the pain is gone

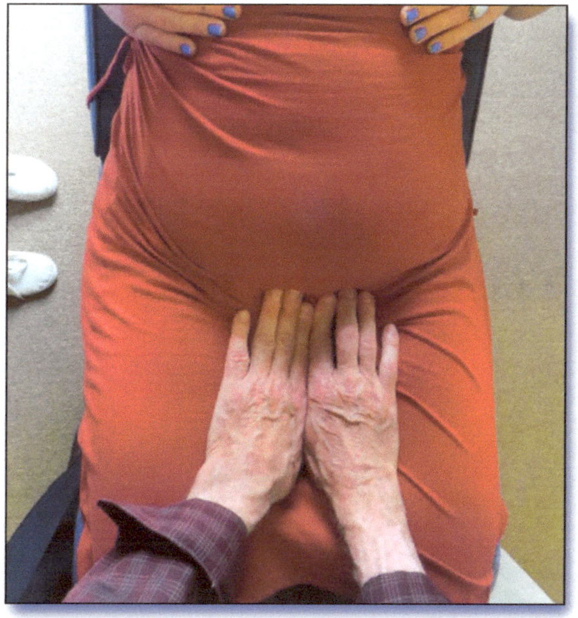

FIGURE 2-31A EVALUATING, POST ADJUSTMENT

The aligned pubic bones, the doctor's hands go over an aligned, smooth, non-tender joint. The goal here is to align the pubic bones. Be thorough, get rid of as much pain as possible. We need "dead level" at both the top and front parts of the pubic bones. In this view the patient is being evaluated for front to back or anterior-posterior subluxation. This shows an aligned pubic symphysis, with no tenderness, big difference from her presenting condition.

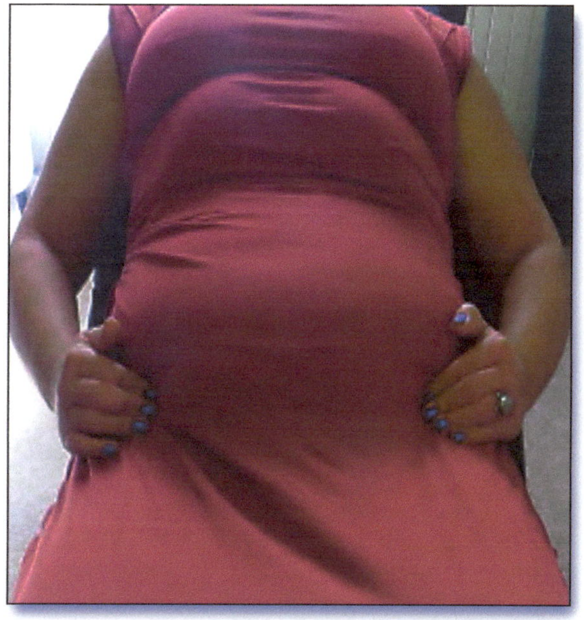

FIGURE 2-31B EVALUATING THE HIGH OR SUPERIOR SIDE

Compare this to Figure 2-

This is critical, since the slipping up of the hip bone is the most painful of the subluxation patterns. When the pubic bones are level across the top there is a relaxation of the abdominal wall. Also the mother can often feel the baby shifting back to the midline. In this view, we have a level pubic symphysis and no pain.

The patient's pattern here was high on the left. A recent Ultrasound study showed the baby all pulled over to the left side. Upon adjusting the mother, she felt the baby shift to the middle of her abdomen.

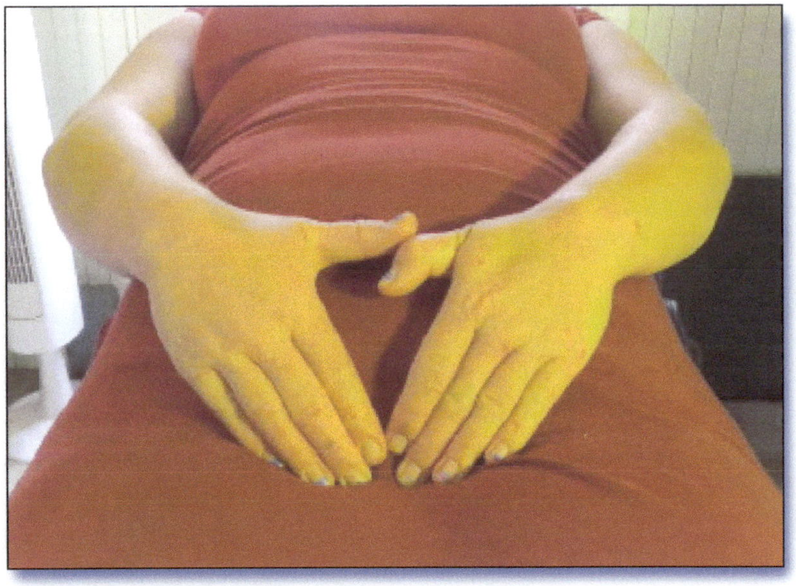

FIGURE 2-32A ANTERIOR PUBIC SYMPHYSIS SELF EVLUATION

The patient can contact the anterior surface of her pubic symphysis for tenderness or pain and signs of misalignment

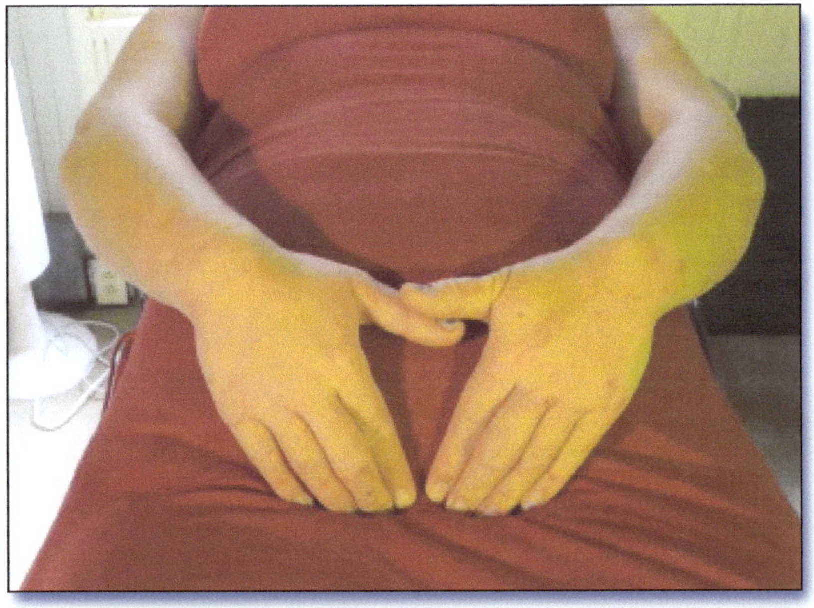

FIGURE 2-32B SELF EVALUATION OF THE SUPERIOR PUBIC SYMPHYSIS

The patient can self evaluate the superior displacement of her pubic symphysis, she might not be able to do this in late stage pregnancy.

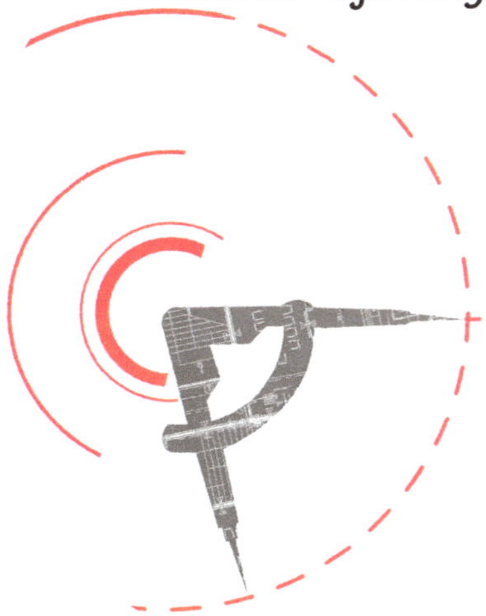

CHAPTER THREE

Evaluating, Adjusting, and Managing the Rib Cage

One of the main things I find about injuries sustained in a motor vehicle accident (MVA), stroke or traumatic brain injury is that the anterior joints of the chest or rib cage can also be injured. The axilla is painful to touch and hyper-responsive to any palpation. In the anatomy lab, I would find osteophytes on the posterior aspects of these joints that are on the inside of the chest wall. Sometimes the osteophytes were so large as to impinge on the aorta or vena cava. This indicates they suffered injury.

Speaking anatomically, if the costosternal joints are disturbed, the costovertebral and the costo-transverse joints are disturbed. In my view, the rib cage is a vital cavity, and the guarding response will be mediated by the spinal cord and thus be global in its impact. Guarding mechanisms will then involve all the musculature that arises off of it. This would include all of the muscles that go to the head, neck and shoulders. The rigidity of these muscles is usually regarded as tightness that needs to be stretched. Muscle testing will indicate the muscles are weak instead of fatigued and exercise will be prescribed. I feel most of us misread the guarding mechanisms as misbehaving muscles that need to be changed with exercise and stretching regimens instead of providing the patient with joint relief and stabilization.

Use of pain medications by the population when other therapies have failed is a very frequent occurrence. More people die now from pain medication overdoses than from heroin. I believe that since most have been in motor vehicle accidents, using pain medication is really quite understandable. Since most of our professions do not adequately evaluate the full extent of the injuries sustained, therapeutic intervention is less than helpful. This leaves patients with few options for relief but pain medications. It has been shown in numerous studies that X-ray or MRI studies cannot predict pain and disability. There is no way to predict from radiographic findings what symptoms will be present. Normal MRI findings of the cervical spine will sometimes be found with someone in terrible pain. The rib cage is never evaluated in these studies. If the upper ribs are subluxated, there will be pain and distress patterns in the head, neck and shoulders. When I have had my patients evaluated by medical specialists, they tell the patient there is no connection between the rib cage and the neck or shoulder. This is anatomically incorrect and clinically not supported by exam findings, if a full exam is performed.

In more than 30 years of practice, I have found the most common source of injury to the rib cage is the motor vehicle accident. The exposure of our population to this type of injury is huge. In this country, currently there are more than 16 million motor vehicle accidents per year. Most of them are multiple-vehicle, multiple-occupant events. Most of my patients coming in for initial care have a history of motor vehicle accidents. We also find these types of injuries from other crashing events such as skiing, skateboarding, snowboarding and falls. I've also had a number of patients forget to tell me about their history of airplane crashes, which belong in this category as well. Another source of these types of injuries are open-heart surgeries and breast cancer surgeries, where the rib cage is distressed in positions necessitated by the surgical procedure, usually with the arm or arms dropped off the table. During the surgery, the use of general anesthesia and the length of time, usually hours, leaves the rib cage injured after the surgery. Persistent difficulty breathing, tightness of the chest, stiff and painful neck muscles, limited shoulder motion, entrapment of neurological and vascular structures leading to upper extremity complaints are not uncommon post-surgery.

A stroke can also leave the rib cage disturbed, with terrible pain and the loss of motion of the arm, hand and neck. In my experience dealing with stroke victims, it appears that for a lot of these patients, the cerebral accident causes a loss of ligament tone as well as muscular tone and function. The weight of the arm and shoulder can pull the ribs out of place. This can cause entrapment of the neurological and vascular structures that involve the arm and hand. If I encounter a stroke victim with rigid musculature, especially of the upper extremity, I know that motor firing has returned to the spinal cord and other neurological components. The rigidity of the musculature guarding patterns is trying to hold the subluxated joints together. This can leave the patient with debilitating pain and, of course, loss of function (We will be covering these issues in more detail later in this book).

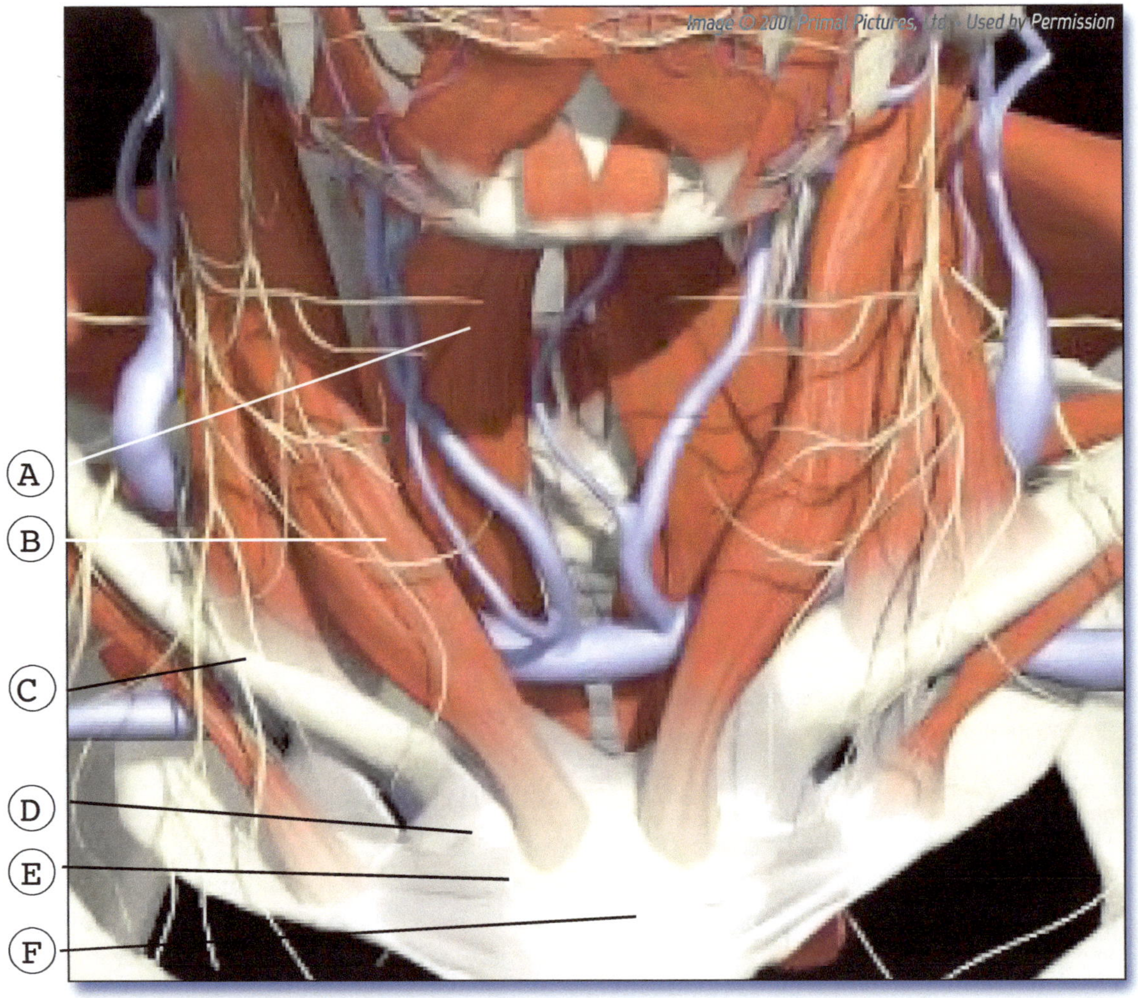

FIGURE 3-1 THE UPPER ANTERIOR JOINTS OF THE CHEST

These joints control the tone and function of the throat, neck and shoulder muscles.

A) Sternohyoid muscle
B) Sternocleidomastoid muscle
C) Clavicle
D) Sternoclavicular joint
E) 1st costosternal joint
F) Sternum (manubrium)

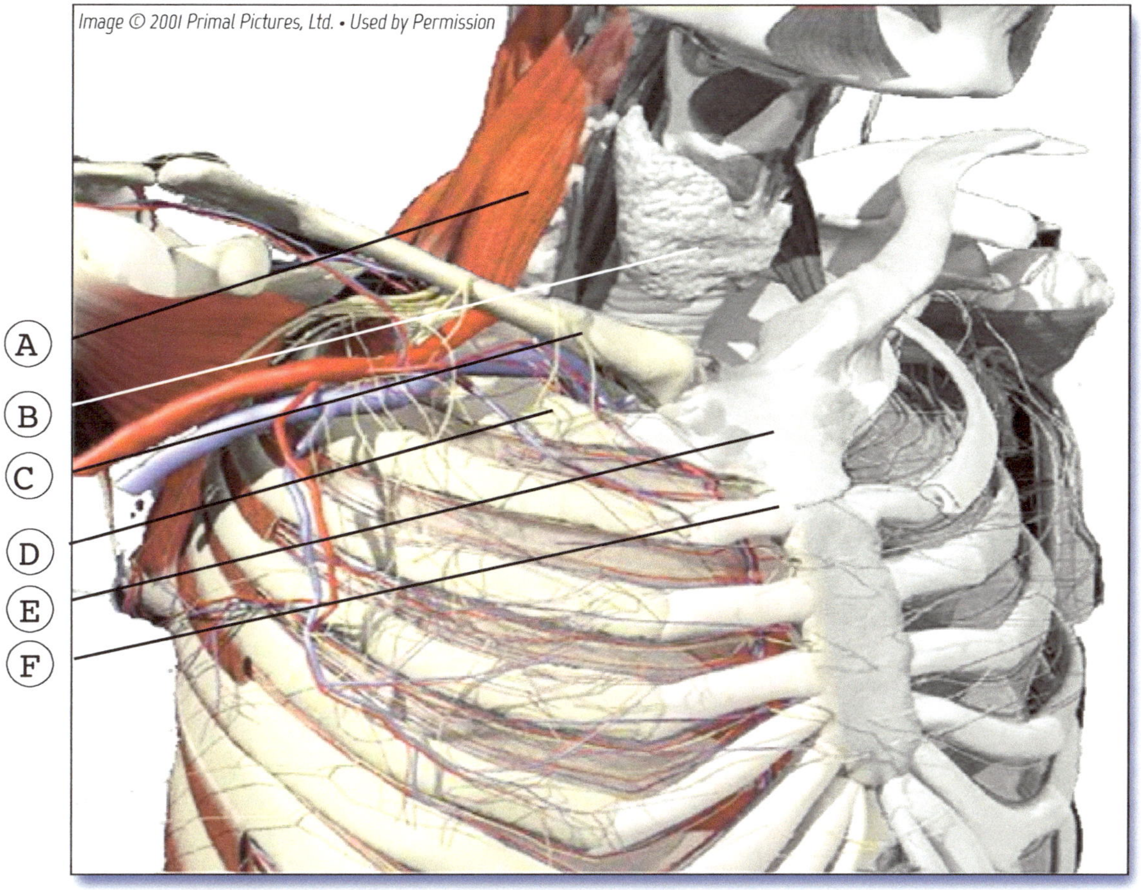

FIGURE 3-2 THE ANTERIOR AND LATERAL VIEW OF THE RIB CAGE.

It should be apparent that rib subluxation at the sternum should be perceived as distress in the axilla region.

A) Scalene muscle

B) Throat

C) Clavicle

D) Ist rib

E) Sternum (manubrium)

F) 2nd costosternal joint

THE RELEVANT ANATOMY OF THE RIB CAGE

The anterior joints of the chest are integral structural components of the rib cage. Injury to these structures can be devastating to the patient's head, neck and shoulders *(See Figures 3-1 and 3-2).* Few patients will direct you to these injuries. These injuries appear not to give conscious pain signals to most patients. This is why a thorough exam by palpation is necessary. The pectoralis major and minor muscles originate at the costosternal joints. Subluxation of the costosternal joints will cause the pectoralis muscles to become tight, which will internally rotate the humerus.

The subluxation of the ribs from the sternum will also cause the serratus anterior muscle to tighten as part of this guarding mechanism. This tightening will translate the scapula away from the midline. This displacement of the scapula, along with the internal rotation of the humerus will leave the shoulder joints in a compromised position. This will leave the patient's body irritated, inflamed and producing a dull, achy shoulder with a limited range of motion. For some people, this is the etiology of adhesive capsulitis or, as some would call it, frozen shoulder syndrome.

The sternoclavicular joints have attached to them the sternocleidomastoid muscle (SCM) *(See Figures 3-1 and 3-3).* The sternoclavicular joints control the tightness of the SCM. When injury has occurred and these joints are subluxated, the SCM tightness can produce headache and head pain at the insertion at the parietal, temporal and occipital bones.

The SCM has a close relationship to the external jugular vein. In Figure 3-3, this vein is shown lying externally on the SCM, but most people have the vein in the SCM. The external jugular vein drains the orbit of the eye, nasal sinus, inner ear, TMJ and scalp on that side of the head. Over the years I have found many cases of sternoclavicular joint injury causing tension headaches, throbbing behind the eye, severe sinus pain, vertigo, loss of hearing and aching teeth. Also, the muscles of the throat attach to the posterior aspect of the sternoclavicular joints. Injury to these joints can produce a complaint of difficulty swallowing or pressure on the throat and loss of normal vocal function.

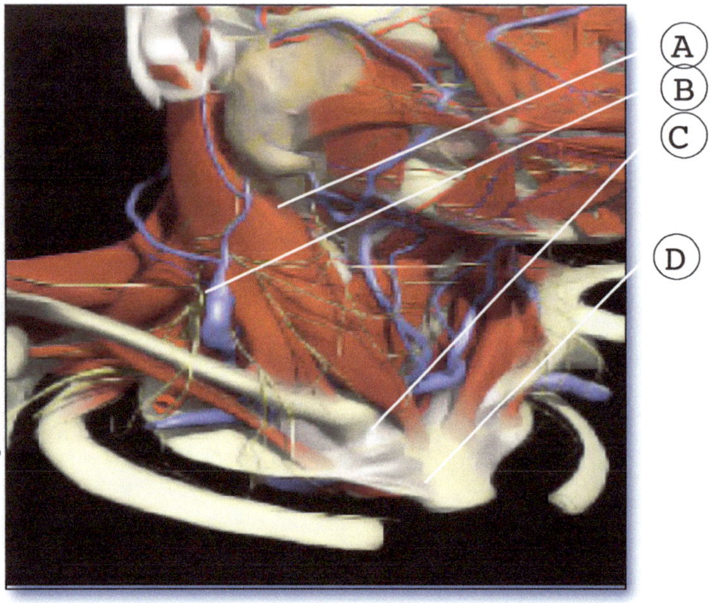

FIGURE 3-3 THE NECK AND THROAT MUSCULATURE WITH NEUROLOGICAL AND VASCULAR STRUCTURES

Subluxation of the ribs and clavicles in the thoracic regions can cause significant dysfunction of the face, head, neck and shoulders.

A) SCM
B) External jugular vein
C) Sternoclavicular joint
D) Ist costosternal joint

The scalene muscles attach to the ribs and the cervical vertebrae *(See Figure 3-2)*. Subluxation of the ribs at the sternum will cause the scalene muscles to tighten, restricting the range of motion of the head and neck and producing pain in the neck, most commonly in the lateral aspect.

When the costosternal joints are subluxated, costovertebral and costotransverse joints will also be subluxated. This type of injury is a global event – front, lateral and back of the rib cage. This will have an adverse effect on the sympathetic chain, leading to insidious and chronic health problems that are subtle and difficult to diagnose. Chest wall pain and panic attacks have a high correlation in emergency room studies. Persistent subluxation of the ribs can lead to chronic anxiety disorders from constant sympathetic simulation. Exhausted adrenal glands can be from a chronic state of "flight or fight" *(See Figure 3-4)*. The alignment of the ribs to the spine are critical

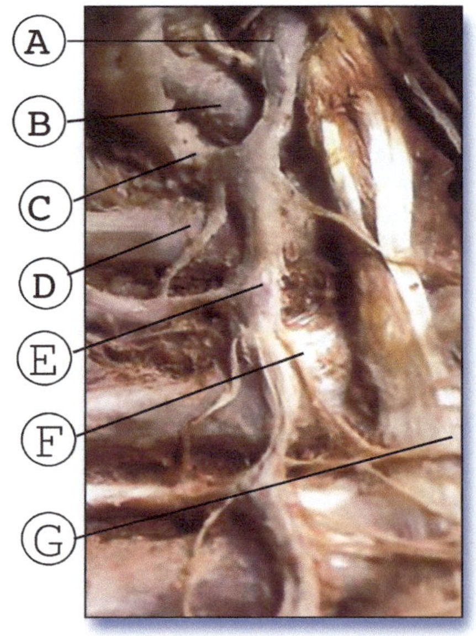

FIGURE 3-4 ANTERIOR VIEW OF THE UPPER THORACIC SPINE

A) Inferior Cervical Sympathetic Ganglion
B) First Rib
C) First Thoracic Nerve Root
D) Second Rib
E) Sympathetic Chain Ganglion
F) Costovertebral Joint Ligaments
G) Anterior Longitutinal Ligament of the Vetebral Column

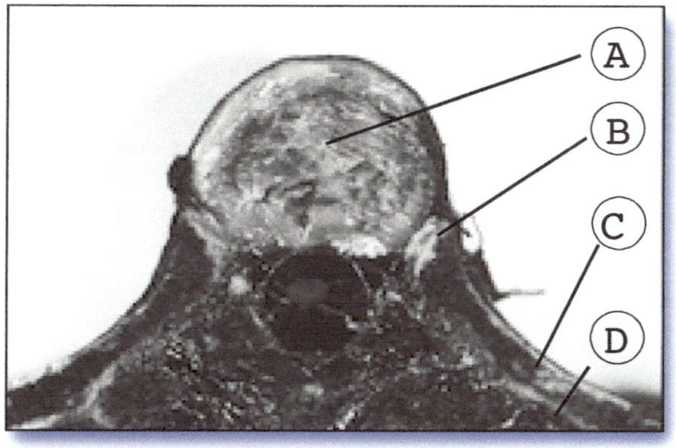

FIGURE 3-5. THE NORMAL RIB-VERTEBRAL RELATIONSHIP

Note the closeness of the rib neck and head to the transverse process and vertebral body.

A) Vertebral body
B) Rib head
C) Rib neck
D) Transverse process

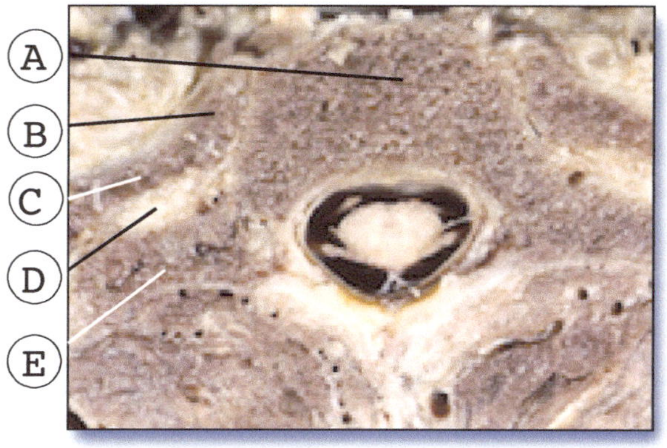

FIGURE 3-6. SUBLUXATION OF THE RIBS TO THE VERTEBRA

Note how the ribs are separated from the transverse processes and vertebral body.

A) Vertebral body
B) Rib head
C) Rib neck
D) Gap between rib and transverse process
E) Transverse process

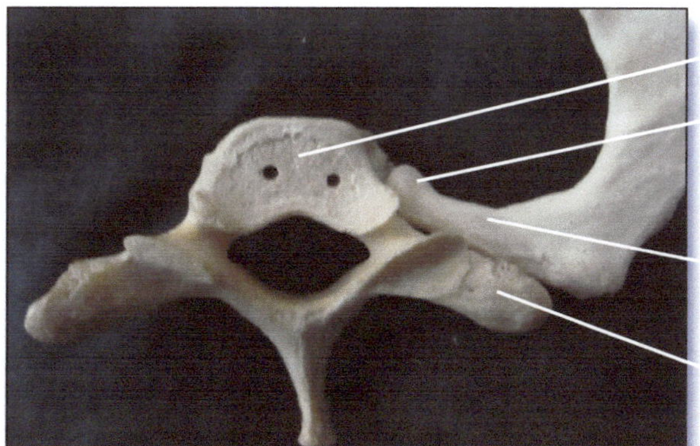

FIGURE 3-7 NORMAL ALIGNMENT FOR THE COSTOVERTEBRAL AND COSTOTRANSVERSE JOINTS

A) Vertebral body
B) Rib head
C) Rib neck
D) Transverse process

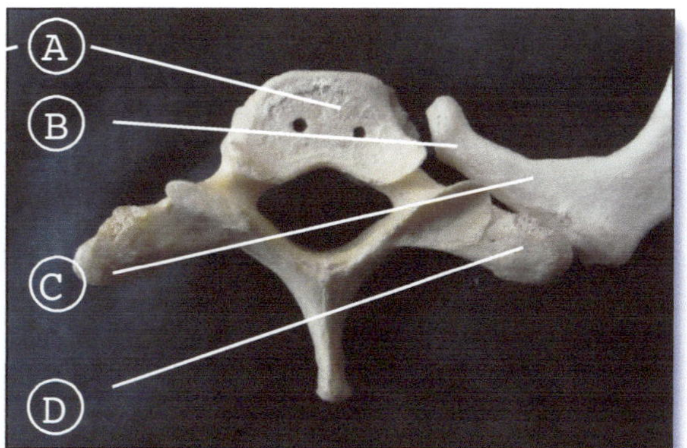

FIGURE 3-8. SUBLUXATION OF THE COSTOVERTEBRAL AND COSTOTRANSVERSE JOINTS

A) Vertebral body
B) Rib head
C) Rib neck
D) Transverse process

joints to a vital cavity: the rib cage. We use the term "subluxation" but the central nervous system view is "impending luxation". The neurological guarding response to rib subluxation can be a serious health problem. The rib joints to the spine have ligaments and joint capsules with very sensitive proprioceptors and mechanoreceptors *(See Figures 3-5 to 3-8).* Subluxation of the ribs can be subtle but serious, interfering with breathing, sleep and digestion.

THE IMAGING ANALYSIS OF THE RIB CAGE

The appearance of subluxation of the rib cage on imaging is not something the radiologists, either medical or chiropractic, investigate. I have made numerous attempts to get radiologists to recognize these radiographic features as subluxations and injuries. These injuries need full care and recovery time. For Worker's Compensation and personal injury cases, often the word "normal" in the radiographic report undermines the case and the need for care.

Nerve path patterns differ from person to person. This could explain why people with normal appearing X-rays and MRIs of the cervical spine can have terrible pain, entrapment syndromes and debilitating symptoms, while others who have degenerative changes of the cervical spine yet have little in the way of symptoms. This can lead to confusing and confounding observations. If the rib cage injuries are never evaluated, it will always remain a mystery why some people with no apparent pathology of the cervical spine have very painful symptoms.

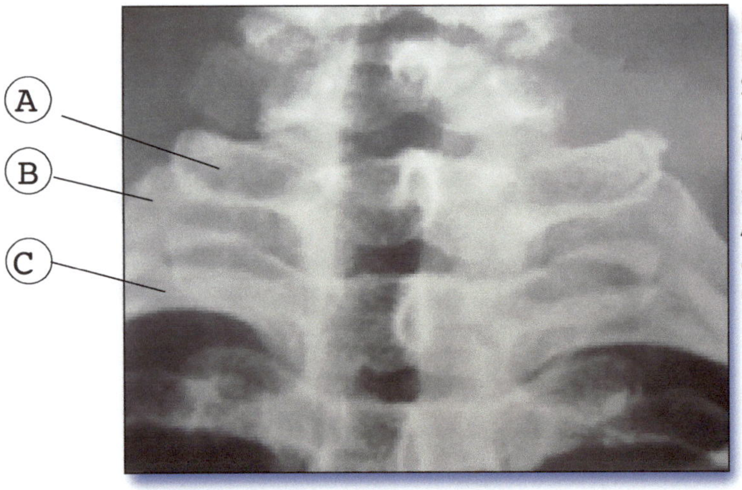

FIGURE 3-9. NORMAL A-P VIEW OF UPPER RIB CAGE AND THORACIC SPINE

Note the overlapping of the ribs over the transverse processes and the proximity of the rib heads to the vertebral bodies.
A) Transverse process
B) Overlap of transverse process and rib
C) Rib neck

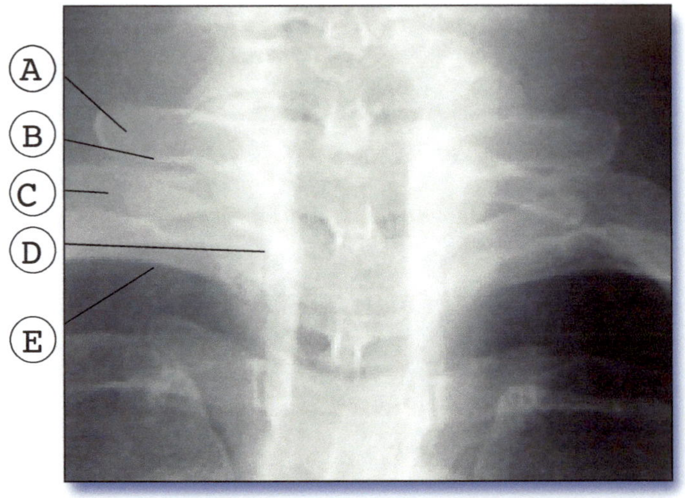

Figure 3-10. SUBLUXATION OF THE UPPER RIBS FROM THE THORACIC SPINE

Note the lack of overlap the ribs have with the transverse processes and the gaps the heads of the ribs have with the transverse processes and the vertebral bodies.

A) Transverse process
B) Gap between rib and transverse process
C) 1st rib
D) Gap between rib head and vertebral body
E) 2nd rib

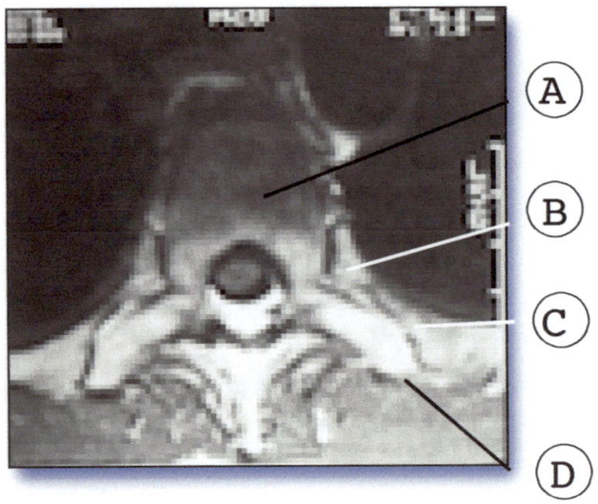

FIGURE 3-11. MRI OF THE THORACIC SPINE SHOWING ALIGNED RIBS WITH THE VERTEBRA

Note that the ribs fit snugly up against the vertebra.
A) Vertebral body
B) Rib head
C) Rib neck
D) Transverse process

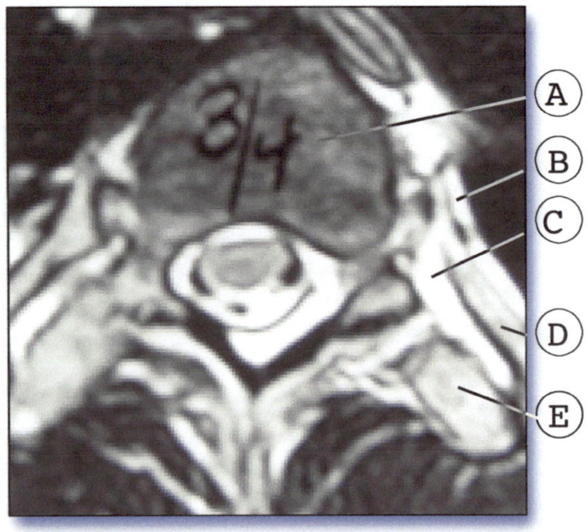

Figure 3-12 MRI OF THE THORACIC SPINE SHOWING RIB SUBLUXATION

Note that there is a gap between the ribs and the vertebra. The patient had terrible chest pain, keeping him awake.
A) Vertebral body
B) Rib head
C) Gap between rib neck and transverse process
D) Rib neck
E) Transverse process

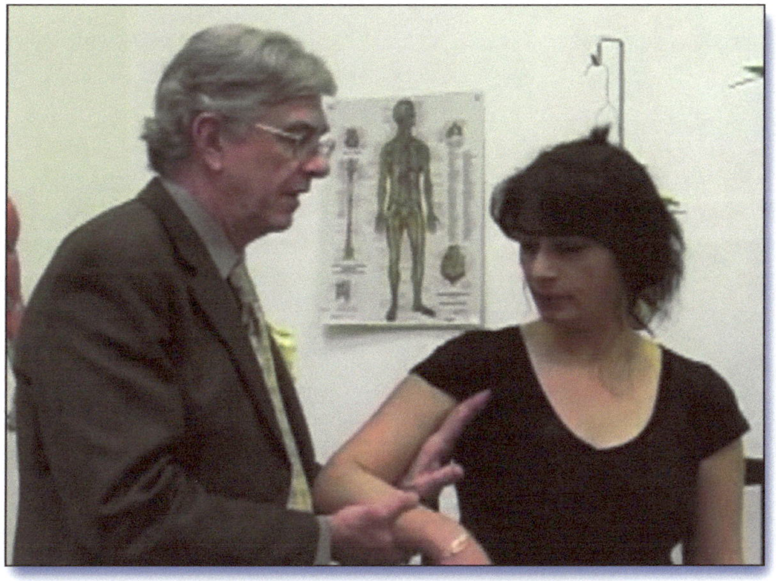

FIGURE 3-13. EXAMINATION OF THE AXILLA.

With the doctor on the side of the patient, palpate for a tender pectoralis major tendon insertion. Ask female patients to move breast tissue forward. Evaluate both pre- and post-adjustment.

The X-ray findings are subtle to distinguish *(see Figures 3-9 and 3-10)*, but on careful inspection, the loss of the overlap of the ribs on the transverse processes is apparent. In a normal X-ray, the rib neck is in contact with the transverse processes and in the lower X-ray, the rib necks are separated from the transverse processes. The MRI findings are subtle as well, but the subluxations must be searched for, or they will never be found. All of this is secondary to the physical examination *(See Figures 3-13 to 3-15)*.

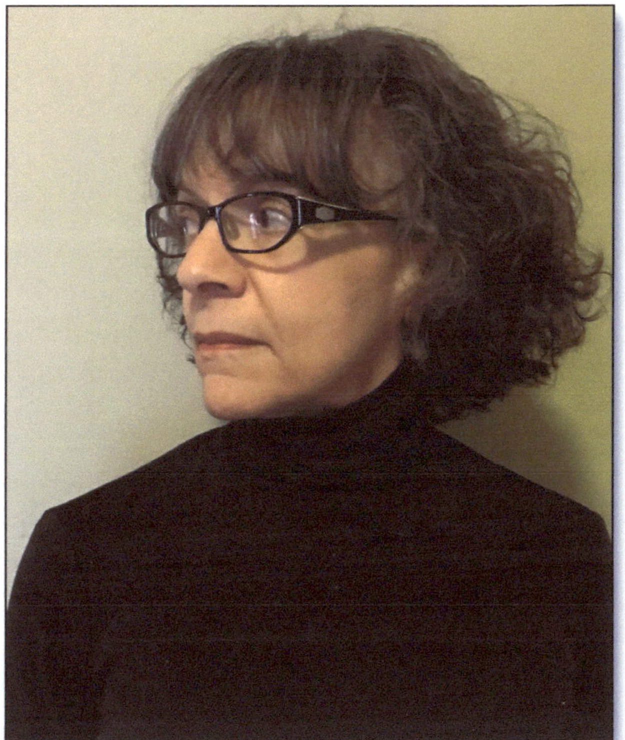

FIGURE 3-14. EVALUATE RANGE OF MOTION FOR THE NECK, HEAD, AND SHOULDERS

This test can be performed for pain. Direct the patient to provoke the worst part of their neck pain and then perform the test. This example shows loss of rotation in the neck.

FIGURE 3-15 RIB CAGE COMPRESSION TEST WITH INCREASED RANGE OF MOTION

Note the increased range of rotation of the cervical spine while the ribs are being compressed.

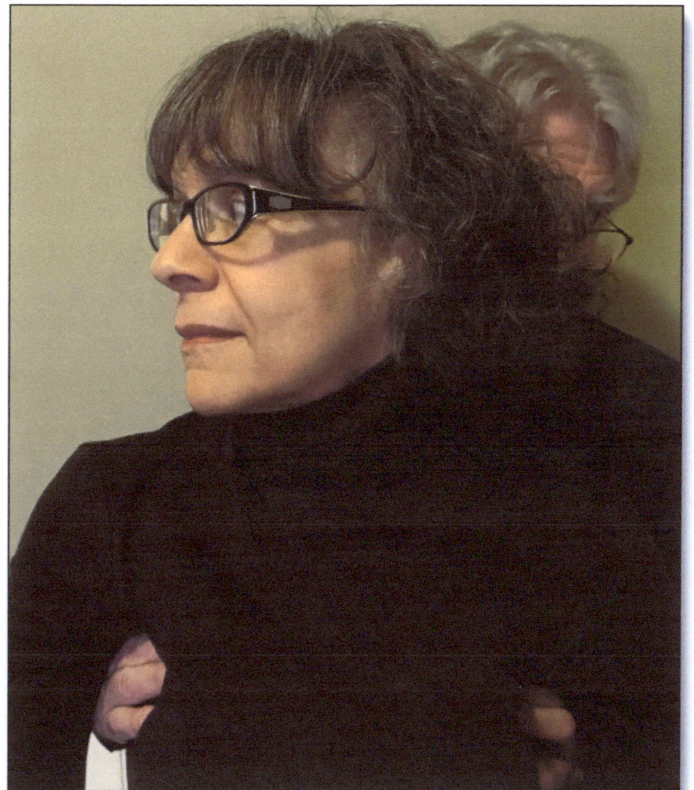

THE EVALUATION AND PALPATION OF THE RIB CAGE

In evaluating the anterior joints of the rib cage, I use direct palpation of the costosternal, sternoclavicular joints and the axilla *(See Figure 3-13).*

The costosternal joint can be palpated by placing the doctor's hand on the ribs and slide toward the sternum. If the hand moves forward or anterior to the ribs, then the ribs have moved posteriorly. The physical structure and curvature of the rib cage indicates that the ribs must also move laterally in order to be posteriorly (to the sternum) subluxated. This can also be palpated by placing the doctor's hand on the sternum and gently gliding laterally onto the ribs, noting any dipping or posterior subluxations.

The doctor can also hold the weight of the patient's arm in one hand while palpating the pectoralis major tendon insertion into the humerus underneath the humeral head. If this tendon is taut and tender to palpation with the arm weight removed, there is a high probability the rib cage is subluxated.

Palpate for muscle/tendon relaxation following the adjustment. In addition, evaluate patient tenderness in these areas before and after the adjustment.

After evaluating the range of motion of the neck, head and shoulders, then perform the rib cage compression test *(See Figures 3-14 and 3-15, and further description in the next section).* While the ribs are being compressed, re-evaluate the range of motion of the neck, head, and shoulders. Noting any changes in symptoms while the ribs are held in place.

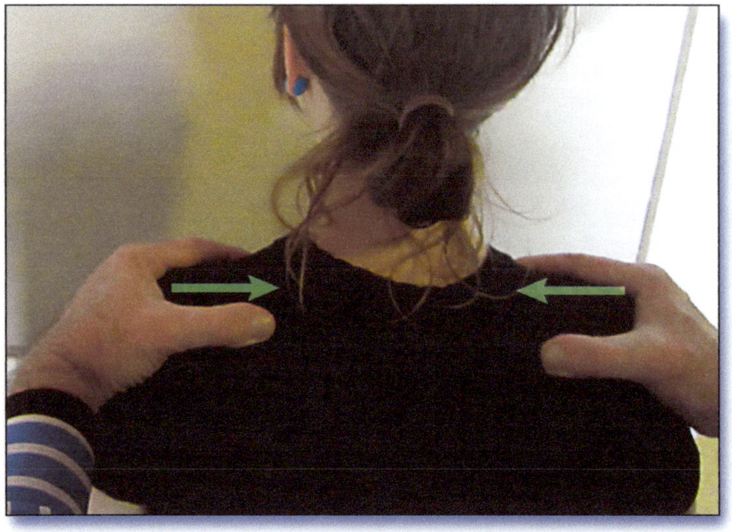

FIGURE 3-16 POSTERIOR VIEW OF THE SHOULDER SQUEEZE TEST

The Sternoclavicular joints are being pushed together in the Shoulder Squeeze Test. You can see the SCM and throat muscles attach to these joints. See Figure 3-1

THE RIB CAGE COMPRESSION TEST

The Rib Cage Compression Test is performed to demonstrate the effects of the injured, subluxated rib cage on shoulder function, entrapment syndromes and other associated complaints.

The Rib Cage Compression Test can be very uncomfortable for the patient if the ribs are subluxated. The doctor's hands should go up underneath the arms into the axilla. The doctor's fingers are pointed up with the hands compressing the rib cage from lateral to medial. Have the patient demonstrate their cervical range of motion and then perform the rib cage compression test and have them redo their range of motion. Note any differences *(See Figures 3-14 and 3-15).* In Figure 3-14, we see minor loss of cervical range of motion, while in Figure 3-15, we see the increased range of motion while the ribs are being compressed.

In the majority of cases, this can be done with the doctor standing behind the patient. Both hands are used, one on each side of the patient, and a squeezing or compression of the ribs from lateral to medial is performed. The compression should be maintained for 20 to 30 seconds. If the doctor is much smaller than the patient, the patient can be seated and, if needed, only one side at a time is treated. If the patient is in a hospital bed or wheelchair, perform the adjustment one side at a time.

This test is dual-purpose:

1. The doctor needs to see how much the restriction or pain with shoulder activity is related to the subluxated rib cage.
2. The patient can see that any positive changes from having their ribs compressed reveals that the rib subluxations are part of their injury and diagnosis.

Managing a rib cage injury that is restricting shoulder function or creating entrapment syndromes needs to be fully understood by the patient. The more the patient can see these relationships, the more the patient can assist in managing their own injuries.

THE SHOULDER SQUEEZE TEST

For the Shoulder Squeeze Test, the doctor takes the patient's shoulders and compresses them both, lateral to medial. This brings the sternoclavicular joints back towards a normal alignment. This test should be done for at least 20 to 30 seconds, while noting any improvement in the patient's headache, sinus pain, loss of hearing, vertigo or aching teeth.

To test for this condition, stand behind the patient and place your hands on the outside or lateral aspect of the shoulders. Squeeze them together, aiming to bring the clavicles into the sternum or manubrium. Count to 20 and then ask the patient if they feel any changes (i.e., reduced of headache or dizziness) *(See Figure 3-16)*.

ADJUSTING THE RIBS WITH THE SLI.

Rib compression adjusting can be done with an adjustive instrument or drop table. The adjustive instrument should be used when the patient is so highly distressed that they may not be able to lie supine or prone or tolerate the drop table *(See Figures 3-17, 3-18, 3-19 and 3-20)*.

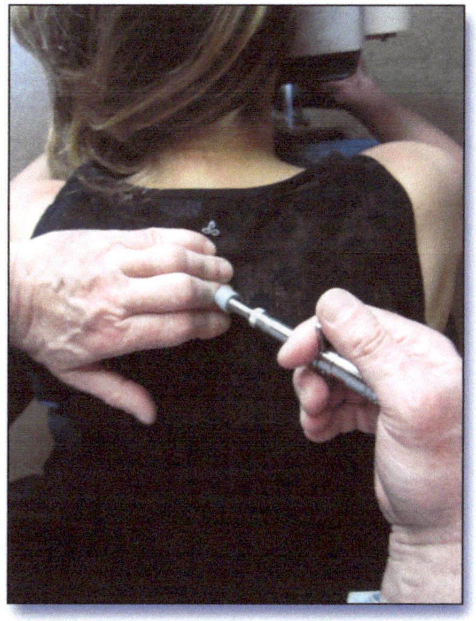

FIGURE 3-17 RIB ADJUSTING WITH A SPRING LOADED ADJUSTING INSTRUMENT AS THE PATIENT LIES PRONE.

Note firm contact with the fingers pressing the rib into the desired position.. The SLI is applied through the finger.

For adjusting the highly distressed patient, use the adjusting instrument for the following adjustments.

- In correcting the posterior subluxation, cross an arm over the patient's chest to move the scapula away from the angle of the ribs.
- Then use the adjusting instrument posterior to anterior (PA) over the angle of the ribs *(See Figure 3-18)*.

For the lateral rib subluxations, have the individual seated or standing with the doctor located laterally and placing the fingers in the patient's axilla. If this is too painful or sensitive for the patient, have the patient put their hand over the axilla and do the adjusting through the doctor's hand on top of the patient's hand.

- Contact the first/second rib and have the patient laterally flex toward you.
- Have the patient take a deep breath and the doctor pushes toward midline.
- Place the adjustive instrument over the doctor's contact fingers and tap repeatedly *(see Figure 3-19)*.

Note: This adjustment can be used all the way down the ribs *(See Figure 3-20)*

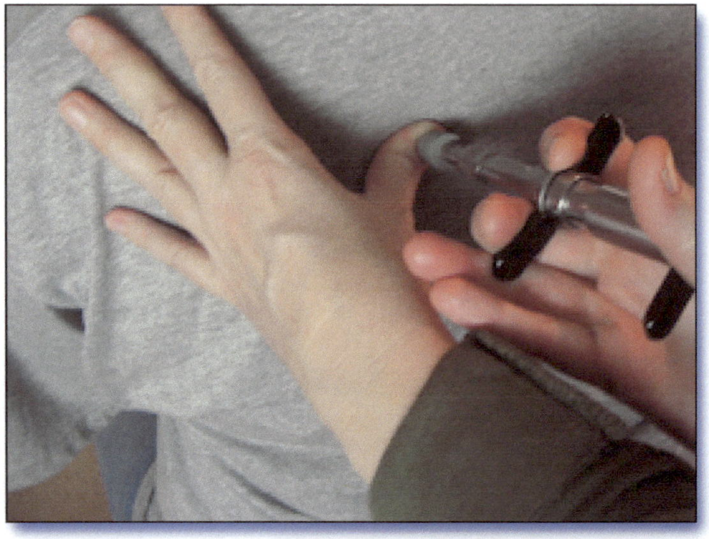

FIGURE 3-18 RIB ADJUSTING WITH THE SPRING LOADED ADJUSTING INSTRUMENT WITH THE PATIENT PRONE.

Note the SLI does not contact the patient. The force of the fingers pressing the rib is combined with the force of the SLI to make the correction.

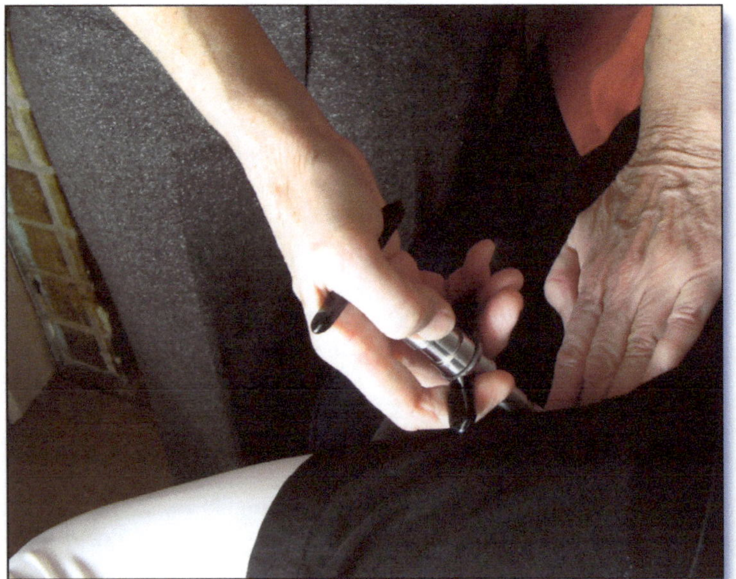

FIGURE 3-19 RIB ADJUSTING WITH THE SLI

Note the broad hand contact by the doctor. This can be more comfortable to the sensitive and acute patient.

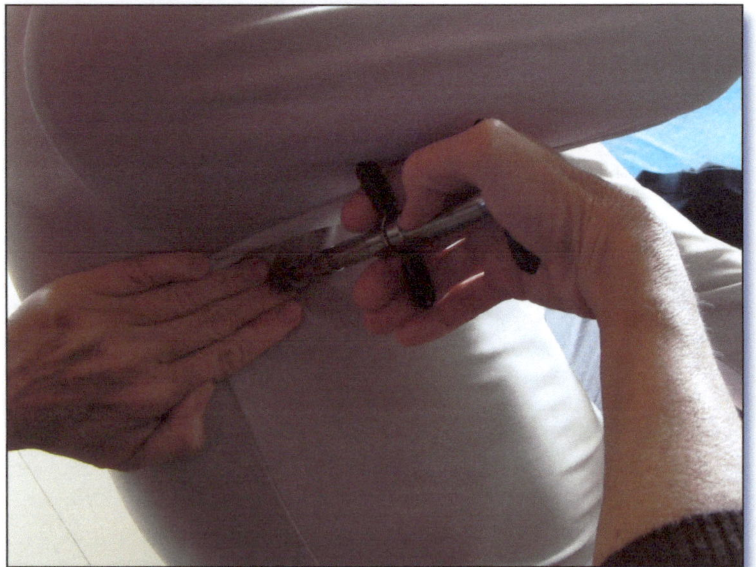

FIGURE 3-20 ANOTHER VIEW OF RIB ADJUSTING IN THE AXILLA WITH THE SLI

Note the lateral contact on the ribs; this can be done whether the patient is sitting or recumbent. Some patients are so distressed that lying down is painful.

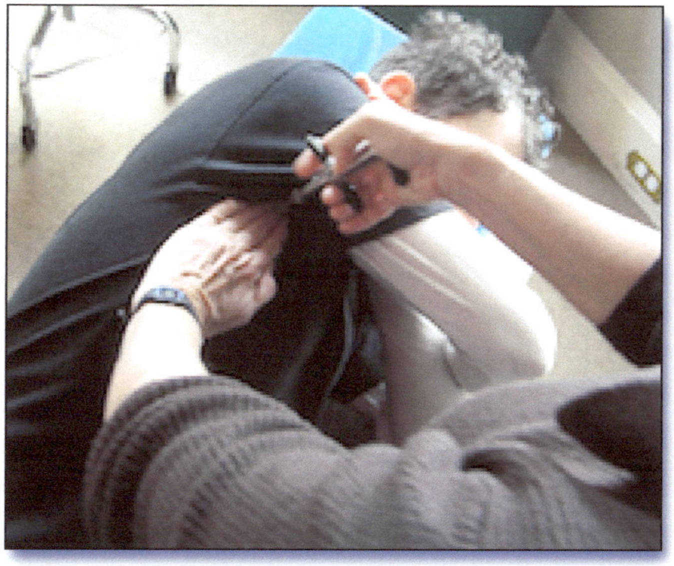

FIGURE 3-21 ADJUSTING THE RIBS FROM THE AXILLA WITH THE SLI.
Using broad hand contact, pushing medial or anterior, contact Doctor's fingers with SLI

This maneuver with the adjustive instrument can be done with a patient seated, recumbent or standing. It is done repetitively and gently. It is performed until the patient' tenderness and flinch response are reduced and the muscles of the shoulder girdle and neck muscles soften.

By firmly holding the instrument in the doctor's hand, with no recoil, the procedure should be painless for the doctor. The broad contact of the doctor's hands to the patient's torso should be more comfortable than contacting a specific subluxated rib *(see Figure 3-21)*.. If the patient's flinch response or ticklishness is too great to perform the maneuver, the doctor can take the patient's hand, put it where the doctor's hand needs to be and then place the doctor's hand over the patient's hand. The adjustment should be done in this manner until the hypersensitivity fades. When that happens, do the procedure with the doctor's hand in direct contact with the patient's rib cage.

ADJUSTING THE RIB CAGE WITH THE DROP TABLE

Have the patient lie supine over the thoracic drop piece. Place a small roll on the patient's sternum and take the same side arm across the body over the top of the roll. This helps to facilitate the rib adjustment that is about to take place by moving the scapula away from the spine and opening up a location for the doctor's contact. The doctor stands on the same side of the patient being adjusted and

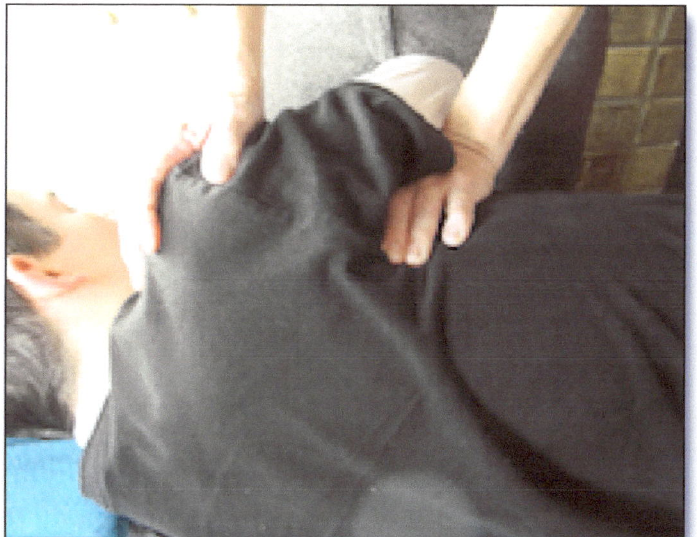

FIGURE 3-22 DROP TABLE ADJUSTING OF THE RIBS
Note the broad contact the doctor has, all the way into the upper axilla..

FIGURE 3-23 DROP TABLE ADJUSTING LATERAL TO MEDIAL

Broad hand contact, pushing medial or anterior

Set up with cushions to accommodate the other shoulder. Ribs and lower rib cage can be adjusted as well.

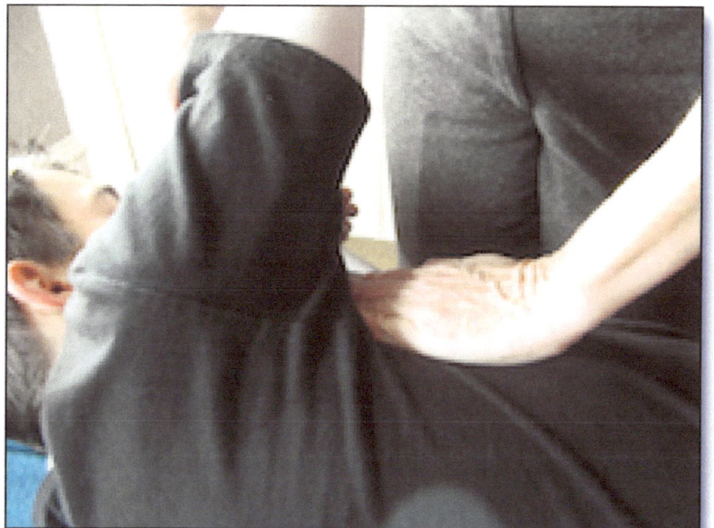

places the superior hand in a fist on the posterior rib cage between the spine and the medial scapular border. The inferior hand is placed gently on the sternal roll with a light anterior to posterior (AP) sustained contact. The thoracic drop piece is cocked and the patient inhales deeply and holds their breath during the procedure. The superior hand pulls from posterior to anterior as the table simultaneously drops with the patient's body dropping away from the doctor. The doctor should release the drop piece by using their superior knee. The majority of effort is by the superior pulling hand. Start with the doctor's contact at the superior posterior ribs and work down.

Next, take the superior hand and place it flat along the lateral ribs on the same side where the doctor is standing *(See Figures 3-22 and 3-23)*. Then, take the patient's inferior hand and place it across the body on their other arm to help stabilize the upper torso. Have the patient take a deep breath and thrust lateral to medial while the doctor triggers the drop piece with the superior knee. Repeat several times and then place the fingers deeper into the axilla, contacting the first/second rib. Repeat the adjustment and reevaluate.

Please note all procedures should be gentle and firm. Don't expect the first drop to complete the correction.

There can be the need for as many as 15 or 20 drops. With additional office visits, the goal is to reduce the amount of adjusting because the body is healing and the alignment is improving. Regular patients should be less work than people that only come in for a flare-up.

THE FROZEN SHOULDER

In my clinical experience, the rib cage involvement in a frozen shoulder or adhesive capsulitis is 100 percent. In the case of a frozen shoulder, most of the ribs on the affected side are subluxated. Subluxation of the sternal joints will cause the pectoralis muscles to contract, which will internally rotate the humerus. The serratus anterior muscles contracting will cause the scapula to translate laterally away from the spine. The humerus rotating internally and the scapula translating laterally stress the rotator cuff, creating an inflammatory response. If this condition persists, the fibrinogen in the exudate (swelling) will coagulate inside the rotator cuff, adhering the humeral head to the rotator cuff. The winged scapula is a result of the subluxation of the rib cage and it is a guarding response to hold the chest together. The adjusting must focus on the rib subluxations. This can be difficult in well-established cases where the patient cannot move their arm away from their body.

THE ERGONOMICS OF MANAGING THE INJURED RIB CAGE

The human rib cage has variations in shape. The distance between the spine and the sternum can vary between individuals, creating shapes that differ in anterior to posterior dimensions and left to right dimensions. There are no studies that show what portion of the population has a narrow chest and how many have barrel chests *(See figure 3 – 24)*. The tendency for the population to get more barrel shaped as they age is documented. Injury to the thoracic spine altering the kyphosis is another complicating factor. My clinical experience is that the narrow chested individuals have injuries that are harder to manage.

After adjusting the rib cage and gaining some relief, it is necessary to have the patient get up and walk around for a few minutes. Then a re-evaluation of the rib cage and guarding mechanisms should be done. As stated earlier, this is a test to determine if the rib cage can handle the weight of the shoulder girdle. If distress patterns start to return, then bracing of either the rib cage or the shoulder should be considered. Each shoulder girdle can weigh from 12 to 24 pounds or more depending on the size of the individual. So the rib cage has to have some ligamentous integrity to withstand the weight and motions of the arms. If the rib cage starts to become distressed after a few minutes of walking, then operating a motor vehicle, grocery shopping and other activities of daily living could easily cause a setback in the patient's recovery.

Sleeping positions can be a big problem for the injured patient. For some people, no matter which way they turn or what positions they get into, their chest and neck or shoulders are distressed. The pain patterns can result in chronic sleep deprivation. I counsel the patient to use multiple pillows for side sleeping. One pillow underneath the torso, above

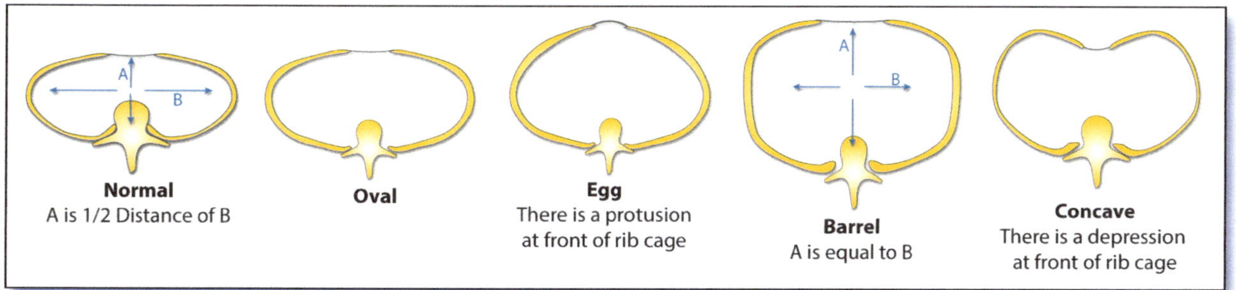

FIGURE 3-24 SHAPES OF THE RIB CAGE

There is a variation in the population in the shape of their rib cage. I find the oval rib cage to be the most difficult to manage. Adjusting is easier than managing the injuries.

the hipbone and below the axilla. Leave a space for the shoulder and then rest the head and neck on two pillows. This way the injured shoulder and upper rib cage are not being compressed. If the patient sleeps on their back, a pillow under each shoulder to keep them slightly forward can give relief. Stomach sleeping should be stopped. These changes can be very difficult for some patients.

Dressing with an injured rib cage can be painful. Women have to stop fastening and unfastening the bra strap from behind. They need to develop new habits to put the bra on, namely, clasping the fastener in the front, and then spinning the bra into its proper position. Changing the habits of these repetitive daily motions is necessary for the rib cage injury to recover. One sleeve of a blouse or shirt goes on easy, the other arm has to do an extension and rotation to put on the clothing. Choose which shoulder should be favored, then it's on first and off second for that shoulder.

The patient's habits of operating a motor vehicle have to be reviewed and modified once the shoulder injury has occurred. They should avoid reaching into the backseat, and all items should be placed in the car before the patient gets in. The only thing in the patient's hands when they get into the car should be the car keys. When getting out of the car, the patient should follow the same protocol. Any extra weight carried during these motions can destabilize an injury. Grabbing a seatbelt with the opposite hand is necessary to manage the rib cage and shoulder injury. So the driver should not reach backwards for the seatbelt with the left shoulder and hand, but instead should reach across the body with the right hand.

Patients with rib cage and shoulder injuries need to be interviewed about their activities of daily living regarding children, animals and any duties they routinely perform. I will ask if there are any doors, windows and gates that are difficult to close or open. Sometimes a weather change can alter the function of doors, sliding doors or gates, and cause additional injury to the rib cage and shoulder.

A large dog walking the patient can interfere with recovery of a shoulder injury. So will a three-year-old child. All pertinent factors should be reviewed with the patient, and alternatives should be implemented as much as possible.

BRACING AND EXERCISE FOR THE INJURED RIB CAGE

In the initial office visit, after assessing the rib cage involvement in the patient's complaints, adjusting the ribs and determining that guarding patterns have been relieved, then it should be determined if the ribs can stay in place with normal weight-bearing activity, such as walking. If the guarding pattern and the rib cage subluxation pattern are starting to return after a few minutes of walking, then driving and other activities could also cause the ribs to go back out of place.

At this point, the patient should be fitted with a simple rib brace and asked to walk around for a few minutes *(See Figures 3-25 and 3-26)*. Then, remove the brace. Usually, the patient will feel a difference and want to put the brace back on. If the rib belt provides relief from the neck pain or other symptoms, then the patient will be able to determine this usually fairly quickly. Some women will not respond to using the rib belts for very long due to the discomfort it causes their breasts. So various supportive, thicker-banded bras or sports tops can provide some relief. As mentioned earlier, sometimes the weight of the arm and shoulder is too much for the injured rib cage, and using an arm sling can provide relief.

Once the stabilization of the rib subluxations has begun, the exercise regimen should be limited, but effective. The first exercise is to put the hands together like in prayer, bring the forearms together and then squeeze. This is an isometric exercise. Direct the patient to engage all the shoulder and chest muscles with maximum or near maximum effort for ten seconds, and if there is pain, stop – it's too soon for the patient to start exercising. Once it is no longer painful, the patient can do sets of progressive repetitions of resistance band exercises. These are all exercises that cross the costosternal joints with none of the motions pulling them apart. The Shake Weight is a common piece of exercise equipment and, when used for the purpose of strengthening the costosternal joints, can be very helpful. Push-ups, bench presses, butterfly exercises are all to be avoided as they tend to pull the ribs away from the sternum if there is ligament injury to the structures.

Do remember: in designing exercise and rehabilitation protocols for the injured and unstable rib cage, avoid reproducing the mechanism of injury. I feel that exercise, repetitive motion with resistance, should not be done on unstable and inflamed joints. It is necessary to have some time elapse after initiating treatment to allow inflamed processes to resolve. This will never happen if subluxations are allowed to persist. Tissue repair and inflammation cannot happen at the same time in the same place.

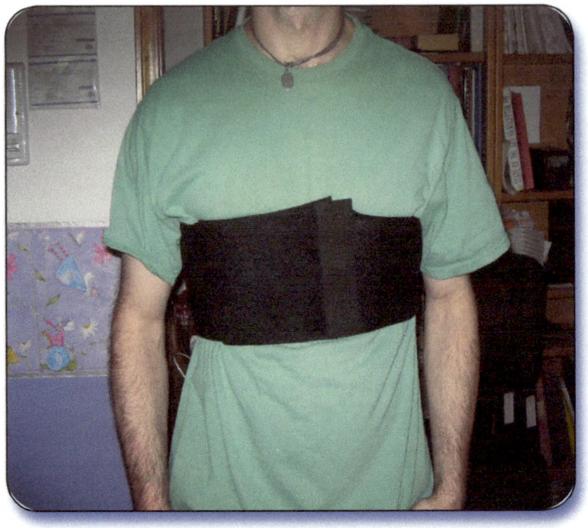

FIGURE 3-25 WIDE NEOPRENE RIB BELT

This is a 6 inch wide neoprene rib belt. 2 inch and 4 inch sizes are most commonly used, according to the patient's needs.

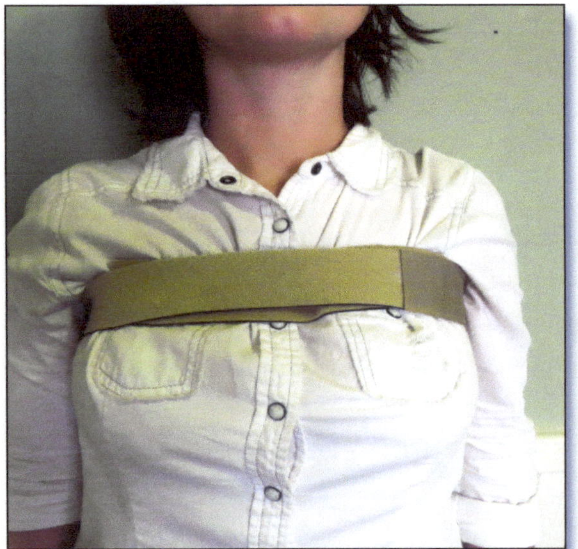

FIGURE 3-26 NARROW NEOPRENE RIB BELT

For women a 2" rib belt can be very helpful with unstable upper rib cage injury. These can be worn under clothing, but over some undergarment.

CHAPTER FOUR

Evaluating, Adjusting and Managing The Cervical Spine, Head and Temporal Mandibular Joint

In evaluating the injured neck and head, it is best to start the evaluation at the upper thoracic and anterior joints of the chest. The vast majority of patients, including those evaluated for motor vehicle accident injuries, stroke, and traumatic brain injury, have suffered moderate injuries to the anterior joints of the chest, including the clavicular joints. These injuries can greatly affect the head, neck and shoulder function of the patient. Ignoring these injuries will give incomplete and unsatisfactory results.

RELEVANT ANATOMY FOR THIS CHAPTER

- *The Sternoclavicular Joint, external jugular vein, swallowing issues, headaches*
- *The Costosternal Joints, Scalenes*
- *The Cervical Spine, Levator Scapulae*
- *The Occiput and Suboccipital musculature*
- *TMJ alignment*

These injuries can mimic disc herniation without a full evaluation and MRI showing a damaged disc (that could be asymptomatic), which would lead to an unnecessary surgery of the cervical spine – leaving the patient with the original symptoms and a fused and degenerating neck.

There are some important relationships between the anterior upper thoracic joints and the face and head. The sternoclavicular joints have the sternocleidomastoid (SCM) and the inferior muscles of the throat attached to them. This is significant in that the injury to the sternoclavicular joints can cause the rigidity of both muscle groups. In a lot of people, the SCM contains the external jugular vein. The external jugular vein drains the nasal sinuses, the orbit of the eye, the TMJ region, the inner ear and the scalp. This relationship might seem remote, but most patients with headaches that are frontal, sinus, and ocular have very tender and painful sternoclavicular joints. When these joints have been adjusted until the pain and tenderness abates or is greatly reduced, the headaches cease.

Vertigo, dizziness, muffled hearing and loss of hearing can be caused by the subluxation of the sternoclavicular joint. An explanation for this is "venous stasis," the blockage or compression of the external jugular vein, in the SCM. This will cause a backup or filling up of the veins higher up in the face, in the sinus, orbit or frontal areas. The resulting feeling of throbbing and engorgement can be very painful. Puffy eyes, swollen sinuses and achy teeth are more possible effects of sternoclavicular joint subluxation. Difficulty swallowing, a constant tickle in the throat and the loss of the full vocal range can also be resolved with adjusting the sternoclavicular joint.

The costosternal joints, when subluxated, can cause the scalenes muscles to become rigid, and reduce the cervical range of motion and create pain patterns in the lateral aspect and base of the neck. The first and second costosternal joint subluxation can also cause dizziness or vertigo.

In dissections of the cervical spine, it has been discovered that some people have the vertebral artery passing through the anterior scalenes muscles, and first rib subluxation can entrap the vertebral artery, causing what I call a pseudo-basilar artery insufficiency. This can manifest itself as vertigo, dizziness or nausea.

Palpation of the cervical spines of arthritic individuals can be relatively free of pain, but the scalene muscles and SCM distress will be the major source of pain patterns for these patients. If the upper rib cage is subluxated, the winging or movement of the scapula away from the midline will cause levator scapulae to tighten and exert constant pulling on the upper cervical spine. Thus, palpating the upper costosternal joints reveals tenderness and makes it likely that the upper cervical joints are distressed and misaligned. With modern injuries, it is common that the occiput is not aligned with the upper cervical spine and the suboccipital musculature is rigid and painful to the touch.

Figure 4-1 is a picture of the upper cervical spine, right lateral structures. The shadow in the upper right-hand corner is from the mandible. "B" is the lateral tip of C1, the muscle descending towards the lower left is levator scapulae. The levator scapulae attach from C1 to C3 or lower. I have found it attached to all seven cervical vertebrae in one individual. That is uncommon, but there certainly are variations among individuals.

The temporomandibular joint alignment is assessed by visualization and palpation. When palpating, contact the mastoid process and determine how far away the neck of the mandible is from the mastoid process. Frequently, there are uneven spaces between the right and left side, indicating a subluxation pattern. If the mandible does not track straight down when the patient opens his/her mouth, this is another indication of TMJ subluxation patterns.

THE ANTERIOR JOINTS OF THE CHEST

In evaluating the rib cage, I start with the anterior joints. The sternoclavicular joints are the only points of bony attachment that the arm and shoulder have to the axial skeleton. All the other attachments are muscular, and they are primarily attached to the rib cage.

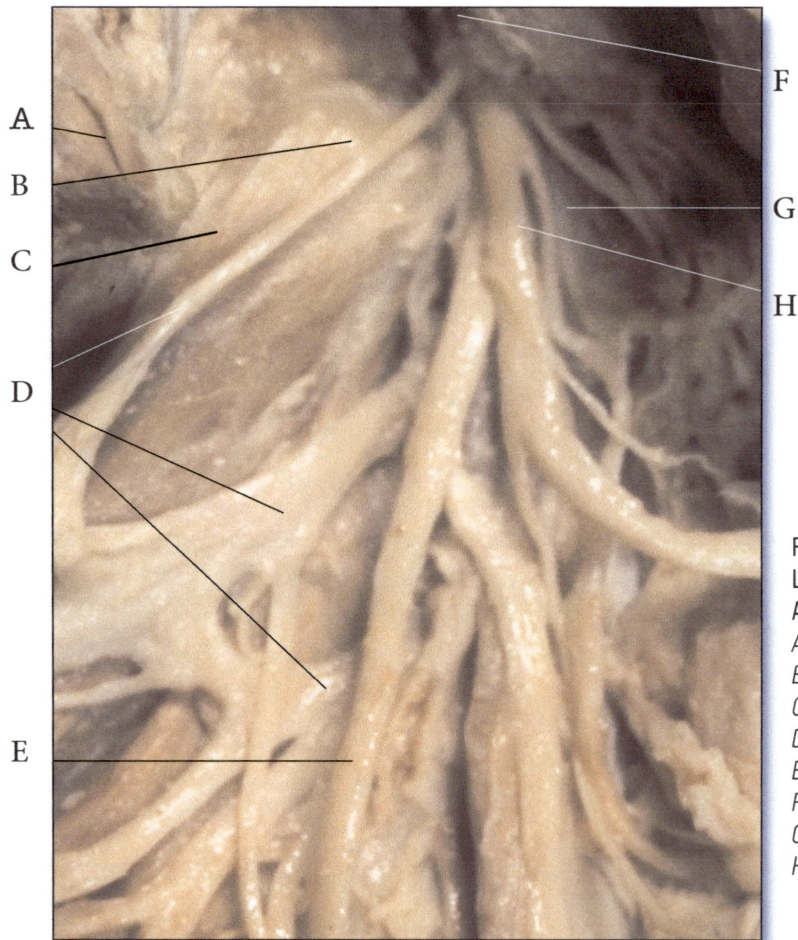

FIGURE 4-1. RELATIONSHIPS IN THE RIGHT LATERAL VIEW OF THE UPPER CERVICAL AREA.

A. Mastoid process
B. Tip of transverse process of C1
C. Levator scapulae
D. Cervical nerve roots 1, 2 and 3
E. Cranial nerve X, the vagus nerve
F. Jugular foramen
G. Superior sympathetic ganglion
H. Cranial nerve IX, the glossopharyngeal nerve

EVALUATION OF THE RELEVANT STRUCTURES

- *Palpation of the anterior joints*
- *Palpation of the axilla*
- *Rib cage compression test*
- *Shoulder squeeze test*
- *Palpation of the cervical vertebrae*
- *Palpation of the occiput*
- *Palpation of the TMJ*

At the sternoclavicular joints, take careful note of any pain or tenderness when palpating. A common sign is rigidity and tension in the SCM. Palpate across the front of the joint and feel if there's alignment or a "step," indicating subluxation. In typical modern injuries (car accidents), the clavicle is positioned posteriorly to the manubrium or sternum. This is the result of the outstretched hands or having a seatbelt restraining the forward movement of the body.

The same protocol is used for the costosternal joints. This includes searching for pain or tenderness along the border of the sternum down into the chest, looking for the same "step" of the ribs from the sternum, posteriorly or anteriorly. Some people will have acute pain in these joints. In most cases, this would not be conscious pain, but pain on palpation only.

THE AXILLA PALPATION (see Chapter 3)

While inspecting the axilla and the flank, a broad contact with the doctor's fingers spread out is suggested. Lift the patient's arm, hold it with one hand and place the other hand up underneath the arm gently, but firmly. You're looking for a pain or flinch response, but also for what feels like "railroad ties" or "speed bumps." The rib cage in this region should be nice and smooth with no bumps or ridges. If you do find these bumps there, they are almost invariably very painful. This is an indication of rib cage subluxation patterns *(See Figure 3-13).*

THE RIB CAGE COMPRESSION TEST (see Chapter 3)

This test is performed to demonstrate the effects of the injured, subluxated rib cage on cervical function, entrapment syndromes and other complaints. It is performed by placing the hands, with fingers oriented superiorly, into the axillary region of the patient and then applying compression *(See Chapter 3, Figures 3-14 and 3-15)*. In the majority of cases, this can be done with the doctor standing behind the patient. Both hands should be used with a squeezing or compression of the ribs from lateral to medial. The compression should be maintained for 20 to 30 seconds. If the doctor is much smaller than the patient, then the patient can be seated, and only one side at a time is performed. If the patient is in a bed or wheelchair, then one side at a time should be addressed.

This test is dual-purpose: the doctor needs to see how much restriction or pain occurs when the shoulder activity is related to the subluxated rib cage. This test also allows the patient to feel any positive changes from having their ribs compressed. This is part of the patient's diagnosis. Managing a rib cage injury that restricts the shoulder function or creates entrapment syndromes needs to be fully understood by the patient. The more the patient can understand these relationships, the easier the management of the case.

THE SHOULDER SQUEEZE TEST (see Chapter 3)

This test is performed if there is sternoclavicular joint distress or if any of the head and face symptoms are present. This is done to evaluate sternoclavicular joint involvement *(See Chapter 3).*

THE EVALUATION OF THE CERVICAL SPINE

The Atlas

With the patient supine, palpate the mastoid processes and move anterior-medial. Move the tragus of the ear to get into the anterior space of the mastoid process, posterior to the mandibular border, superior to the angle of the mandible. Don't go too anterior

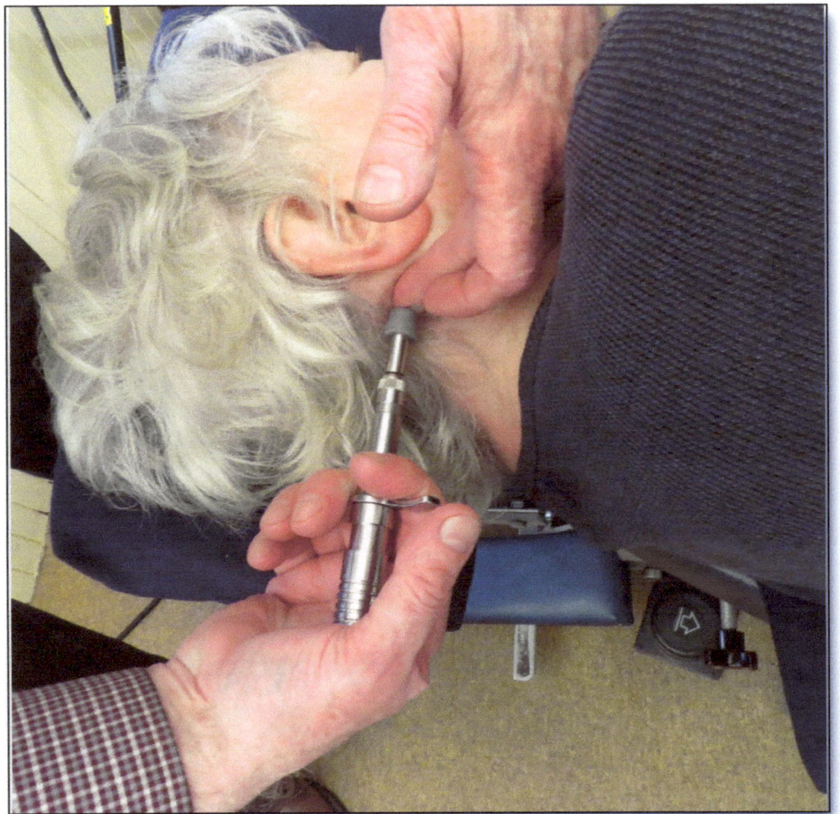

FIGURE 4-2. SLI ADJUSTING OF THE UPPER CERVICAL SPINE

Doctor's finger is pushing on CI in direction of correction, then tapping.

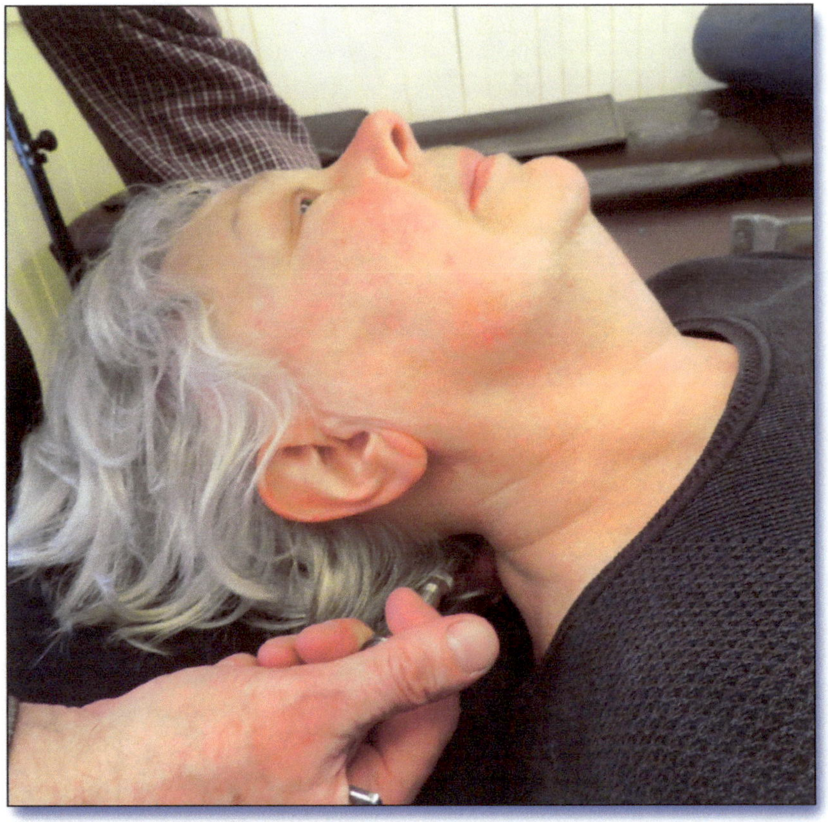

FIGURE 4-3. SLI ADJUSTING OF C2

C2 is rotated to the patients right side, This is a two handed manuever with one finger of my hand pulling on C2 back to midline and tapping the SLI with the other hand.

to avoid the styloid processes. This is approximately lateral to the transverse processes (tp) of C1. Upon palpation, if more of the mastoid can be felt on one side, then the atlas has rotated to the opposite side. One side of the occiput can be more anterior than the opposite side.

The Axis

The taut and tender muscle fibers are usually on the side that the C2 spinous process (SP) has rotated toward. Symmetry and soft muscles of the suboccipital region are normal. Asymmetry and taut muscles indicate subluxations. Find the base of the occiput, then palpate and find that the C2 SP has rotated, for example, to the right of the external occipital protuberance.

The Cervical Spine (C3-C7)

If the SPs of the cervical spine are not aligned on the mid-line, there is a subluxation pattern. This is usually accompanied by tight and tender muscles. Determine the direction of the displacement.

The Occiput

Occiput subluxation is common with motor vehicle accidents. To test for occiput subluxation, the doctor palpates for the C2 spinous process (SP) and its relationship to the occiput while the patient is supine. If there are painful and tender suboccipital muscles, some subluxation patterning has occurred. Test these by gently pushing or pulling the components forward or backwards to determine which direction gives relief. Generally, if I can feel a very prominent C2 SP and even if the top of it is separated from the occiput and it's very painful, I will consider that to be an anterior occiput. If the C2 SP is tucked in or not palpable, and there is pain or tenderness, the occiput has become posterior to the spine.

ADJUSTING THE CERVICAL SPINE WITH THE SPRING LOADED ADJUSTING INSTRUMENT (SLI)

Adjusting the cervical spine with the SLI is most easily done with the patient in a supine position, although this can be done in the seated position as well. Place the fingers of one hand on the segment to be adjusted. Because you've already determined which way the vertebrae have gone, you pull or push each vertebra, either by the spinous process or the lamina, in the direction of correction, even C1. The SLI is placed firmly against the fingernail of the target finger and tapped repeatedly *(See Figure 4-2)*. The tension on the SLI is determined by your judgment about the patient's tolerance for force. Children will need a smaller force or lighter setting than an adult.

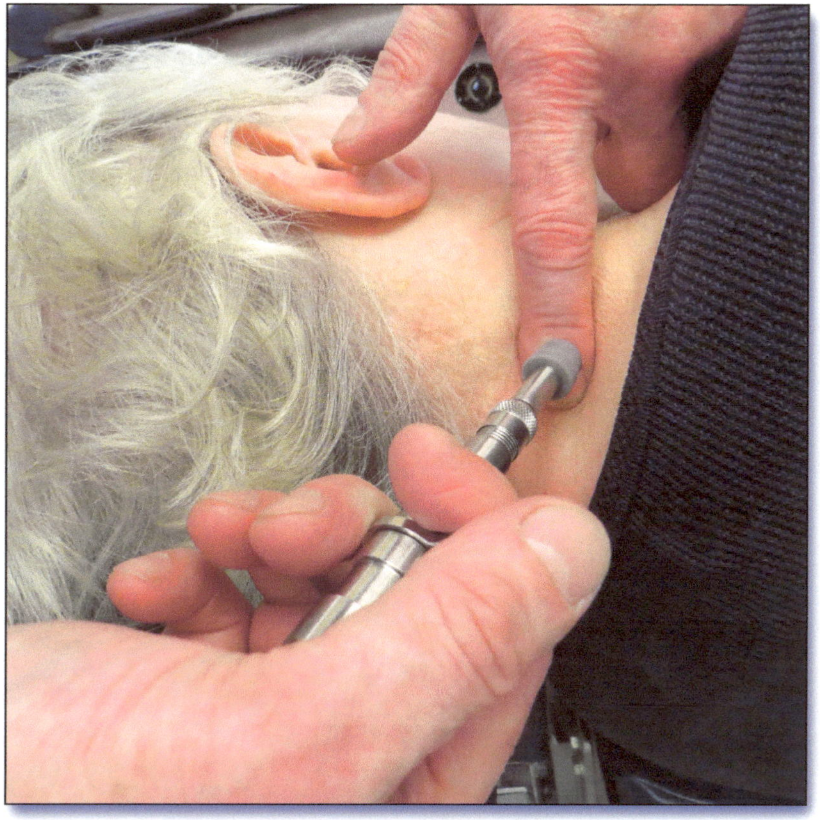

FIGURE 4-4. SLI ADJUSTING OF THE LOWER CERVICAL SPINE

Doctor's fingers are on the various transverse and spinous processes, pushing or pulling in direction of correction, then tapping.

The patient lies supine. For example:

- Place the left index finger on the right side of the patient across the base of their skull and contact the lateral portion of the C2 SP on the right, pulling with the finger back toward the left (A "pull move" in some techniques). See Figure 4-3
- Then slightly rotate the head to the left (which would move C2 to the left) and continue pulling the C2 SP with the finger toward the left.
- Place the adjusting instrument on the left finger over the right border of C2 and tap five to six times. (If the SP is difficult to move, then slightly rotate the head to the right and contact the TPs/lamina on the left with the adjusting instrument).
- Tap over the finger several times to help rotate the vertebrae.
- Put the head back in the neutral position and reevaluate.

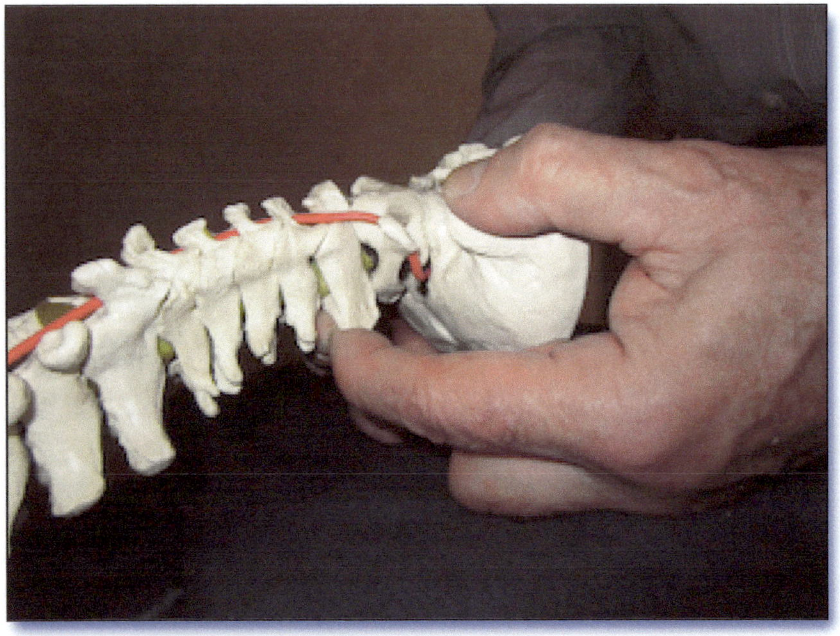

FIGURE 4-5. SET UP ON BONES FOR AN ANTERIOR OCCIPUT ADJUSTMENT.

Contact mastoid processes and posterior, inferior spinous process of C2. Distract, squeeze and drop simultaneously.

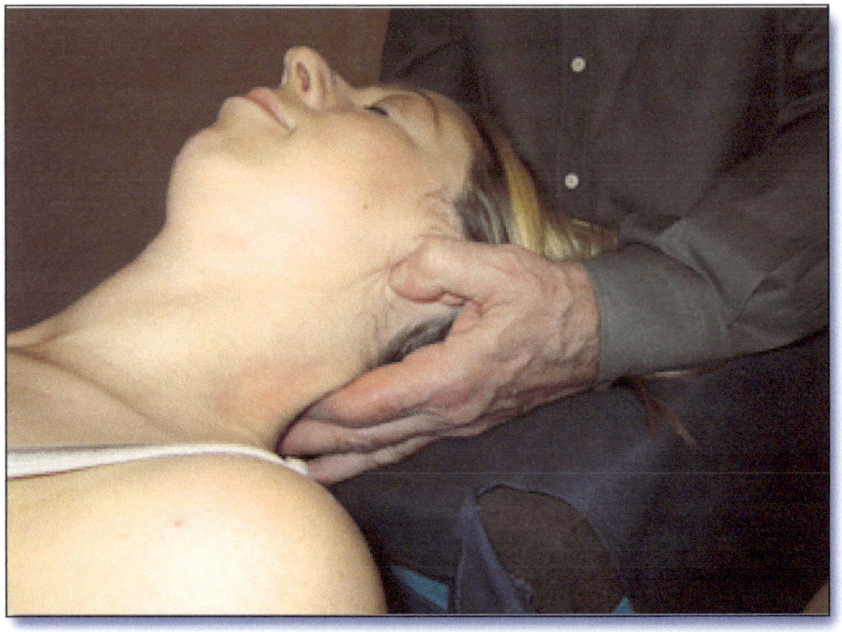

FIGURE 4-6. ANTERIOR OCCIPUT DROP

Thumbs contact the anterior mastoid processes and fingers are under C2 spinous process.

It is common to find C3 counter-rotated in the situation of a C2 rotation. Therefore, repeat the above list.

The procedure of pulling on the SP from the opposite side, tapping through the doctor's finger repeatedly, then rotating slightly and tapping the TP to realign the segments. This should be done down the whole cervical spine *(see Figure 4-4).*

CERVICAL ADJUSTING WITH THE DROP TABLE

Palpate the posterior neck from C2 through C7. If there is a normal lordotic curve present, the doctor should not be able to palpate the spinous processes of C3 to C6. If you can distinctly palpate these vertebrae, there is a loss of lordotic curve and/or kyphotic curve. Confirm this with X-ray findings. When performing prone drop work with a reversal of curve (kyphosis), the doctor must consider that to place the patient's neck in neutral will still maintain the kyphotic curve.

When adjusting in the case of a loss of cervical curve, place the patient in postural extension. This creates a neutral position for the patient and takes the ligaments to tension. Then continue with the drop work. Position the adjusting hand using a double thumb or knife's edge contact inferior to C2 and superior to T1. The exact level is determined upon X-ray analysis. Perform repeated gentle drops to promote a return of the lordotic curve while protecting the spinal cord integrity. This should be modified when a kyphotic cervical spine and a posterior occiput are concurrent.

Note: Using multiple gentle drops is preferred over a

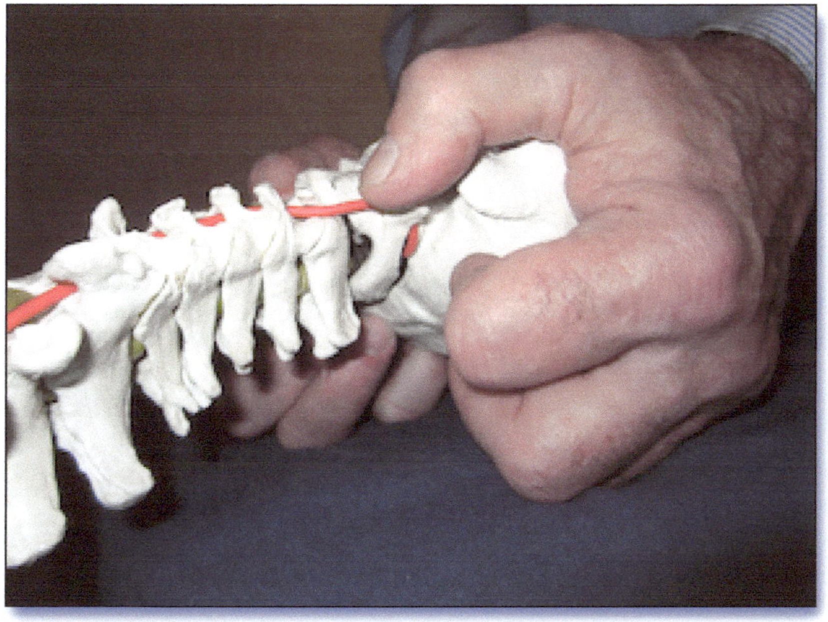

FIGURE 4-7. THE SETUP FOR A POSTERIOR OCCIPUT ADJUSTMENT

Contact the posterior occiput with fingers and anterior CI and C2 transverse processes with thumbs; distract, squeeze and drop simultaneously.

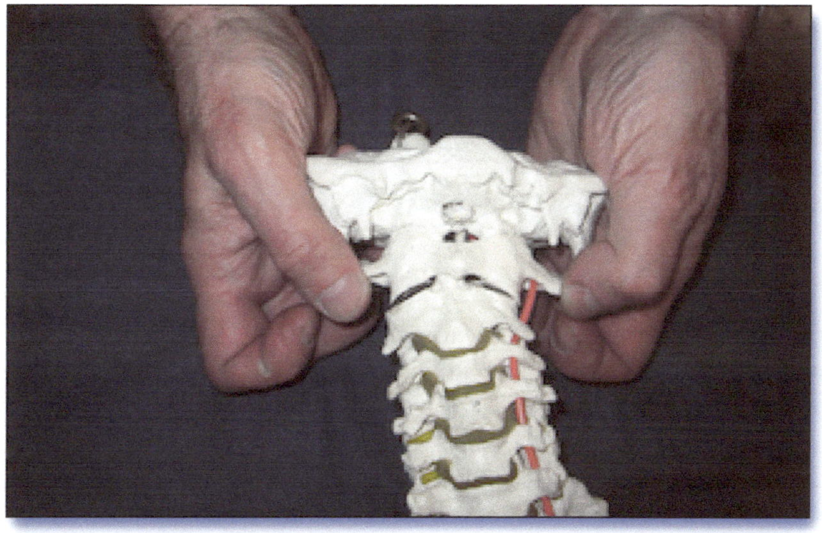

FIGURE 4-8. ANOTHER VIEW OF THE SET UP FOR POSTERIOR OCCIPUT ADJUSTMENT

Thumbs contact anterior CI and C2 transverse processes, fingers are on posterior occiput.

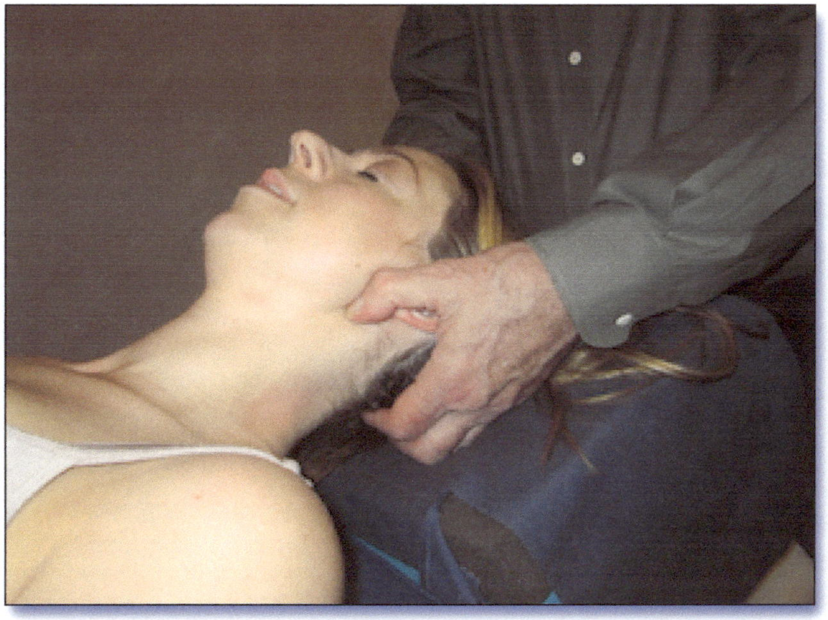

FIGURE 4-9. POSTERIOR OCCIPUT DROP

The posterior occiput adjustment is to contact the base of the occiput with the fingers and the anterior transverse processes of CI with the doctor's thumbs.

more forceful single thrust, considering the patient's multiple traumas and joint distress. Our goal is to change the shape of the ligaments, creating a normal lordotic cervical curve. I recommend post X-rays only if a full compliance has been achieved by the patient. Intermittent or occasional tractioning is not sufficient to make any changes.

OCCIPUT ADJUSTING

Occiput subluxation is common with motor vehicle accidents. To test for occiput subluxation, the doctor palpates for C2 spinous process and its relationship to the occiput while the patient is supine. If there are painful and tender suboccipital muscles, then some subluxation pattern has occurred. Test by gently pushing or pulling the components forward or backwards to determine which direction gives relief. Generally, if I can feel a very prominent C2 spinous process (if even the top of it is separated from the occiput and it's very painful), then I will consider that to be an anterior occiput.

The adjustments described here can be done on the drop headpiece of any drop table or with a portable drop piece. The drop action will be performed with the doctor's wrist or forearm in contact with the drop piece. The occiput is cradled in the doctor's hands and will usually not have contact with the drop piece.

Anterior Occiput: The maneuver for an anterior occiput is to contact the anterior mastoid processes with the thumbs, and the posterior, inferior spinous process of C2 with index fingers *(See Figures 4-5 and 4-6)*. The adjustment is done with a slight superior distraction and then a squeezing of the fingers on both sides simultaneously. The doctor's arms rest on the head piece and the drop is initiated by the doctor's arms.

Posterior Occiput: The posterior occiput adjustment is to contact the base of the occiput with the fingers and the anterior transverse processes of C1 with the doctor's thumbs. With a slight superior distraction, a drop is initiated by the doctor's arms with a squeeze or pinching of the doctor's thumbs and fingers together *(see figures 4-7 through 4-9)*.

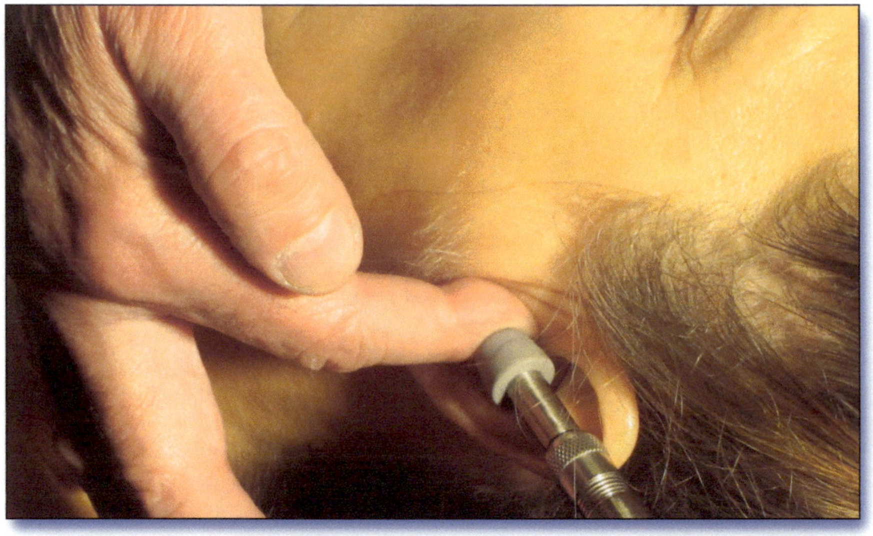

FIGURE 4-10. ADJUSTING THE HEAD OF THE MANDIBLE THROUGH THE EAR.

Gently press down on the mandibular head through the ear, tap your finger with the SLI multiple times.

TEMPOROMANDIBULAR JOINT ADJUSTING

The evaluation of the temporomandibular joint (TMJ) motion and palpation should lead to a determination of laterality and posteriority. There are four separate maneuvers that I use to adjust the TMJ. In every part of the procedure, the patient keeps their mouth open.

1. On the posterior side, contact the head of the TMJ through the ear of the side to be adjusted. Have the patient open their mouth and tap through the doctor's finger repeatedly with the SLI *(See Figure 4-10)*.

2. On the posterior side, contact the neck or rami of the mandible with the doctor's finger. With the patient's mouth open, pull forward and tap through the finger

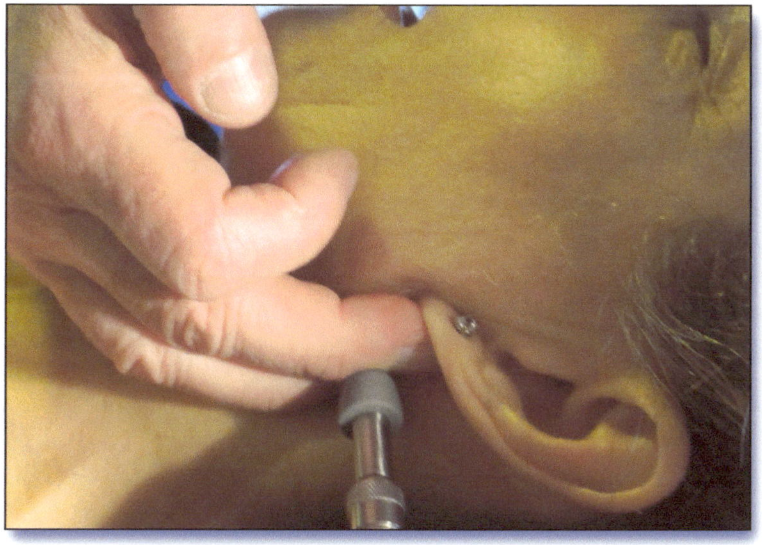

FIGURE 4-11. WITH THE PATIENT'S MOUTH OPEN, CONTACT THE POSTERIOR PART OF THE MANIBULAR RAMI WITH YOUR FINGER, AND TAP WITH THE SLI.

This is performed on the side of posteriority. If you find both sides are posterior, then both sides should get this adjustment.

FIGURE 4-12. WHEN THE MANDIBLE IS LATERAL, CONTACT THAT SIDE, PRESS LATERAL TO MEDIAL AND TAP YOUR FINGER WITH THE SLI.

All these adjustments are performed with the patient's mouth open.

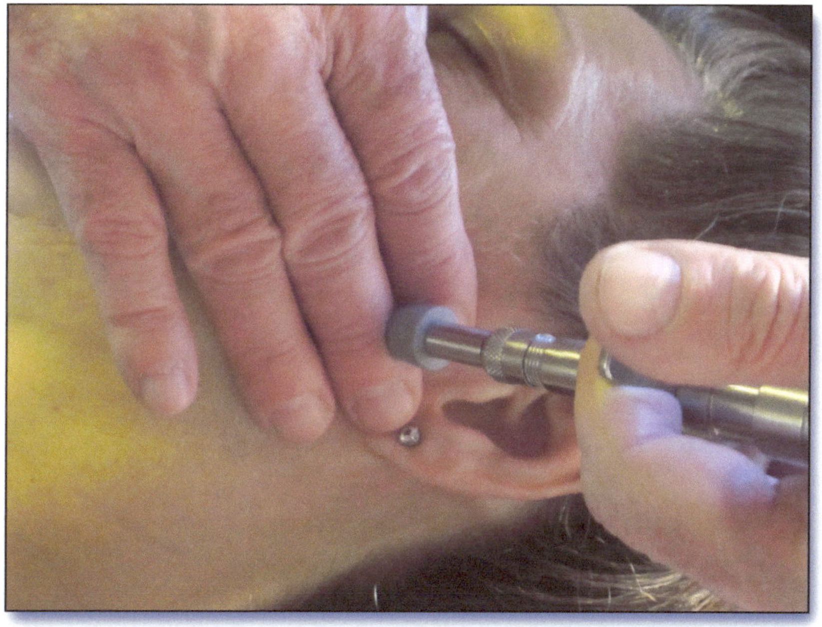

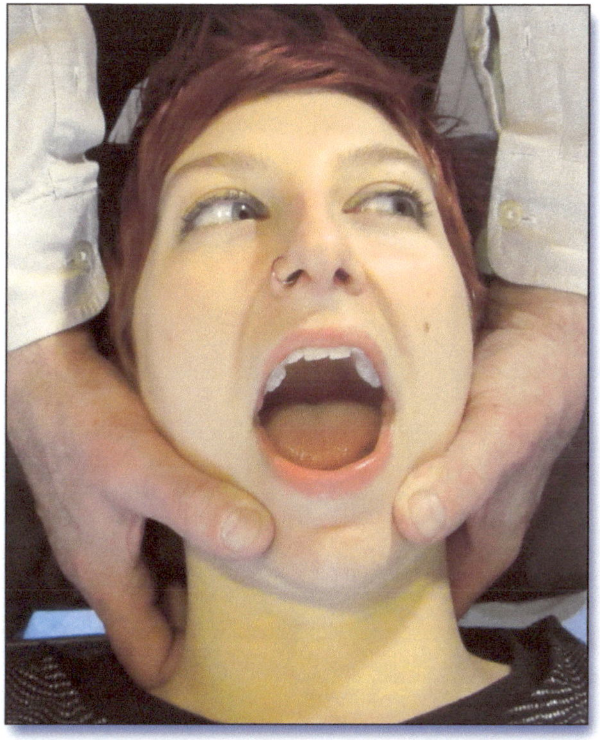

FIGURE 4-13. THE MANDIBLE DISTRACTION ADJUSTMENT.

The last maneuver in this series is to perform a gentle drop on the inferior part of the mandible, bilaterally. This is performed repeatedly.

repeatedly with the SLI *(See Figure 4-11).*

3. If you evaluate a lateral displacement of the mandible, have the patient open their mouth and tap on the lateral side from lateral to medial, repeatedly, using the SLI *(See Figure 4-12).*

4. With the patient's mouth open contact each side of the lower mandible (mental foramen) with the thumbs and drop straight inferiorly, repeatedly *(See Figure 4-13).*

Note: all maneuvers should be done gently. Even with the most gentle touch, there will be, in some cases, extreme sensitivity. If you are making the correct adjustments, the region should get less sensitive. Note and monitor the motion of the mandible. Asymmetric mandibular motion should start to become symmetrical with continued adjusting.

Online lessons at:
https://youtu.be/GUH5orLq8qs
https://youtu.be/BrU61G_F-Kk

CHAPTER FIVE

Evaluating, Adjusting, and Managing the Shoulder

An injured rib cage dramatically influences the shoulder's function and should be carefully and thoroughly evaluated. Almost every patient I have treated with a spinal cord injury has had a dislocated humerus and clavicle, in addition to an injured and subluxated rib cage. In every one of these cases the "peripheral injuries," not the spinal cord injury, was the cause of the pain and dysfunction of the arms, hands and shoulders.

Every case of adhesive capsulitis has had an injured rib cage. I feel it is likely to be the etiology of the capsulitis and the subsequent adhesion of the humeral head to the rotator cuff. The guarding mechanism of the injured rib cage will internally rotate the humerus by acting on the pectoralis major and minor muscles by causing them to tighten. This tightening from chest wall distress will leave the humerus in a position of internal rotation relative to the scapula. The rib cage distress will also cause a tightening of the serratus anterior which will leave the scapula lateral to the spine, or as it's termed, "winged."

This change in position of the scapula from the midline will also alter the position of the rotator cuff relative to the humerus.

The combination of the internal rotation of the humerus and the winging of the scapula, both products of neurological guarding patterns from rib cage injury, will cause in some people an inflammatory response of the rotator cuff. If this condition persists, then the fibrinogen in the inflammatory exudate will coagulate and adhere the humerus to the rotator cuff. This would happen in a slow, insidious manner, which fits most people's description of the development of their frozen shoulder. I have also dealt with shoulder replacement surgeries and in these cases, the rib cage is involved with the injury, as well as the subsequent dysfunction. Following surgery, managing the rib cage injury and clavicle injuries has kept the patient active. In fact, the patients can continue to play tennis, even though the replacement is in their racquet-arm.

RELEVANT ANATOMY IN THIS CHAPTER

- *Sternoclavicular joints*
- *Costosternal joints*
- *Acromioclavicular joint*
- *Glenohumeral joint*
- *Musculature of the shoulder*

THE STERNOCLAVICULAR JOINTS

The sternoclavicular joint is the only bony or joint complex that holds the pectoral girdle to the axial skeleton. Injury to this joint and the joints of the ribs to the sternum, can cause the body to have a neuromuscular guarding response of the upper chest musculature. This guarding response will affect the shoulder's range of motion and possibly create entrapment syndromes that cause pain in the shoulder and arms. *(See Chapters 3 and 4.)*

THE COSTOSTERNAL JOINTS

The axillary and brachial plexuses are attached to the upper rib cage, thus, displacement of the ribs can cause symptoms radiating into the shoulder, arm and hand. *(See Chapters 3 and 4.)*

THE ACROMIOCLAVICULAR JOINT

The distal clavicle, when it is subluxated, can cause discrete pain to the acromioclavicular joint, pain with certain positions or motions or can entrap neurovascular structures and create symptoms radiating into the hand.

THE GLENOHUMERAL JOINT

The glenohumeral joint has been subjected to deforming forces in the typical car accident or other crashes. The rotator cuff can be injured in these events. Unfortunately, there are no solid orthopedic tests that give definitive findings on rotator cuff injuries. The MRI is the only way of knowing if there is tearing of the rotator cuff. What I recommend is an evaluation of the rib cage, and if it is injured, perform a rib cage compression test, and while the ribs are held in place redo the motions or tests that were positive, noting any changes.

THE MUSCULATURE OF THE SHOULDER

The musculature of the shoulder is directly attached to the ribs, scapulae and clavicles, and they will become tight and sometimes painful with subluxations of the clavicle, humerus or ribs. So the resting tone of the musculature of the shoulder tells me if there are distress patterns that need to be treated *(see Figure 5-1).*

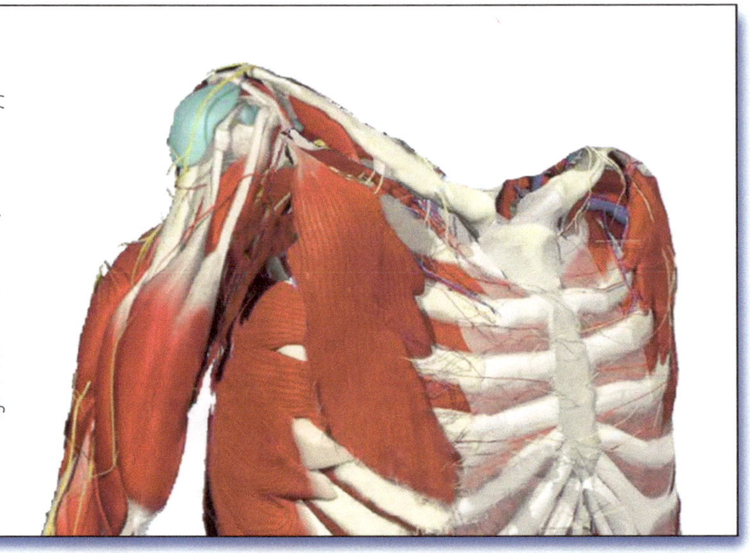

FIGURE 5-1. THE CHEST AND PECTORAL GIRDLE

Note the attachments pectoralis minor and serratus anterior have on the ribcage. Ribcage injury can cause these muscles to tighten and change the position of the humerus and scapula.

Costosternal joint subluxations can cause the rib cage to be altered in its normal position and cause the pectoralis major and minor to tighten, internally rotating the humerus. This can produce a dull, achy shoulder. The same rib cage injury will cause serratus anterior to tighten, winging the scapula. This combination of the displacement of the humerus and scapula will reduce the range of motion and give a wide variety of symptoms and complaints, especially the very common posture of rolling the shoulders forward, which make it difficult for the patient to stand up straight. A head forward carriage should also be noted since the scalene muscles will tighten as well.

THE EVALUATION OF THE PECTORAL GIRDLE

- ***Inspect the sternoclavicular joints.***
- ***Inspect the costosternal joints.***
- ***Inspect the axilla and flank.***
- ***Examine the muscles of the chest.***
- ***Examine the SITS muscles.***
- ***Inspect the acromioclavicular joints.***
- ***Inspect the position of the humeral head.***
- ***Inspect the rotator cuff.***
- ***Perform the Rib Cage Compression Test.***
- ***Perform the Shoulder Squeeze Test.***
- ***Perform the Acromioclavicular Compression Test.***

Inspect the sternoclavicular joints. Begin by noting any pain or tenderness on palpation. I want to discover if the SCM muscles are tight and rigid. Palpate across

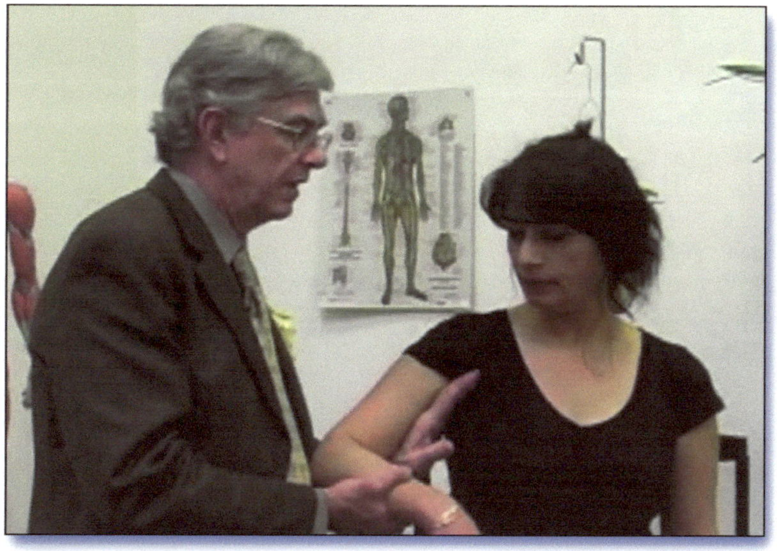

FIGURE 5-2. THE EXAMINATION OF THE AXILLA.

With the patient's arm still at rest in your hand, palpate the SITS muscles, these are Supraspinatus, Infraspinatus, Terres major and minor and Subscapularis.

the front of the joint to feel if there's alignment or a "step," which would indicate misalignment. In typical modern injuries, the clavicle is displaced posteriorly to the manubrium, or what we call the sternum. This is the result of the outstretched hands or a seatbelt restraining the forward movement of the body during an accident.

Inspect the costosternal joints. Similarly, look for pain or tenderness along the border of the sternum down into the chest. Search for pain posteriorly or anteriorly that the ribs may have from the sternum. Some people will have severe pain at these joints. This will not, in most cases, be conscious pain, but pain on palpation only.

Inspect the axilla and the flank. The doctor should use a broad contact with the fingers spread out while lifting up the patient's arm and holding it with one hand – while placing the other hand up underneath the patient's arm gently, but firmly. Look for a pain or flinch response, but also for what feels like railroad ties or speed bumps. The rib cage in this region should be nice and smooth with no bumps or ridges. If you do find these bumps, they are almost invariably very painful. This is an indication of rib cage subluxation patterns. *(See Figure 5-2.)*

Inspect the chest wall muscles: This will require the doctor to stand or be on one side. While holding the patient's arm up, try to have the patient relax so the doctor can feel the whole weight of the arm, then palpate the tension on the pectoralis tendon and serratus anterior muscle. If there is rigidity and tightness in these muscles, this should be assumed to be a guarding reflex of the subluxated rib cage.

Inspect the SITS muscles (supraspinatus, infraspinatus, teres major/minor and subscapularis). If these muscles are sore and tight, this could be another sign of rib cage subluxation patterns. To prove this, have the patient contact the supraspinatus muscle with the opposite hand while the doctor presses firmly up underneath the axilla. This is a unilateral rib cage compression test. In most cases, this compression of the rib cage will cause the supraspinatus to relax.

Inspect the acromioclavicular joints. The acromioclavicular joint should be flat or even – any bump or elevation should be suspected to be an injury to the joint *(See Figure 5-3)*. My test for AC joint separation, called the AC Compression Test, is to palpate the triceps muscle and, in particular, the medial tendon just above the capitulation at the base of the humerus. If there is tightness and tenderness at this site, and maintained pressure provokes discomfort or pain when pressing down on the distal clavicle, maintain the pressure for 20 to 30 seconds. If there is a change in the tone of the triceps and the tendon, the AC joint is distressed. *(See Figure 5-4.)*

Inspect the position of the humeral head. The humeral head should be partially exposed in front of the acromion process when the arm is at the patient's side and in a neutral position. This should be about one finger's width for the average size person. If the doctor can put two fingers or more on the humeral head, it is displaced anteriorly. In stroke victims, the doctor might even find a gap between the top of the humeral head and the underside of the acromion. This is a sign of a dislocation, probably a Grade 2 but at least a Grade 1. Grade 3 is when the whole humeral head can be felt, free of the shoulder. Sometimes, the top of the humeral head cannot be felt in front of the acromion at all. This would indicate that the humerus has gone superiorly and posteriorly, and has slipped behind the glenoid fossa.

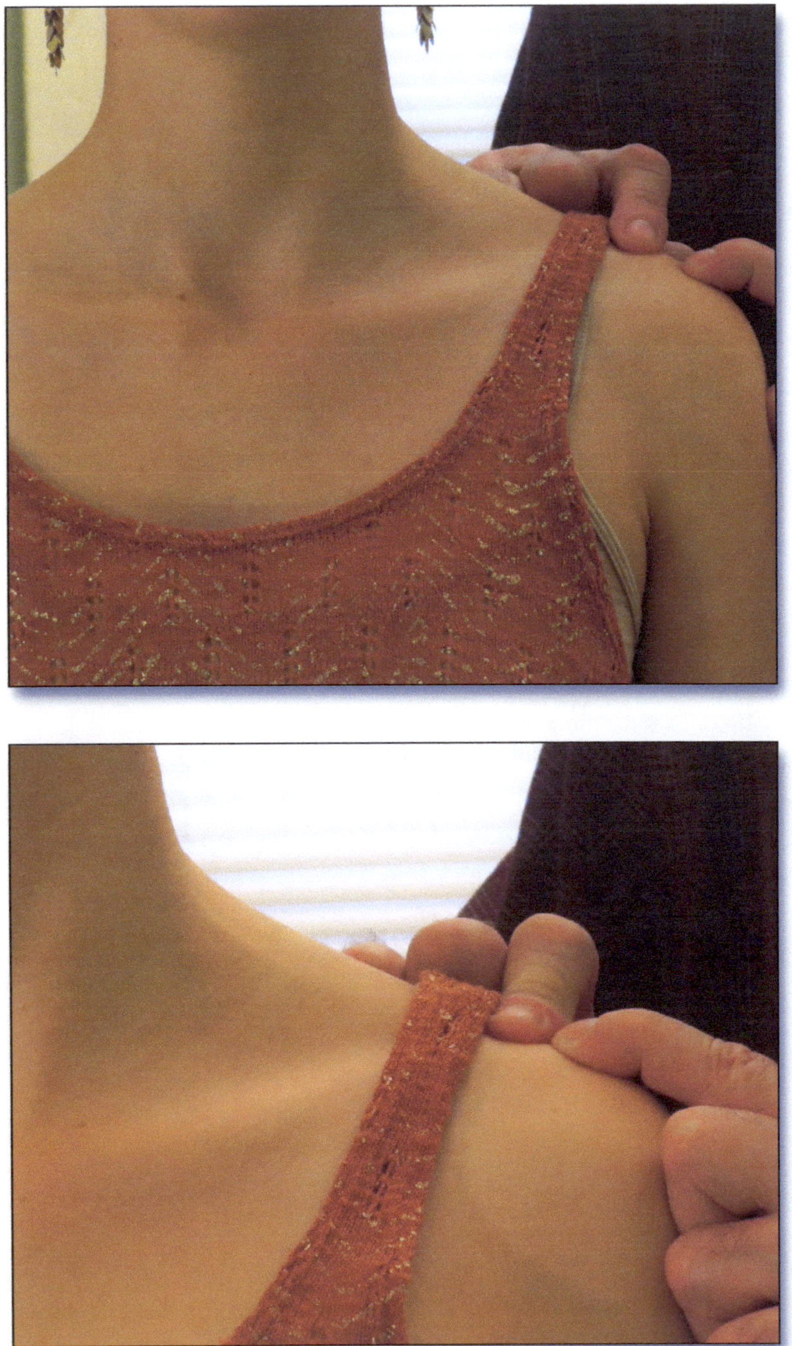

FIGURE 5-3A & B. EVALUATION OF THE AC JOINT.

Note the slight elevation of the Clavicle above the Acromion.

The acromioclavicular joint should be flat or even, any bump or elevation should be suspected to be an injury to the joint. (See Figure 5-3.) My test for AC joint separation, called the AC Compression Test, is to palpate the triceps muscle and, in particular, the medial tendon just above the capitulation at the base of the humerus. If there is tightness and tenderness at this site, and maintained pressure provokes discomfort or pain when pressing down on the distal clavicle, maintain the pressure for 20 to 30 seconds. If there is a change in the tone of the triceps and the tendon then the AC joint is distressed. (See Figure 5-4.)

FIGURE 5-4 A & B. THE AC COMPRESSION TEST.

The distal Clavicle is depressed while holding the arm, if the AC Joint is separated the tone of the Triceps and Deltoid muscles should soften and become less tender.

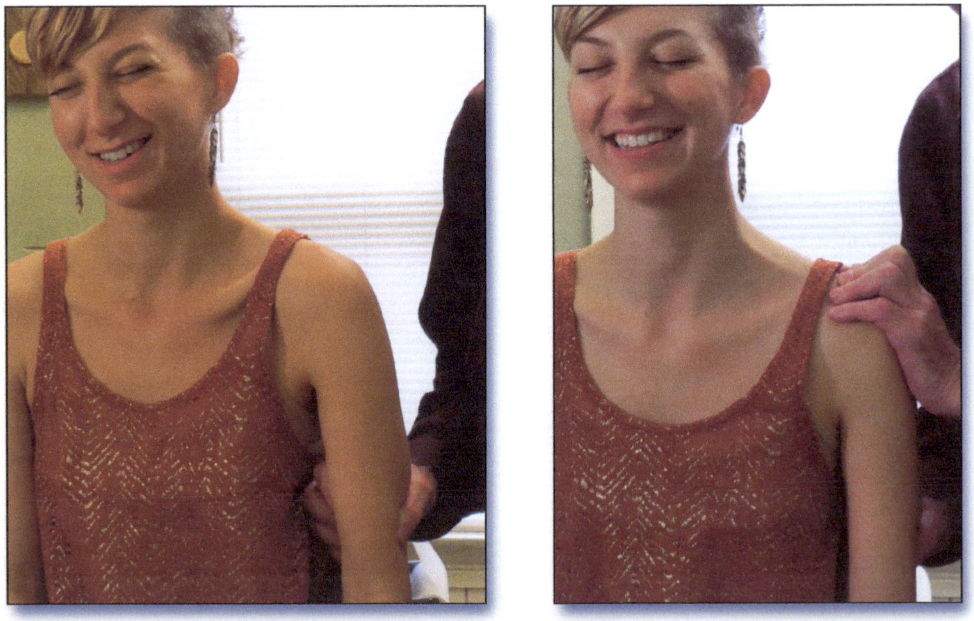

Inspect the rotator cuff. This requires the doctor to extend the patient's arm behind the coronal plane, exposing more of the top of the humeral head. With a slight rotation of the patient's arm, the doctor can feel with the fingers the top of the rotator cuff, while palpating the humeral head.

The rib cage compression test is performed to demonstrate the effects of the injured, subluxated rib cage on shoulder function, entrapment syndromes and other complaints. The test is performed by placing the hands and fingers oriented superiorly into the axillary region of the patient, and then applying compression lateral to medial for 20-30 seconds. In the majority of cases, this can be done with the doctor standing behind the patient, as well as on one side of the patient only. *(See Chapters 3 and 4.)*

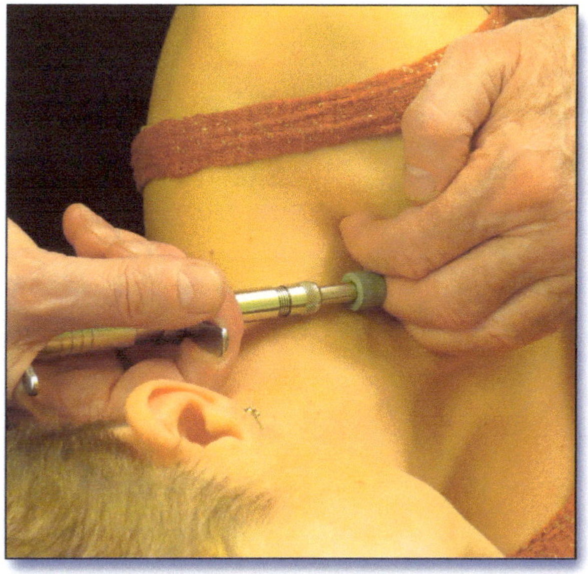

FIGURE 5-5. USING THE SLI TO ADJUST THE STERNOCLAVICULAR JOINT

A recumbent adjusting procedure using the hand to pull the Clavicle anterior and then tapping the fingers with the SLI.

ADJUSTING THE STERNOCLAVICULAR JOINT USING THE SLI

Posterior to Anterior on Clavicle (seated, standing, supine and lateral decubitus)

> *Broad hand contact on the clavicle*
> *Contact doctor's fingers with SLI*

Contact firmly on the desired spot, then use the SLI, see Figure 5-5.

ADJUSTING THE STERNOCLAVICULAR JOINT WITH THE DROP TABLE

The patient is prone on the drop table, the doctor's thumbs contact the posterior aspect of the Clavicles and drop down or anteriorly. (This can be very painful for the patient.) See Figure 5-6.

ADJUSTING THE SHOULDER WITH THE DROP TABLE

> *AC joint*
> *Consideration of additional injuries*
> *Glenohumeral joint (superior and inferior) The setup looks the same for the AC Joint and the Humerus. (See Figures 5-8, 5-9.)*
> *Contact doctor's fingers with SLI*

This can be done with the patient seated or supine. The doctor's hand has firm contact while cupping the whole shoulder. Sometimes a wedge is needed under the shoulder when the patient is supine to keep the thrust in front of the coronal plane. The thrust is done with two hands: one hand over the shoulder and thrusting inferior, gently. The lower hand has a hold of the arm using a slightly superior thrust. See Figures 5-8 and 5-9.

ADHESIVE CAPSULITIS

Adhesive capsulitis, as mentioned previously, has a significant rib cage component to its etiology. I've treated dozens of these cases over more than two decades and I have not found one that had a happy rib cage. The guarding mechanism of the rib cage will rotate the humerus internally, and the winging of the scapula causes a distress pattern of the rotator cuff. This distress pattern will gradually produce an inflammatory response, and adhesions will develop between the humeral head and the rotator cuff. The condition will commonly develop weeks or months after a trauma or an event, so the patient's recollection usually doesn't reveal any details.

ADJUSTING ADHESIVE CAPSULITIS

> *Restore the alignment to the rib cage.*
> *Adjust the clavicle, acromioclavicular and sternoclavicular joints.*
> *Adjust the humeral head to its proper position.*
> *All mobilizing should be done in front of the coronal plane.*

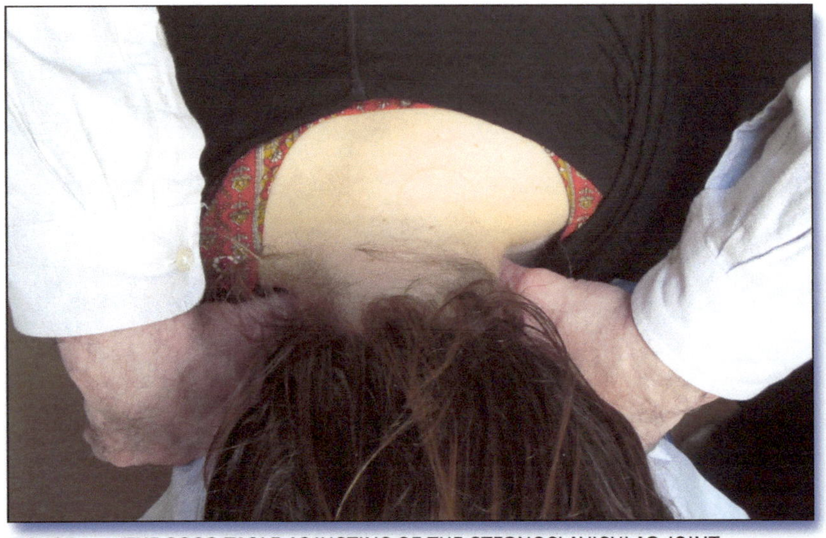

FIGURE 5-6. THE DROP TABLE ADJUSTING OF THE STERNOCLAVICULAR JOINT

The patient is prone on the drop table, the doctor's thumbs contact the posterior aspect of the Clavicles and drop down or anteriorly. (This can be very painful for the patient.)

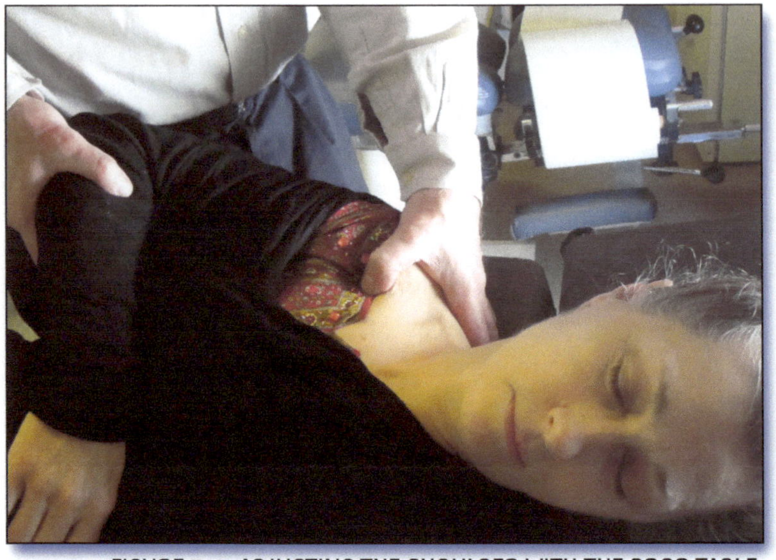

FIGURE 5-8. ADJUSTING THE SHOULDER WITH THE DROP TABLE.

The patient has their affected-side up. The doctor grips the shoulder and lower arm. Thrust is inferior with the upper hand and superior with the lower hand.

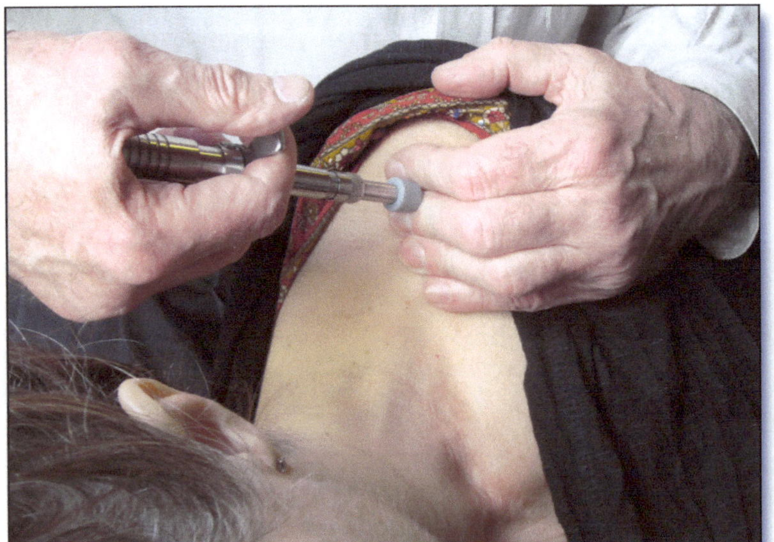

FIGURE 5-7. ADJUSTING THE A/C JOINT WITH THE SLI

This can be done with the patient seated, laying on their side or supine.

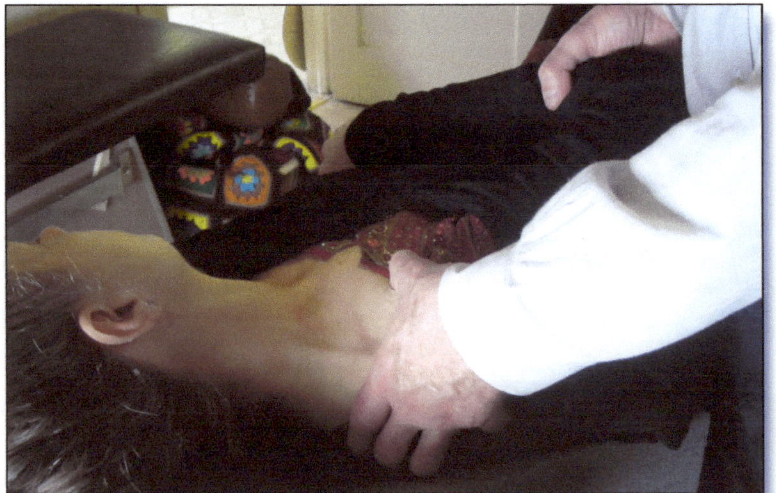

FIGURE 5-9. ANOTHER VIEW OF THE DROP TABLE SET UP

Note the wedge under the shoulder to keep the thrust in front of the coronal plane.

The adjusting is similar to the other conditions we have been discussing. It is important to get the rib cage aligned and free of distress. Adjust the clavicular joints, get the humerus in its proper position and then start the mobilization. The mobilization should not stress the rib cage or clavicle joints; all the activity is in front of the coronal plane.

These are tough cases to manage and most patients have let the effects of the injury become very well established before they come in for care. As in so many other types of injuries, the longer the patient waits, the more work the patient has to do to get back to normal. Some important factors in recovery are the age of the patient, how much motivation and understanding they have, as well as how well they manage their injury.

MANAGING THE SHOULDER INJURY

> *Determine if the rib cage can support the shoulder's weight (ligament stability test).*

> *Ergonomics:*
- *Car behavior should be very limited.*
- *Limit ROM to the "window" in front of you*
- *Regarding the injured arm, use the "Goes on first and off second" rule of dressing.*

> *List of questions for the patient:*
- *Are there any children and how old?*
- *Are there any pets, what are your interactions?*
- *Are there any doors, windows or gates that you struggle with?*
- *What are your sleeping positions?*

A ligament stability test for the shoulder is necessary. As advised earlier, after all the adjusting and the guarding response has abated, direct the patient to get up and walk around to see if gravity adversely affects the position of the adjusted joints.

The shoulder girdle and arm can weigh between 12-24 pounds or more, depending on the size of the person. If any of the joints don't stay in place while the patient walks, then I expect the patient to be adversely affected by operating motor vehicle and other activities of daily living, so using braces, taping and supports should be considered.

The ergonomics of managing a shoulder injury can be a complete inconvenience for the patient and will take some getting used to before they fully participate. Pain can be a great motivator. I have not found any literature that talks about being pain-free after a period of chronic pain. The return of pain patterns because of activities of daily living is considered likely with shoulder and rib cage injuries. Restricting activity is necessary to manage these injured joints.

The limited range of motion for the arm and hand and shoulder would be basically a "window" in front of the patient. They can operate their hands inside the window, so simple things like keyboarding or chopping vegetables can be done with both hands directly in front. If they go outside that space, like above the "window" or behind the "window," all those motions can become provocative. Therefore, no reaching to the back of the car. I even have patients put all their stuff in the car first, so the only thing in the patient's hands, when they get in the car or get out of the car, are the car keys. This is especially tough if there are child safety seats in the back of the car.

I can't repeat this enough: getting dressed and undressed can be challenging for a shoulder injury. When putting on a shirt and coat, the injured shoulder and arm need to go into the sleeve first, and off second when removing the garment. So the injured shoulder and arm basically remain in front of the patient during the acts of getting dressed and undressed.

In a further attempt to manage shoulder injuries, I review with the patient a list of concerns I have about their activities of daily living and their injured shoulder. Remember that carrying children, picking them up, putting them in car seats can cause a re-exacerbation of a shoulder injury. I want to know the age and the children's level of development so I can make recommendations about how to interact with the children while protecting the injured shoulder.

Pets can be a challenge for someone with an injured shoulder. Letting the dog take the patient for a walk will not help resolve a shoulder injury.

I want to know if there is any difficulty operating doors, windows or gates. This can be an especially relevant question if there have been any changes in the weather, and the previously easy use of doors has now become difficult.

Sleeping positions can also be an issue, especially if you hear any statements about pain at night or if the patient feels worse in the morning and improves in the course of the day. Sleeping with arms over the head will not be helpful, neither will sleeping on their stomach with one arm up over their head. Often sleeping positions that were normal and not provocative before the injury, become a problem after it.

DO'S AND DON'TS OF MANAGING THE SHOULDER INJURY FOR PATIENTS

- *Don't reach for the driver's seatbelt with your left hand.*
- *Don't reach into the backseat of the car.*
- *Don't reach behind you.*
- *No push-ups, no bench presses.*
- *No butterfly exercises.*
- *No yoga.*
- *Don't sleep on your stomach or your back with your arms up over your head.*
- *No Pilates or rowing machines.*
- *Don't lean on your elbows while in the car, at your desk or on the couch or while lying in bed.*
- *Sleep on your sides with a pillow underneath your waist, above your hip bone, leaving a space for your shoulder, and use two pillows for your head and neck.*
- *You can perform light activities directly in front of you, while keeping your arms and hands in the "window."*

BRACING FOR THE INJURED SHOULDER

Bracing and supporting an injured shoulder can be necessary for some patients whose injuries have left the upper extremity joint unstable. Remember, a patient's arm and shoulder can weigh between 12 and 24 or more pounds. If the rib cage, AC and/or glenohumeral joints are injured and unstable, the weight of the arm and shoulder can be provocative and painful. The braces I use are applied, if necessary, after all the adjusting has been performed, when I have the patient walk around the office for five minutes as a "ligament stability test" to examine the effects of gravity on the injured joint.

There are many approaches to aid in the initial phases of recovery from these injuries. I find the AC splint to be helpful when the distal clavicle joint is completely unstable. This brace has a component that comes across the top of the clavicle and can be cinched down until providing the patient relief or comfort *(see Figure 5-10)*.

The shoulder sling is useful when there is glenohumeral joint instability *(see Figure 5-11)*. The Sully brace *(see Figure 5-12)* is a sports device meant for keeping an athlete on the field. I have used this brace myself. The rib belt can be helpful for any of the neck or shoulder problems that are related to the types of modern injuries that we have been describing *(see Figure 5-13)*.

There are some innovative taping procedures with new types of tape; these can be very helpful. Taping for some people must be temporary because of the dermal responses, and the tape's use must be monitored *(see Figures 5-14a through 5-14c)*. Job descriptions and personal activities should be considered when prescribing these devices. Keeping somebody at work is of paramount importance and these devices can be very helpful. The rib belt and the Sully brace can be worn under the clothing and are completely inconspicuous. There are so many braces on the market now that the focus should be on the proper diagnosis so that appropriate bracing can be provided/recommended.

EXERCISE FOR THE INJURED SHOULDER

- *Do not repeat the mechanism of injury!*
- *Start with isometrics.*
- *Pray with "emphasis."*
- *Perform isotonic exercises with a resistance band in the "window."*
- *Use the Shake Weight.*

There are exercise and rehabilitation practices I find to be questionable. I've had patients prescribed exercises in the emergency room. In my experience, patients recover best when exercises are used only after the inflammation and joint instability have decreased. Doing exercises, (i.e. repetitive motion with resistance), on unstable and inflamed structures can be counterproductive.

I need to remind you: rule number one in exercises

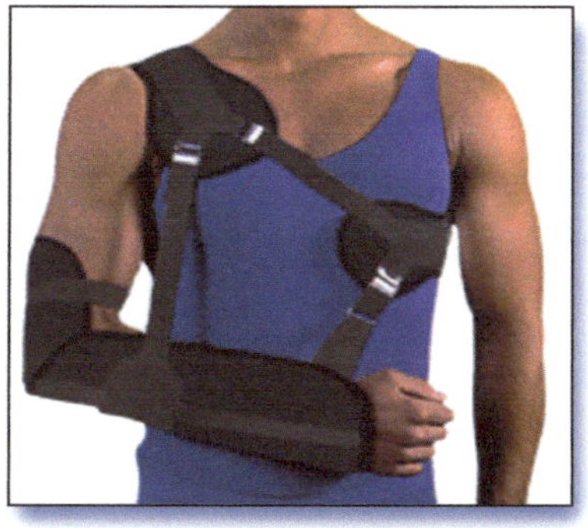

FIGURE 5-10. AC SPLINT (STABILIZER)

This brace requires two people for initial fitting.

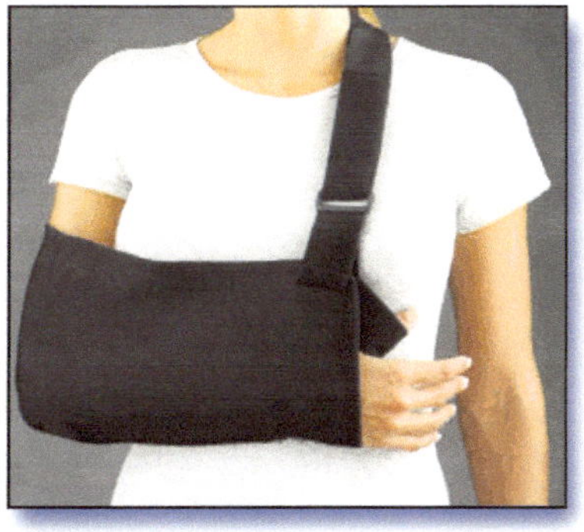

FIGURE 5-11 SLINGS

There are various types. This is needed when the weight of the arm provokes pain.

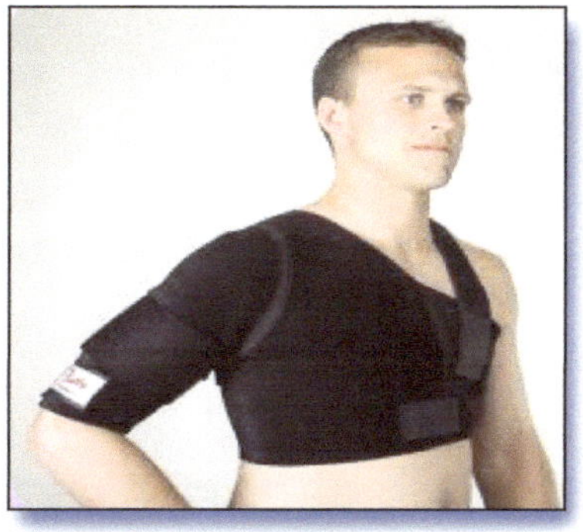

FIGURE 5-12 SULLY BRACE

This neoprene brace is custom fitted and it comes with a set of straps . It is used mainly for sports injuries but can be used for industrial injuries, including the performance of manual medicine.

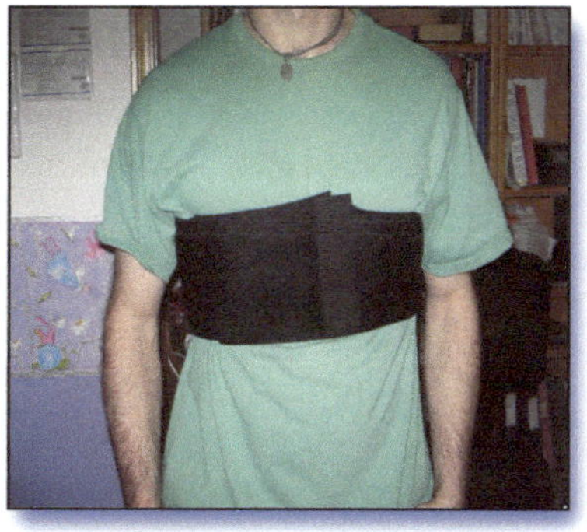

5-13 RIB BELTS

Compression of the rib cage with a neoprene strap can give relief to sprains and strains of the shoulder girdle ands chest. The compression helps pectoralis, serratus and the shoulder muscles relax.

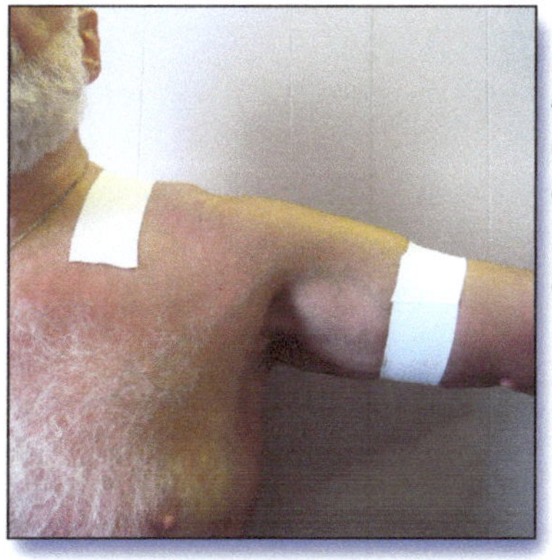

5-14A INNER ANCHOR TAPING

Arm is laterally extended and held by an assistant. Place one anchor at the base of the neck. The second encircles the arm at deltoid tuberosity.

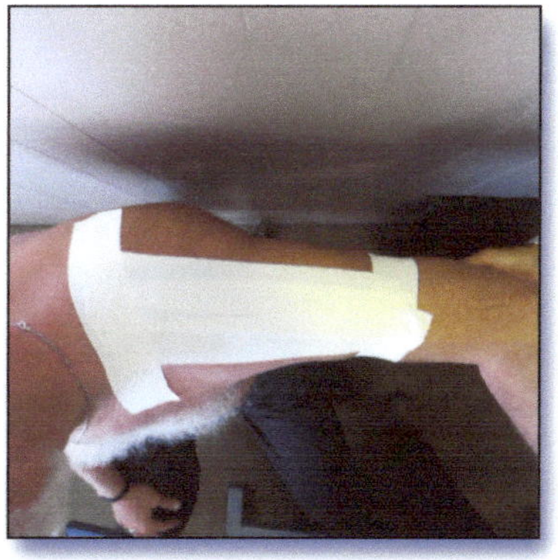

5-14B STABILIZATION STRAPS

The taping acts as a strap, spanning both inner anchors and mimics the deltoid muscles

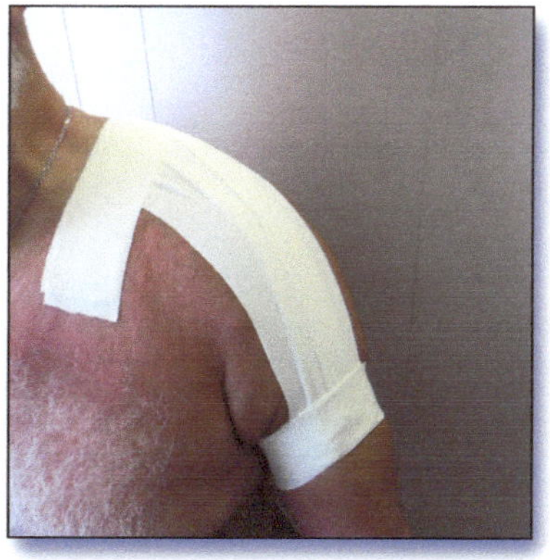

5-14C FINISHED AC SUBLUXATION TAPE

The inner anchor taping is repeated to reinforce the straps

should be to NOT reproduce the mechanism of injury. An example of this is the seatbelt, hands-on-the-steering-wheel type of injuries, especially the rib cage, where a large anterior to posterior force was applied to the body – and then doing push-ups and bench-presses. I found many patients over the years confused about why they're getting worse with exercises. Some exercises that were being performed prior to the injury can now be inflammatory and destabilizing to the new injury. This can make matters worse and create confusion and frustration for the patient.

Starting with isometrics is a beginning point and can be helpful when there are multiple injuries. I follow this with limited resistance band exercises and have found some success with a device called Shake Weight, which is a consumer device and can be very helpful for stabilizing the anterior joints of the chest after injury.

NOTES:

• • •

Online lessons at:
https://youtu.be/A0OafS9hIBY
https://youtu.be/dalze0p6S_o

CHAPTER SIX

Evaluating, Adjusting And Managing The Elbow, Forearm, Wrist And Hand

In patients with advanced arthritis and joint replacements, the arms are often injured and can cause disability and constant pain. In motor vehicle accidents, the patients often have their hands on the steering wheel or outstretched to the dashboard. Other types of crashes commonly occur with skateboards, skiing and other "rapid deceleration" accidents. These instinctive motions, to reach out with the hands to protect the head, can cause injuries to the forearm, elbow, hand and wrist. These arm injuries usually occur simultaneously with shoulder and rib cage injuries in a rapid deceleration event.

Arm and hand pain can be debilitating and not only keep someone from employment, but can interfere with activities of daily living. Bottom-line, they can impair someone's ability to continue living independently.

The common assumption by medical and chiropractic providers is that arm pain and hand pain are actually cervical problems and the pain patterns are diagnosed as radiating pain patterns. This is usually done without examining the arm, hand or elbow. I have seen cases where surgeries were performed on the cervical spine because of an MRI study of the cervical spine. The assumption that the disk problems seen on the MRI study was the source of the arm and hand pain was made without examining the arm. During my contacts with patients and other health care providers, I frequently encounter their belief that the elbow and forearm are considered to be separate from the wrist and hand in the evaluation and diagnosis. I intend to show that the anatomy of the region makes this common belief wrong and is the basis for continued hand and wrist problems.

The ulna and radius have joints at the humerus, and form the base of the wrist and articulate with the carpal bones. If the ulna and radius are misaligned at the humerus, they must be misaligned at the wrist. *(See Figure 6-1.)* I cannot think of a case in my 28 years of practice that did not have elbow involvement with the chief complaint of wrist and hand pain.

It is common for me to encounter patients who have a history of being cared for by previous providers who have ignored the distress of the forearm and elbow in their treatment for the wrist and hand pain. They either ignored or assumed the elbow and forearm pain was unrelated to the complaint. I can only say this is based on a poor understanding of the anatomy of the region. If a thorough understanding of the anatomy and the injury together is not applied, then failure of treatment and possibly harm to the patient are the expected outcomes.

A quick review of the anatomy of the upper body is necessary to make sense of the evaluation procedures

RELEVANT ANATOMY FOR THIS CHAPTER

- *Cervical spine, Brachial/rib/clavicle/ shoulder review*
- *Humeroulnar joint*
- *Humeroradial joint*
- *Forearm musculature*
- *Wrist and hand*

that will follow. *(See Chapters 3, 4 and 5.)* The cervical spine and upper thoracic spine are the source of the neurological structures that operate the arm and hand. A cervical disc injury could produce hand complaints, but so can an entrapment of the brachial plexus by a subluxation of the clavicle. A displaced humerus can entrap neurovascular structures, creating hand pain.

The forearm itself is an amazing structure, especially with respect to the integrated anatomy of the elbow and forearm to the wrist and hand. *(See Figure 6-1.)* The ulna articulates with the humerus, as well as the radius. These two joints comprise a structure we call the elbow. Either one of these joints suffering misalignment can have profound effects on the wrist and hand. *(See Figures 6-2 and 6-3.)* Most of the muscles that operate the fingers and hands originate at or above the elbow. The neuromuscular guarding reflex of these muscles caused by displaced humeroulnar or humeroradial joints will interfere with hand and finger function, including "Trigger Finger," De Quervain's, and other hand and finger patterns of dysfunction. It is impossible to have a subluxated radius and/or ulna at the elbow and have alignment at the wrist.

Almost all of the muscles that attach to the elbow region are the muscular structures that operate the hand and fingers. Most of these muscles are attached to the interosseous ligament as well. When the ulna subluxates at the humerus, the interosseous ligament is injured as well as the joint capsule of the humeroulnar joint. *(See Figure 6-4.)* This type of injury will cause a neuromuscular guarding reflex of

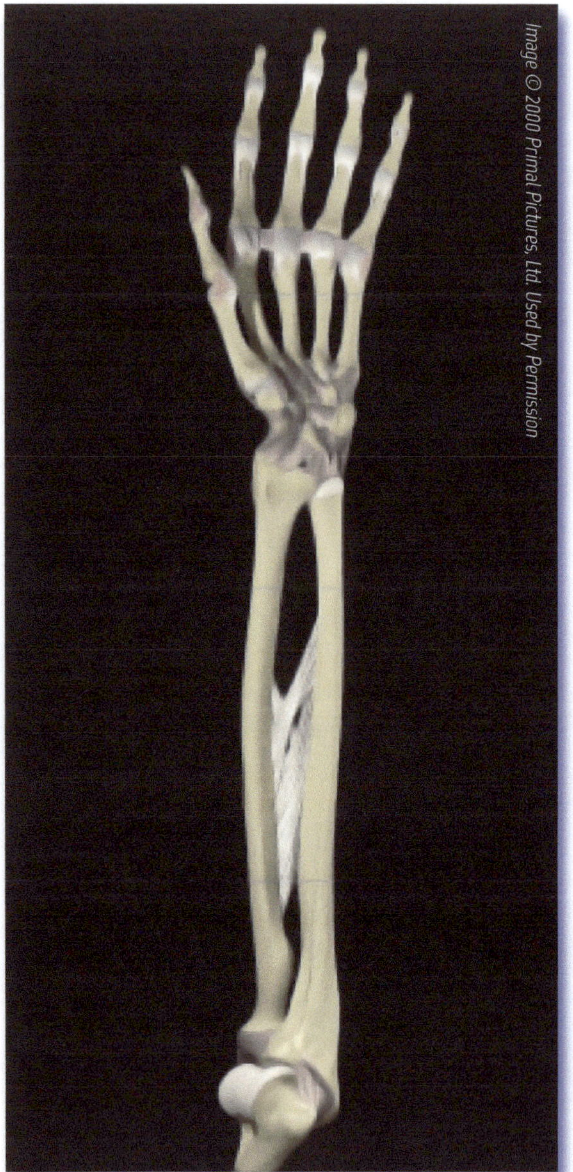

FIGURE 6-1. THE BONES OF THE ELBOW, FOREARM, WRIST AND HAND.

Note the Radius and Ulna are part of both the elbow and wrist complexes.

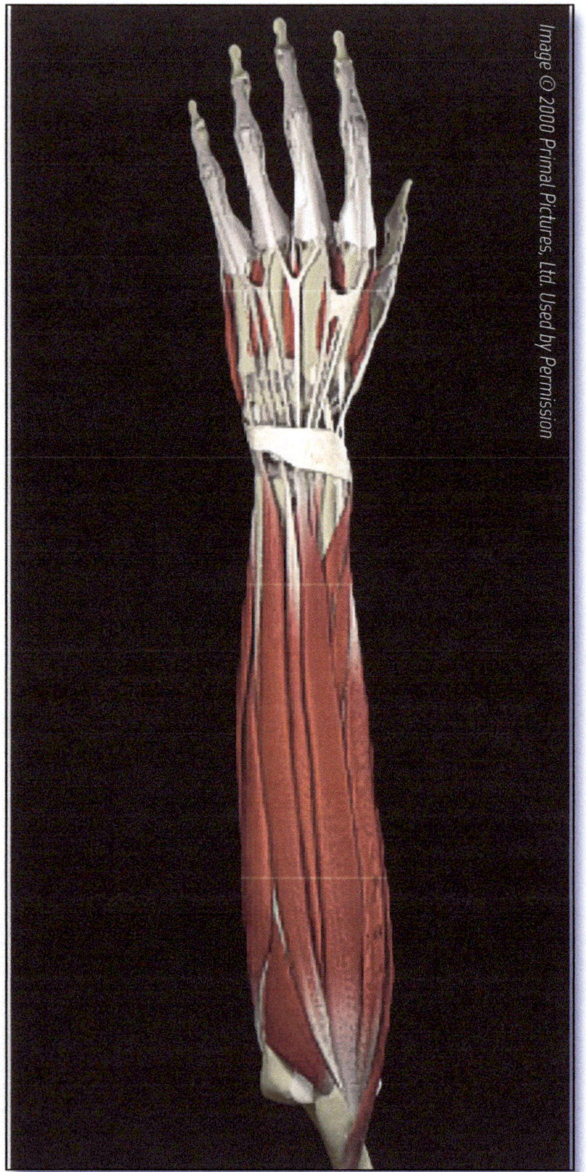

FIGURE 6-2. DORSAL VIEW OF FOREARM, WRIST AND HAND.

Note muscles of the forearm are the muscles of the hand and fingers. Joint distress at the elbow will mostly be felt in the hand and wrist.

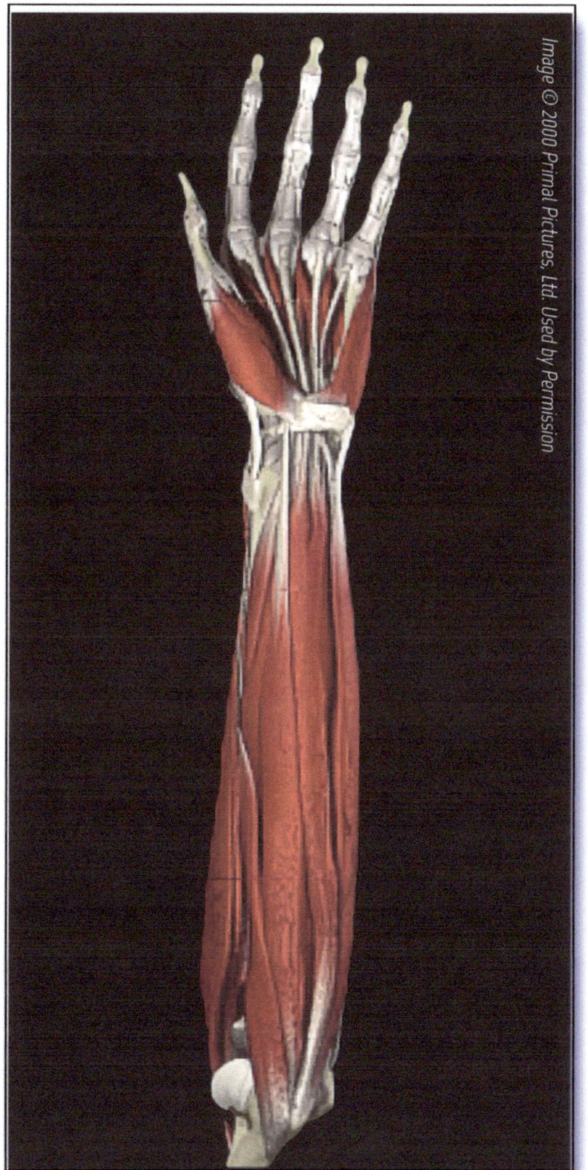

FIGURE 6-3. VENTRAL VIEW OF ELBOW FOREARM, WRIST AND HAND.

This shows the flexors of the hand and fingers. Irritating these muscles leads to painful and inflamed tendons in the wrist and hand.

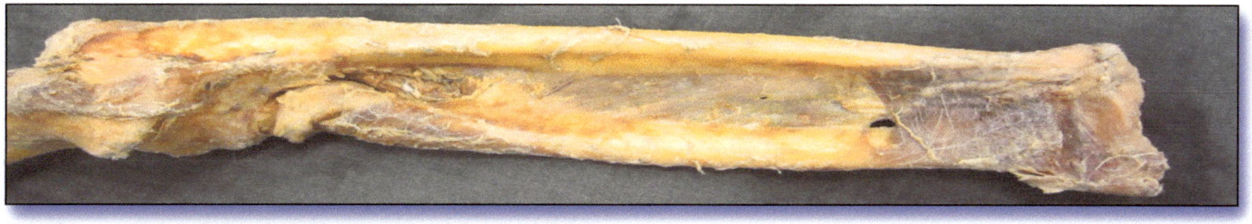

FIGURE 6-4. THE INTEROSSEOUS LIGAMENT OF THE FOREARM.

Injury and instability to this ligament leads to chronic hand and wrist pain.

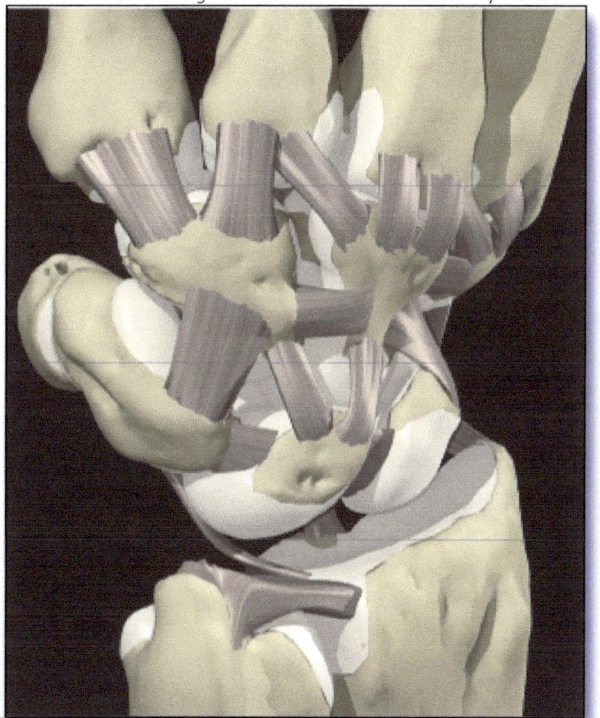

FIGURE 6-5. THE WRIST.

Note the base of the forearm forms a shallow "cup". Any displacement of the forearm bones at the elbow will change the shape of this "cup".

all the flexors and extensors of the hand and fingers. This guarding mechanism will be manifested by rigid, tight, sore and/or painful musculature at the elbow and forearm. The subjective complaints of this type of injury are commonly wrist and hand pain. The injury to the forearm and elbow are routinely missed or ignored. This makes most hand and wrist pain therapies and interventions ineffective at best.

The forearm, elbow, wrist and hand should be considered a functional unit that has an integrated set of structures. When any one component is distressed, it will affect the other components within the structure. The shape of the wrist and alignment of the carpal bones is dependent on the normal alignment of the distal radius and ulna *(See Figure 6-5)*. Subluxations of these bones at the elbow will change this relationship at the wrist, resulting in wrist and hand dysfunction.

THE COMMON MECHANISMS AND MANAGEMENT OF INJURY

> *Look for instantaneous trauma, especially with the fracture of any component of the mechanical chain.*

> *Note the reflexive extension of one's arms to avoid head trauma during a rapid deceleration event.*

> *A persistent and chronic lower extremity and/or low back injury could lead to an upper extremity injury resulting from the use of crutches, canes and walkers.*

> *The combined rib cage, shoulder, elbow, and wrist injuries must be managed simultaneously.*

> *If the patient has lower body injuries, special care is essential.*

> *A review of all life-style factors, (especially employment), must be reviewed.*

Again, a common cause of injury to the upper extremity is stretching out the hands to avoid injuries to the head. Collie's Fracture is the most common fracture in the body. Remember that when the hand contacts a hard surface with the elbow extended, the force of the event can be translated up through the forearm to the elbow, shoulder and rib cage. If the force is sufficient, misalignment of the ulna and radius at the humerus will occur. This is a very common occurrence. Hands on the steering wheel at the moment of impact, or any bracing for an impact will cause disruption of the capsular joints and the interosseous ligament.

The persistent use of a walking-aid post injury can be a continued source of injury to the wrists and hands. In some cases, even though the wrists and hands were not involved with an injury to the patient's lower body, they are now under such constant stress from using walking-aids that the ligaments and joints of the forearm, elbow and wrist fail. I have had a case where a patient's primary low back injury resulted in a diagnosis of bilateral carpal tunnel syndrome. I documented the constant use of her hands and arms. She had to use her hands and arms to get out of bed, out of a chair and into and out of a car.

There were no body position changes that didn't impact her wrists and hands. So within a year of her low back injury, the wrist and hand pain was just as great as the low back pain. These injuries can be common in the patients I examine, even when the accidents occurred decades earlier.

When managing the wrist and hand injuries, assessing the lower body injuries is necessary. The continued use of walking aids and the need to assist body position changes will keep the forearm, elbow and hand injuries unresolved. A review of all activities of daily living and other factors, including their employment, is essential. When lower body injuries are involved, it is necessary to review the use of soft chairs and couches. Sitting for long periods of time, followed by a struggle to get up, will keep the wrist and hand injuries inflamed and unresolved. Recliners and stool high chairs can help in making the transition from sitting to standing much easier and require using the arms much less.

When reviewing employment activities, it is necessary to find out how much time a person is spending at the keyboard. Keyboard use that was pain-free before a car accident or other trauma to the upper body can produce complaints of pain post-trauma. I've had a patient think that 14 to 16 hours of keyboarding a day was normal. These issues have to be addressed – what does a patient consider to be normal? It can vary among individuals quite extensively, and the definition of "normal" needs to change once an injury has occurred. In the age of hand-held devices and gaming consoles, recreational activities must be reviewed as well.

EVALUATING THE ELBOW AND WRIST

> *A thorough evaluation of the spine, rib cage and shoulder should be conducted.*

> *The ulna should tuck into the olecranon process with extension of the arm.*

> *The radius should be under the capitulum of the humerus with pronation and supination.*

> *The forearm muscles should be soft at rest*

> *The wrist should have normal gliding motion with palpation.*

> *If any of this is absent, intervention is required.*

> *If the ulna and radius are subluxated at the humerus, they cannot be aligned at the wrist.*

Like the advice in every examination textbook I've ever looked at, I will also recommend examining the cervical spine and shoulder when dealing with a wrist and hand complaint. However, I also want to include the rib cage and clavicle in this inspection. In dealing with patients that have advanced arthritis and/or histories of surgery, stroke and traumatic injury, assume every aspect of their musculoskeletal system has been injured. With these patients, there are additional complications of adjusting and managing their cases. In many instances, the cervical spine is most likely injured, but it is equally likely that the wrist and elbow also have been. The patient might very well have radiating pain into the upper extremity from the cervical or even thoracic spine, although I find this to be relatively uncommon. But even if they do, it's very likely they have injured the upper extremities as well.

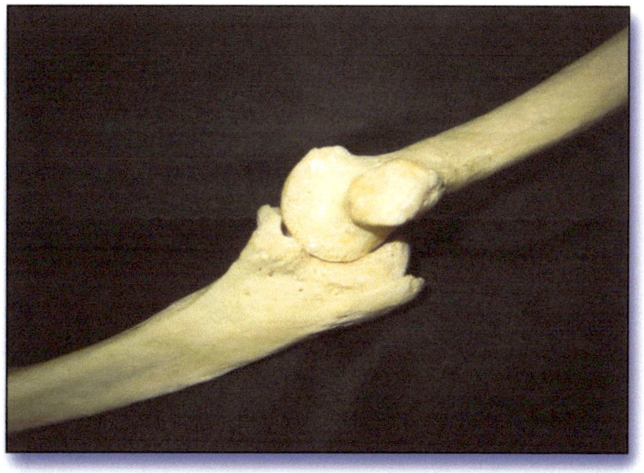

FIGURE 6-6. THE ULNAR HUMERAL JOINT.

The normal elbow should be able to have 180 degrees of extension. Hypermobile ligaments will allow subluxated elbows to extend fully or go into hyperextension.

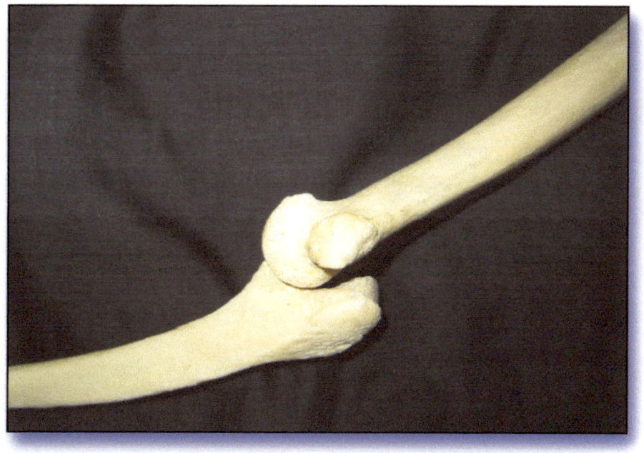

FIGURE 6-7. THE COMMON SUBLUXATION OF THE ULNA AT THE ELBOW.

The subluxated Ulna can cause a neuromuscular guarding response of the flexors and extensors of the hand and fingers, and the elbow will not fully extend.

The orthopedic tests to determine radiating pain from the cervical spine are simple and straightforward: the maximum cervical compression test, Valsalva maneuver, Spurling's test and shoulder depression test can all be done within a brief moment. Firm palpation on the cervical and thoracic spine itself is very important to perform, while noting any increase in complaints. If the sternal joints and axilla are palpated, distress patterns that are more profound than the ones found in the cervical spine will emerge in a lot of these cases. The inspection should also include the humeral joint and the clavicle joint at the shoulder. Each of these joint injuries can give

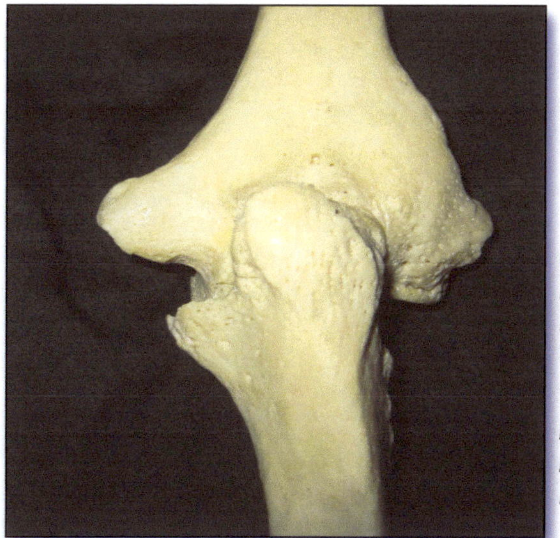

FIGURE 6-8. NORMAL ALIGNMENT OF THE ULNA AND HUMERUS FROM A POSTERIOR VIEW.

The Ulna should be midway between the lateral and medial edges of the Epicondyles.

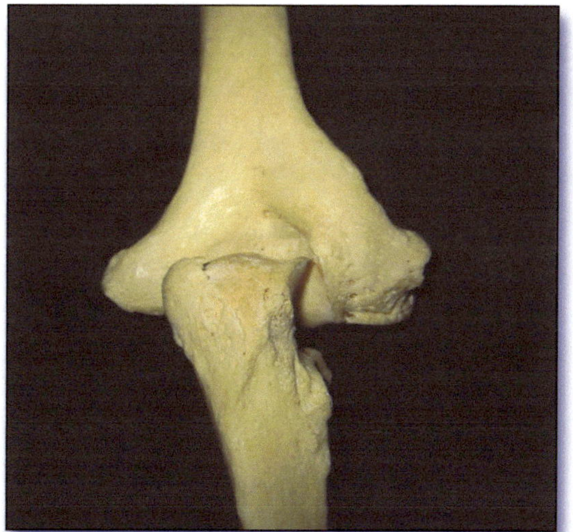

FIGURE 6-9. SUBLUXATION OF THE ULNA, LATERAL TO THE HUMERUS,

This is a posterior view of the elbow. Note the difference in the distance from the edges of the Humerus to the Ulna.

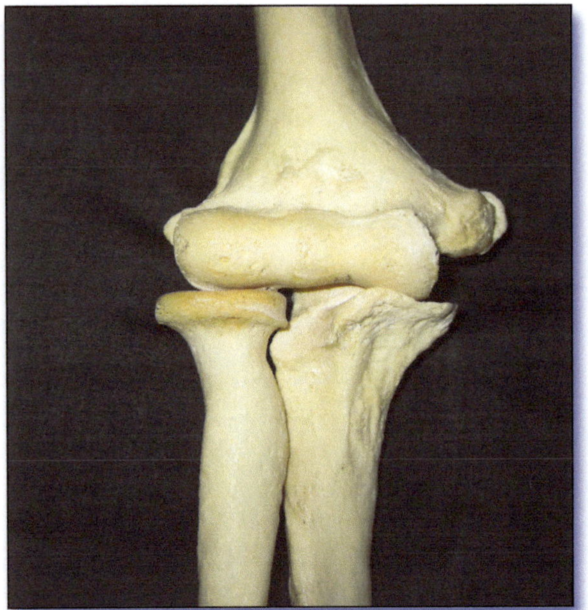

FIGURE 6-10. NORMAL ELBOW ALIGNMENT FROM THE VENTRAL VIEW.

Note the close relationship that the Radius and the Ulna have to each other.

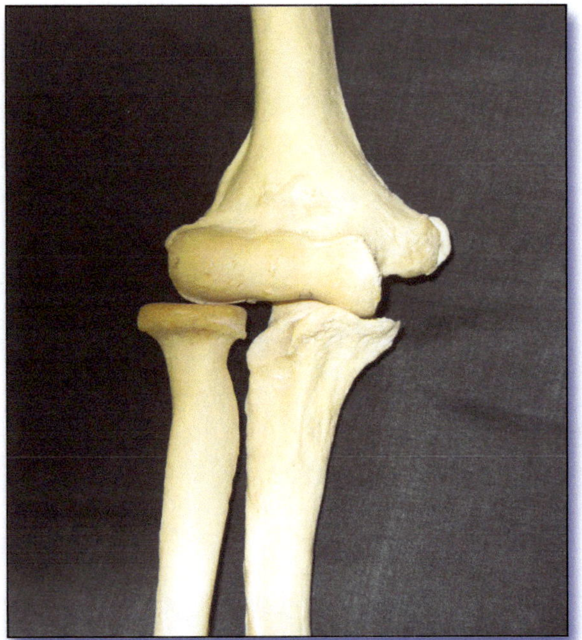

FIGURE 6-11. LATERAL SUBLUXATION OF THE RADIUS.

The top of the Radius is palpable with this subluxation pattern.

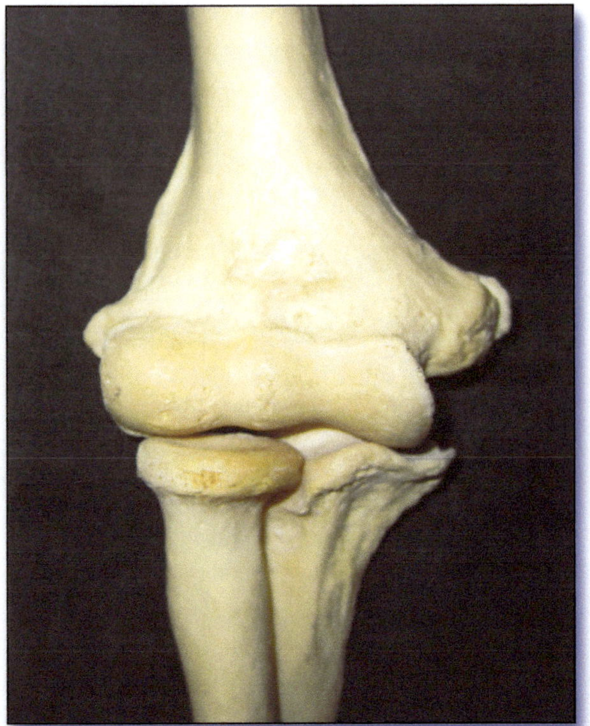

FIGURE 6-12. MEDIAL SUBLUXATION OF THE RADIUS.

The lateral, inferior part of the Humerus is palpable.

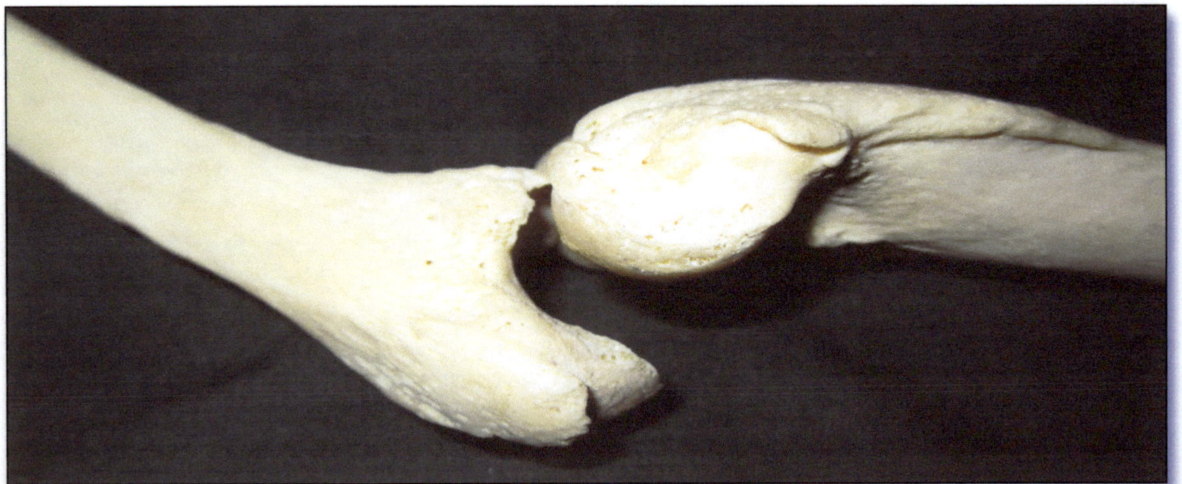

FIGURE 6-13. THE LUXATION OF THE ULNA FROM THE HUMERUS.

If these dislocations are not treated soon after the injury, the tissue will contract, making correction impossible.

pain patterns into the arm. Again, it is likely for a lot of these patients, all of these joints have been injured.

The olecranon process should "tuck" and the elbow should be close to 180 degrees or zero degrees, depending on the system of evaluation. Through the tissue of the triceps and dermis, the doctor should be able to feel the top or superior aspect of the ulna, and it should disappear with full extension of the elbow. *(See Figures 6-6 and 6-7.)*

Here the ulna is set superiorly to the humerus. Note that the elbow is slightly bent, because it cannot go into full extension. Palpation of the olecranon shows that the top or superior aspect does not "tuck" or disappear, thus the ulna has translated superiorly relative to the humerus. This type of injury is consistent with an etiology of outstretched hands at the moment of impact and repetitively using the arms to stand and stabilize the body.

When inspecting the elbow, I am looking for the alignment of the ulna with the humerus from a lateral to medial perspective. The olecranon process should be fairly centered between the two epicondyles of the humerus. *(See Figure 6-8.)* It is common with impact traumas for the olecranon process to be lateral to the fossa. This can be determined by palpating the space between the edges of the epicondyles and the edges of the ulna. *(See Figure 6-9.)* The space between the lateral edge of the epicondyle and the lateral edge of the ulna will be a smaller distance than the space between the medial epicondyle edge and the medial edge of the ulna.

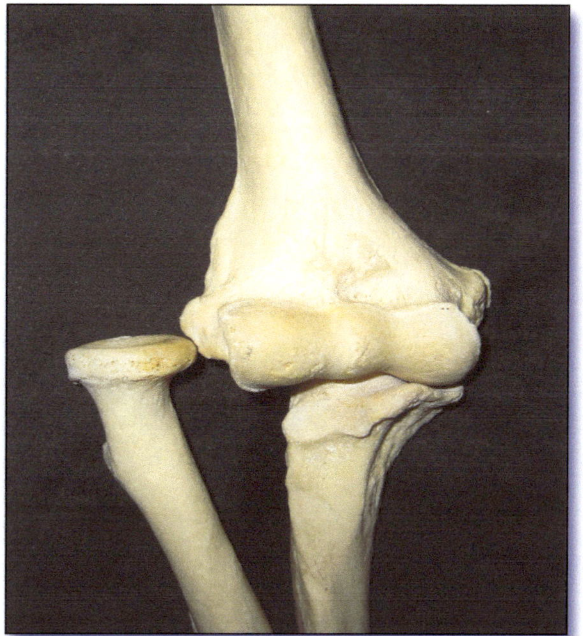

FIGURE 6-14. LATERAL LUXATION OF THE RADIUS.

These injuries are usually associated with other severe injuries and can be over looked.

The humeroradial joint is normal when there is an alignment of the radial head and the lateral aspect of the humerus or the capitulum. If passive supination and pronation are performed upon the patient's arm, there should be a smooth gliding motion of the radial head. *(See Figure 6-10.)*

When the radius has some laterality, the top of the radial head is palpable. *(See Figure 6-11.)* The supination and pronation of the forearm will demonstrate wobbling or uneven motion of the humeroradial joint, and if this is present, the joint itself will usually be painful for the patient due to joint

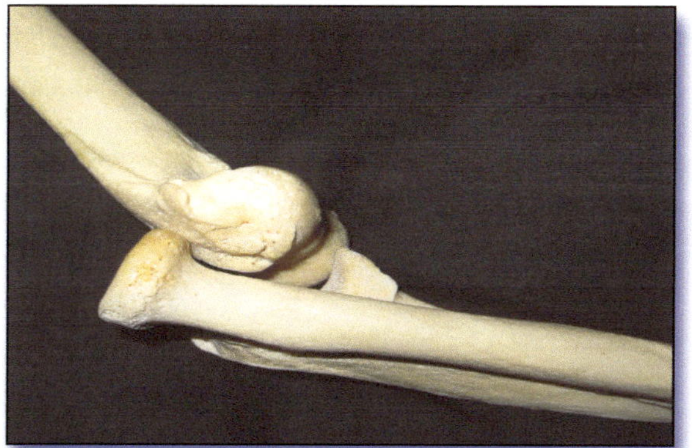

FIGURE 6-15 POSTERIOR LUXATION OF THE RADIUS.

I have seen the dysfunction of the arm in this type of injury as a manifestation of the concommitant brain injury. Usually no one examines additional injuries in TBI or spinal cord injuries.

capsule distress. When the radius has been subluxated medially, the underside or inferior aspect of the lateral epicondyle can be felt. (*See Figure 6-12.*)

In my treatment experience of catastrophic injuries with broken spines and paralysis, I have found the upper extremities to be severely injured. The injuries were mostly ignored by other health care providers and upper extremity dysfunction was blamed on the spinal cord injury, the brain injury or the stroke. In these situations, I've actually found luxated joints; the ulna will be completely pulled away from the humerus, and upon palpation, I can feel the inside of the olecranon process. The elbow is severely bent and extension is impossible. (*See Figure 6-13.*) It is necessary to restore the normal alignment as quickly as possible, especially with this type of injury. All the nerves, arteries, veins and tendons that cross the elbow joint are severely distressed. Their only hope of recovery is to restore the humeroulnar alignment.

I've also found the radius to be completely out from underneath the humerus. The radial head will be completely palpable and even the little dimple on the top of the radial head can be felt. (*See Figure 6-14.*) Sometimes the radial head has slipped up behind the humerus. (*See Figure 6-15.*) Again, I consider this is a luxation of the humeroradial joint. These subluxations will leave the elbow stuck in flexion, and extension will be impossible. The longer this condition persists, the harder it is to restore normal alignment and function, as a contracting of all the tissues will occur. I believe these injuries should be identified in the emergency room, or at least in the intensive care unit.

I've had patients who are in physical therapy with luxated elbow joints, yet in these cases, the arm's lack of function is blamed on the spinal injury or the head injury by the physical therapist. In addition, patients are commonly using the severely injured arms and elbows to push wheelchair wheels or to lean on walkers or canes, thereby causing greater pain and distress.

THE ULNA DRAW TEST

The doctor's hand is on the upper arm, stabilizing it. The other hand takes the patient's elbow at the edge of the olecranon. Have the patient move their hand around, noting any pain or restriction. The hand on the ulna draws it towards the fingers. Have the patient note any changes to the motion of the hand and wrist while the test is being performed. Positive changes during the "Ulna Draw" means the ulna is subluxated superiorly (*see below*).

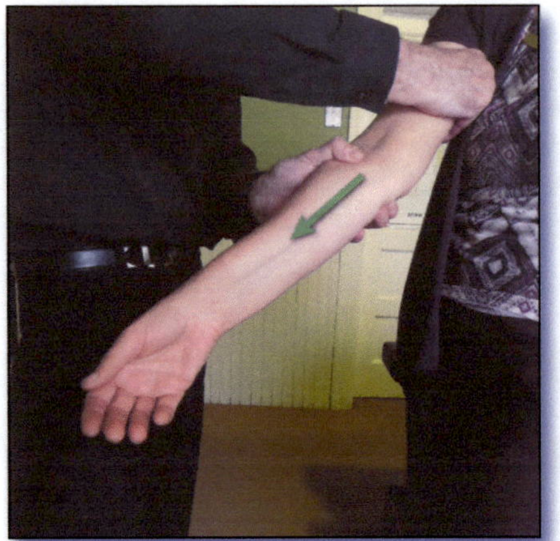

THE ULNA DRAW TEST

The doctor's hand is on the upper arm, stabilizing it. The other hand takes the patient's elbow at the edge of the olecranon, drawing the ulna towards the fingers.

GENERAL RULES FOR UPPER EXTREMITY ADJUSTING

> *With a rib cage injury, always keep the arm in front of the coronal plane. (The ear and the trochanter are landmarks to separate the front from the back halves of the body.)*

> *Using a foam block to raise the elbow and forearm so the adjusting doesn't stress the shoulder and ribcage may be necessary.*

ADJUSTING THE ULNAR HUMERAL JOINT

> *Adjust with the Spring-Loaded Instrument (SLI)*
The Doctor's fingers are contacting the Superior part of the Ulna and pulling it Inferiorly while tapping with the SLI. *See Figures 6-16a and 6-16b.*

> *Adjust the ulna with the drop piece*
The Olecranon Process is placed on the edge of the drop piece and the thrust is on the Humerus. The drop piece is on a block so the adjustment doesn't stress the shoulder or rib cage. *See Figure 6-17.*

> *Adjust the ulna with an Elbow contusion*
The forearm is placed on the drop piece with the Olecranon above or superior to the edge of the drop piece. The thrust, as before, is on the Humerus. *See Figure 6-18.*

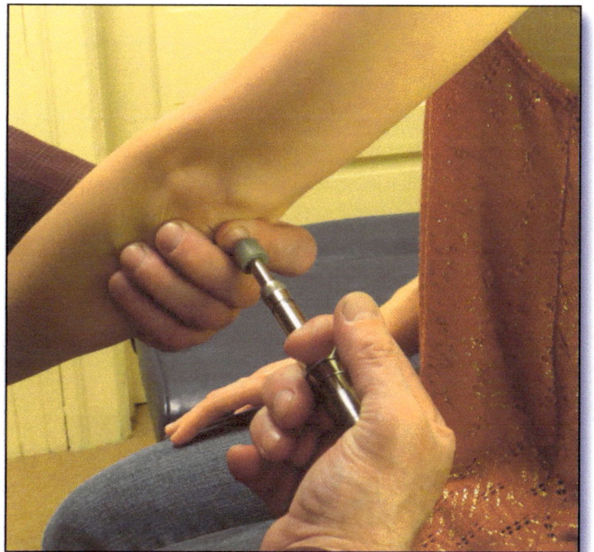

FIGURE 6-16 A. ADJUSTING THE SUPERIOR ULNA WITH THE SLI.

The Doctor's fingers are contacting the Superior part of the Ulna and pulling it Inferiorly while tapping with the SLI.

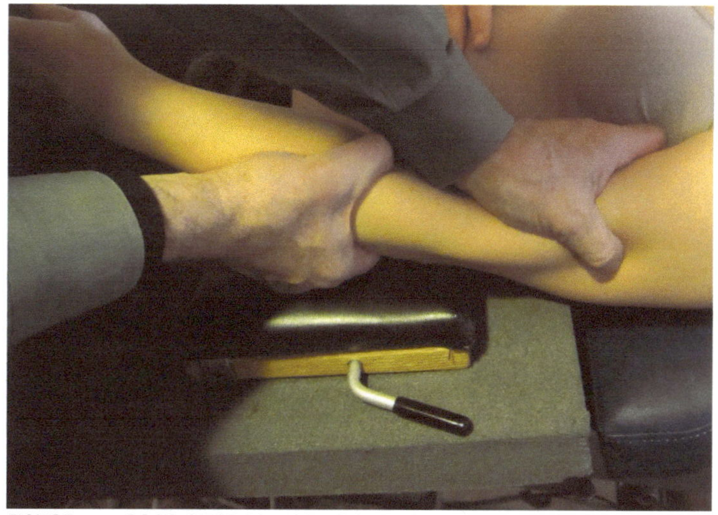

FIGURE 6-17. DROP PIECE ADJUSTING OF THE ULNA.

The Olecranon Process is placed on the edge of the drop piece and the thrust is on the Humerus. The drop piece is on a block so the adjustment doesn't stress the shoulder or rib cage.

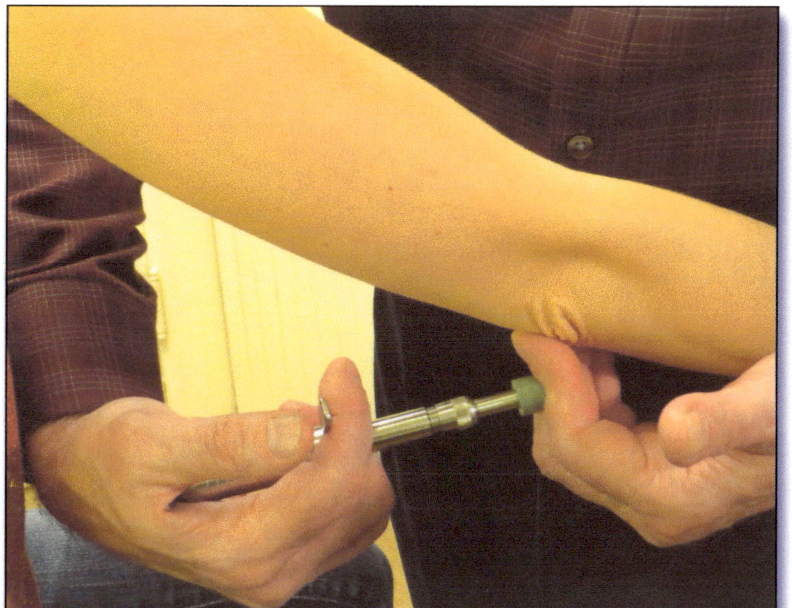

FIGURE 6-16B. ADJUSTING THE SUPERIOR ULNA WITH THE SLI.

Another view.

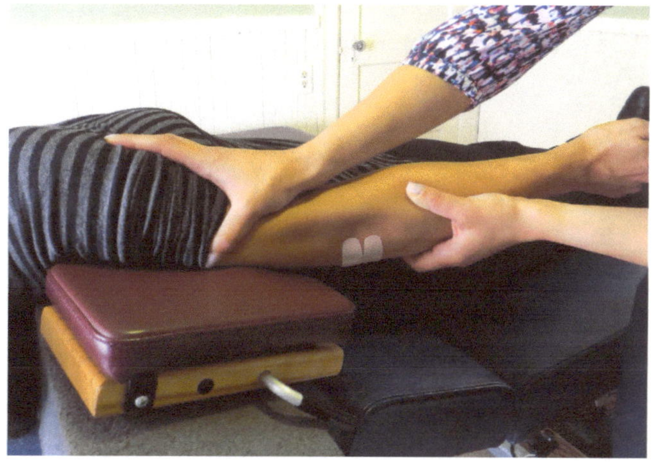

FIGURE 6-18. ADJUSTING THE ULNA WITH AN ELBOW CONTUSION OR FOREARM IN A CAST.

The forearm is placed on the drop piece with the Olecranon above or superior to the edge of the drop piece. The thrust, as before, is on the Humerus.

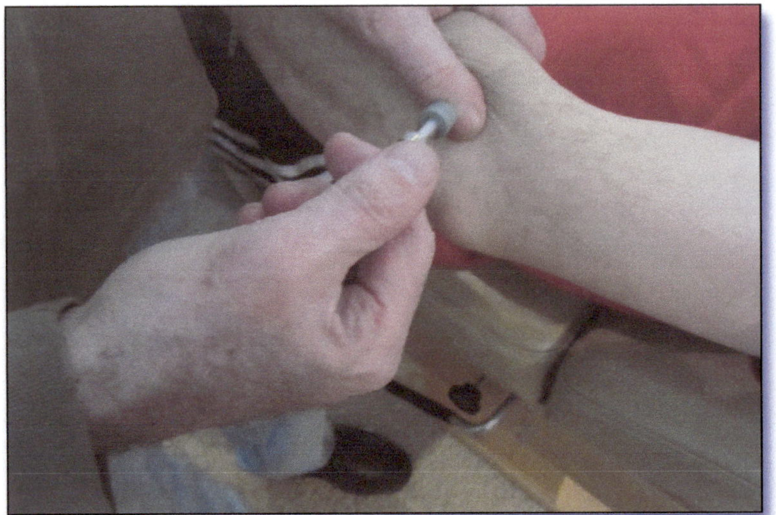

FIGURE 6-19. ADJUSTING THE POSTERIOR RADIUS WITH THE SLI.

The doctor's thumb is contacting the Posterior Radius and initiating a tap posterior to anterior. Repeated taps are usually necessary.

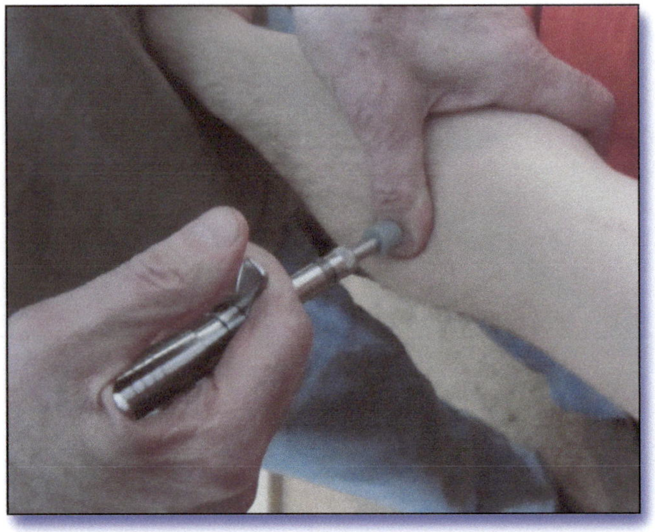

FIGURE 6-20. ADJUSTING THE MEDIAL RADIUS WITH THE SLI.

The Doctor's thumb is contacting the Posterior aspect of the Radius, pushing it into the direction of correction (Posterior to Anterior) and tapping with the SLI.

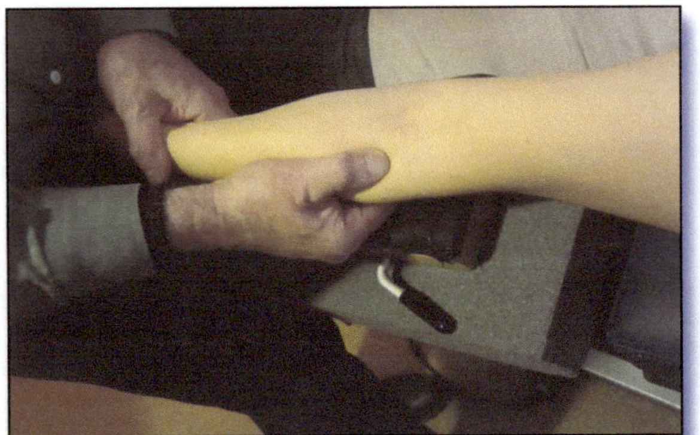

FIGURE 6-21. DROP PIECE ADJUSTING THE MEDIAL RADIUS.

The Doctor's thumb is contacting the Anterior/Medial aspect of the Radius and pressing into the direction of correction (Medial to Lateral) and tapping.

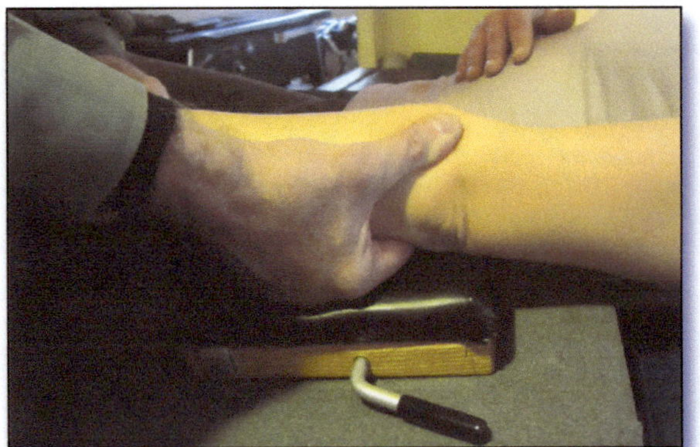

FIGURE 6-22. ADJUSTING THE POSTERIOR RADIUS WITH THE DROP PIECE.

The Doctor's thumb is contacting the posterior aspect of the Radius and thrusting, gently, posterior to lateral initiating the drop piece.

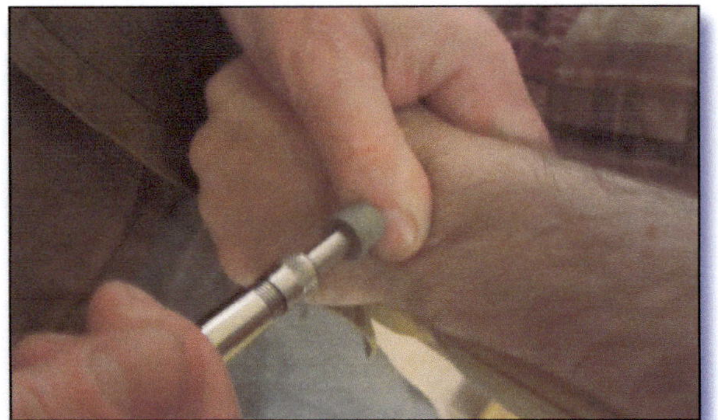

FIGURE 6-23. SLI ADJUSTING OF THE WRIST.

The Wrist is gripped by the Doctor's hand. The Carpal bone or bones that are fixated or misaligned are contacted by the Doctor's thumb and the SLI is tapped through the thumb to the Carpal bones.

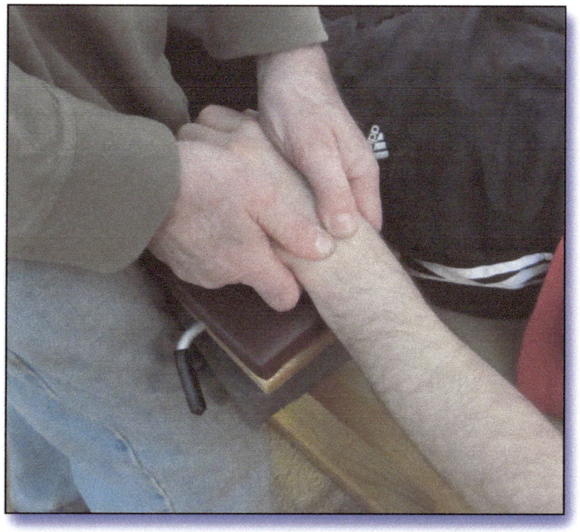

FIGURE 6-24. ADJUSTING THE WRIST ON THE DROP PIECE.

The Styloid Processes of the Ulna and Radius are contacted by the Doctor's thumbs while gripping the Wrist with the rest of his/her hands. While lying on the drop piece, the thumbs and fingers perform a gentle distraction of the Wrist and initiates a drop on the drop piece.

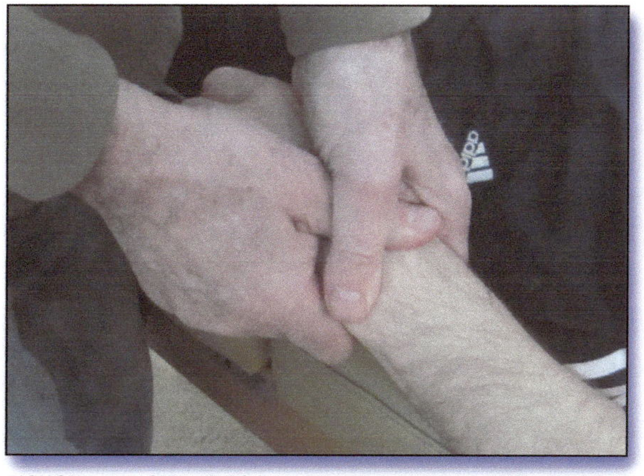

FIGURE 6-25. SET UP FOR A MANUAL MANIPULATION OF THE WRIST.

The crossed thumbs contact the Styloid Processes of the Ulna and Radius. The hands are gripping the wrist. A gentle distraction is performed followed by a pulling (gently) of the hands and a thrust spreading of the Styloid Processes with the thumbs.

ADJUSTING THE RADIO-HUMERAL JOINT

> *SLI adjusting of the Posterior or Lateral Radius*
The doctor's thumb is contacting the Posterior Radius and initiating a tap posterior to anterior. Repeated taps are usually necessary. *See Figure 6-19*

> *SLI adjusting of the Medial Radius*
The Doctor's thumb is contacting the Posterior aspect of the Radius, pushing it into the direction of correction (Posterior to Anterior) and tapping with the SLI. *See Figure 6-20*

> *Drop Piece Adjusting Medial Radius*
The Doctor's thumb is contacting the Anterior/Medial aspect of the Radius and pressing into the direction of correction (Medial to Lateral) and tapping. *See Figure 6-21*

> *Drop Piece Adjusting of the Posterior or Lateral Radius*
The Doctor's thumb is contacting the posterior aspect of the Radius and thrusting, gently, posterior to lateral initiating the drop piece. *See Figure 6-22.*

ADJUSTING THE WRIST

> *With the SLI*
The Wrist is gripped by the Doctor's hand. The Carpal bone or bones that are fixated or misaligned are contacted by the Doctor's thumb and the SLI is tapped through the thumb to the Carpal bones. *See Figure 6-23.*

> *With the drop piece*
The Styloid Processes of the Ulna and Radius are contacted by the Doctor's thumbs while gripping the Wrist with the rest of his/her hands. While lying on the drop piece, the thumbs and fingers perform a gentle distraction of the Wrist and initiates a drop on the drop piece. *See Figure 6-24*

> *By manual release*
The crossed thumbs contact the Styloid Processes of the Ulna and Radius. The hands are gripping the wrist. A gentle distraction is performed followed by a pulling (gently) of the hands and a thrust spreading of the Styloid Processes with the thumbs. *See Figure 6-25.*

The wrist should only be adjusted or manipulated after the elbow has been adjusted. Do not attempt to work on the wrist without assessing and adjusting the elbow joints. Please note: all procedures are gentle and firm, and don't expect the first tap or drop to complete the correction.

MANAGING THE ELBOW/FOREARM/WRIST/HAND INJURY

- *Lifting*
- *Changing positions*
- *Walkers, canes, crutches*
- *Bracing*

Managing the elbow, forearm, wrist and hand injury has its own set of unique challenges. Unfortunately, most of the patients I've worked with also have other injuries. Managing the Activities of Daily Living (ADL) of a patient with multiple impairments requires thorough consideration, especially when the patient has multiple injuries. Methods of ADL that were done before the injuries have to be altered or completely abandoned for new methods.

In discussing ADL with patients, emphasize that lifting and carrying with injured upper extremities should be done cautiously. The most common lifting and carrying actions involve groceries and laundry. So among the management techniques that I recommend, number one is "small and repetitive." For example, when grocery shopping, the patient should have the groceries put in multiple smaller, lighter bags. This will result in more bags and more trips. From the perspective of managing the patient's injuries, this is a better alternative than being "efficient," where efficiency means larger bags and fewer trips. Obviously, in managing these types of injuries, it would be better to have less ambitious shopping trips. Carts with wheels and other devices can be helpful for patients with upper extremity injuries. Laundry is the other typical lifting situation that can cause problems with these upper extremity injuries. So I counsel the patient to do laundry more frequently, rather than waiting until there are large amounts of laundry to be done.

Changing positions is a common source of pain and difficulty for those with multiple impairments. The upper extremity injuries will be challenged, if not continually re-injured by the act of getting up by using the arms. The patients that have lower extremity or low back injuries are usually using their arms and hands to change positions. If the arms and hands are injured as well, this creates a vicious cycle for the patient. Occupational therapy can be helpful, but some people do not have access to these professionals. I have, in extreme cases, made home visits myself to consult with the family and the patient on how to modify furniture, where to place grab bars and possibly ramps. Sitting in a soft chair or couch requires even a normal person to use their arms to get out of a seated position. With these types of upper extremity injuries, soft couches should be avoided altogether. Taking the cushions from the couch and putting them on a standard kitchen chair to boost the height of the seat helps reduce the number of arm assisted position changes.

Walkers, canes and crutches being used by people with upper extremity injuries will also cause continued problems. Usually the walkers, canes and crutches are for lower extremity or other mobility problems, but if the arms and hands are injured as well, using these devices can be a painful and challenging obstacle to recovery.

Bracing the elbow and forearm can help manage the instability of these joints. I have a different view of bracing than the majority of my colleagues. If a brace can keep the patient functional and out of severe pain, I will continue to use the brace as long as the instability of the joints is apparent, to aid in the healing of the ligaments. I have no problem with a patient becoming "dependent" on the brace for however long it takes for the ligaments to heal. If it keeps the patient functional and reduces pain, I will use it.

Some of the injuries that we are treating will be permanent in nature. There will be no full recovery. It is necessary to manage chronically unstable and degenerating joints. The need for activity is great. If functional capacity is improved by using a brace, I feel there is no reason to not wear it. We need our patients to be as active and independent as possible.

Online lessons at:
https://youtu.be/VanSrmPKWLM
https://youtu.be/PBYoImYbuTQ
https://youtu.be/OGWLT1tOZak
https://youtu.be/G54qAYAfFMQ

CHAPTER SEVEN

Evaluating, Adjusting and Managing The Thoracic and Lumbar Spines

The arthritic spine has changes in the articular structures but also in some of neurological structures. There are a number of features of the arthritic thoracic and lumbar spines that should be noted. The joint degeneration can limit mobility. The limited mobility of the vertebral column can lead to decreased blood flow and function of the spinal cord, affecting the health of the entire individual. Osteoarthritis of the spine is caused by trauma, subluxations left uncorrected. The deteriorated joints of the thoracic and lumbar spine are generally devoid of nerve endings. They have been lost with the degenerative changes of the joint tissues. I find most people with severe arthritis of the spine have little or no pain on palpation of the spinous processes. The muscles of the region will still be used to move with altered structures giving them more work and stress and therefore pain. It's not the joints that are gone that's causing the pain, the muscular structures are the source of the pain. This muscle response in part is controlled by the spinal cord reflexes from the altered joint function. With immobility will come muscle atrophy, degenerative changes of the muscle cells themselves and finally infiltration by fat cells rendering the tissue no longer muscle. Osteophytes will become prominent stopping normal motion and impinging on components of the autonomic nervous system. Some of the nerves stretched by the osteophytes i.e. bone spurs will turn the nerves into fiber. Histological changes will occur from persistent deformation. This is end stage degenerative change. *See figures 7-1 to 7-3.* The autonomic nerves are being stretched by arthritic changes. Stretching a nerve decreases it's conductivity. This did not happen overnight, this is a gradual process. Our therapeutic goal should be to reverse this condition or at least manage it and mitigate the effects of the condition. To prevent this we need care of our injuries after they occur and proper rehabilitation.

But the special needs patient, generally, cannot tolerate long axis manipulation. Some of the rib cage injuries or other problems the patients suffer will make prone adjusting contraindicated. Specific vertebral adjusting can be done with the SLI in seated or recumbent positions. When a patient can tolerate prone adjusting, it needs to be gentle. The repetitive, gentle drop table adjusting for the spine can be very helpful for the arthritic spine. Keeping the arthritic spine mobile and the patient active are some of the major goals of chiropractic care. *(See Figure 7-4).*

The management of these conditions becomes very important and will be discussed later. Quite a few patients with advanced arthritis will never have a full correction of their spines. One of the goals should be to prevent severe arthritis from getting worse. This is accomplished in part by trying to take everything back towards the "building code". I use mirror image adjusting as often as possible.

RELEVANT ANATOMY FOR THIS CHAPTER

- *Spinous Processes of the Thoracic Spine*
- *Transverse Processes of the Thoracic Spine*
- *Spinous Processes of the Lumbar Spine*
- *Transverse Processes of the Lumbar Spine*

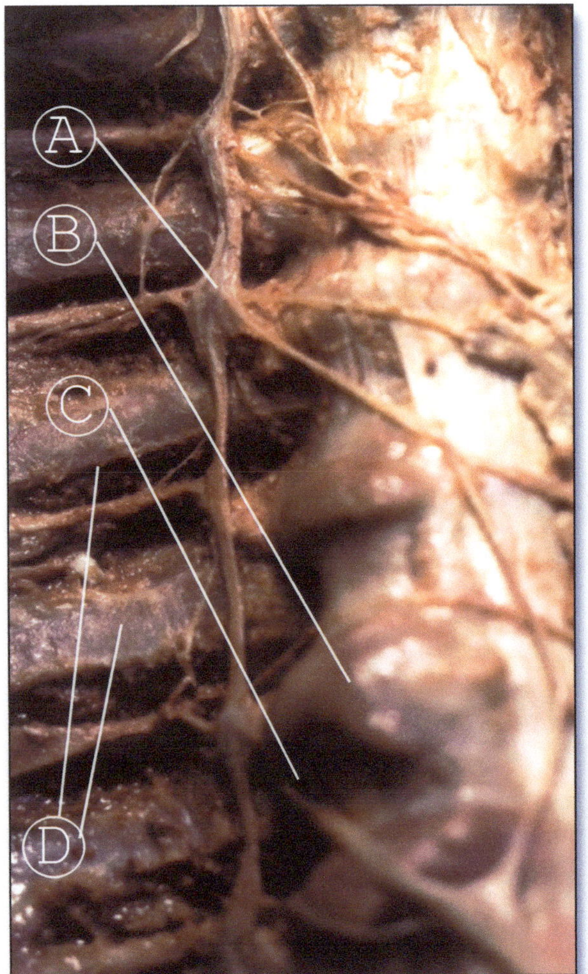

FIGURE 7-1 ANTERIOR VIEW OF AN ARTHRITIC SPINE.

Each of the protrusions are discs that have fused into contiguous osteophytes. Osteophytes are contacting and stretching of autonomic nerves.

A. Sympathetic Chain Ganglion
B. Osteophytes/Disc Bulging
C. Autonomic Nerve in Contact with Osteophyte
D. Ribs

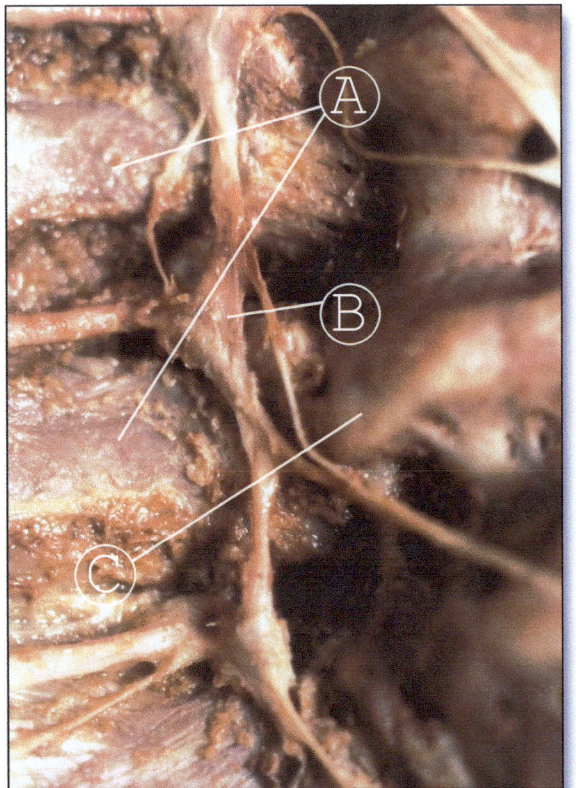

FIGURE 7-2. CLOSE UP VIEW OF THE SYMPATHETIC CHAIN

Note the sympathetic chain next to the rib joints and osteophytes.

A. Rib
B. Sympathetic Chain
C. Osteophyte

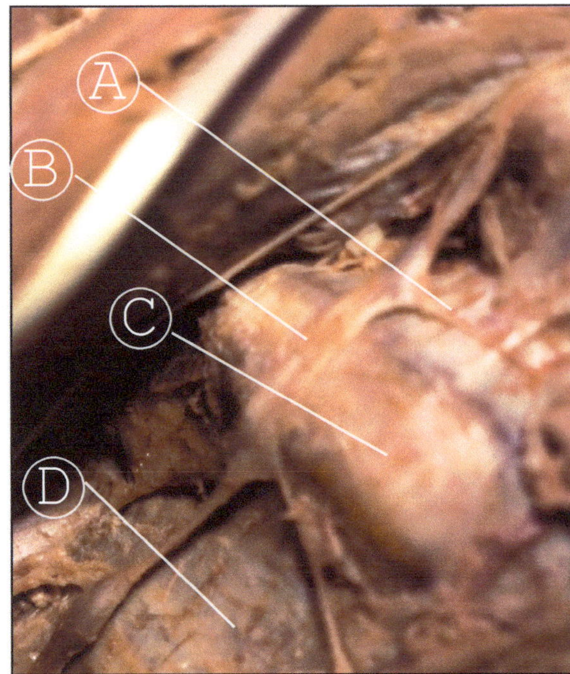

FIGURE 7-3. AN AUTONOMIC NERVE BEING STRETCHED BY A BULGING DISC

This individual's right autonomic nerve has contact with the L5- SI disc, being flattened, possibly interfering with nerve flow.

A. L4
B. Sympathetic Nerve
C. Bulging L5-SI disc
D. Sacrum

As a profession, we in the chiropractic arts have not done long-term studies on the benefits of chiropractic care in reducing arthritic changes. So I have no scientific basis for saying that chiropractic care can reduce arthritic degeneration. However, based on my clinical experience, including my own case, advanced arthritis does not have to be debilitating.

This clinical observation is based on the patients that can afford and continue long-term chiropractic care. It is very difficult to prove a negative. By that, I mean when the prognosis is for someone to develop arthritis and become

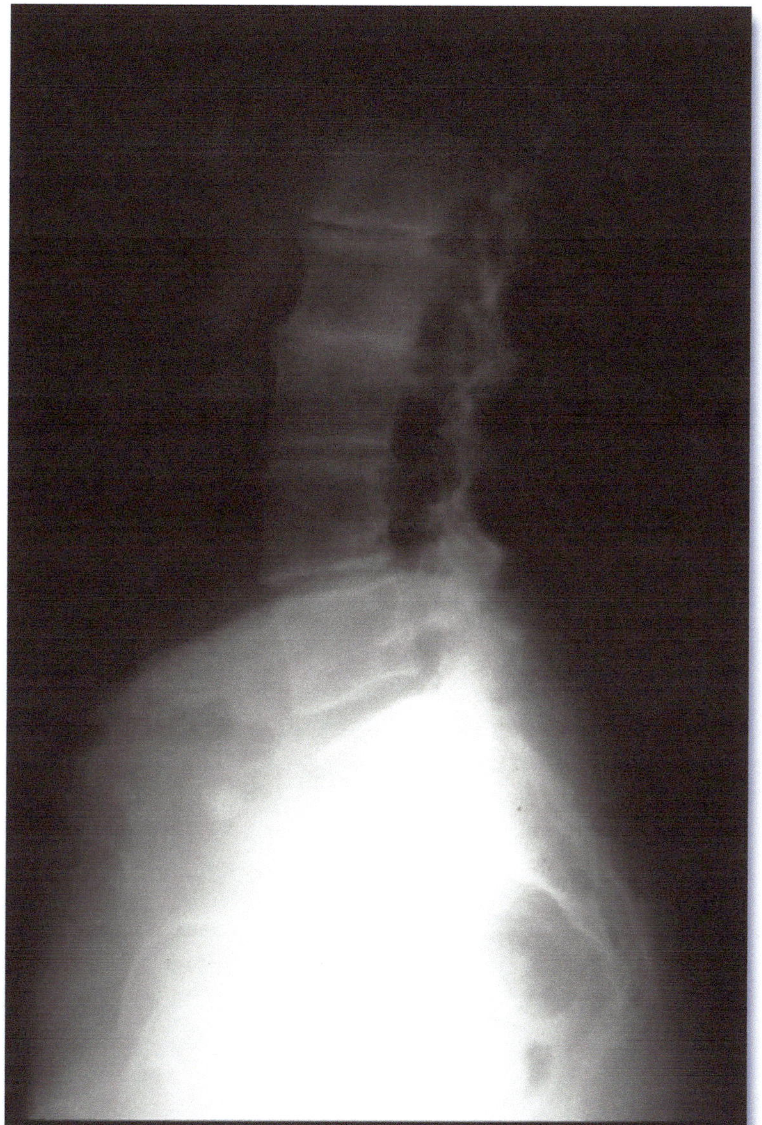

FIGURE 7-4.

This patient has a significant loss of disc height in the mid-lumbar spine. At the time of this film she had been enjoying a high level activity (dancing and gardening) for decades.

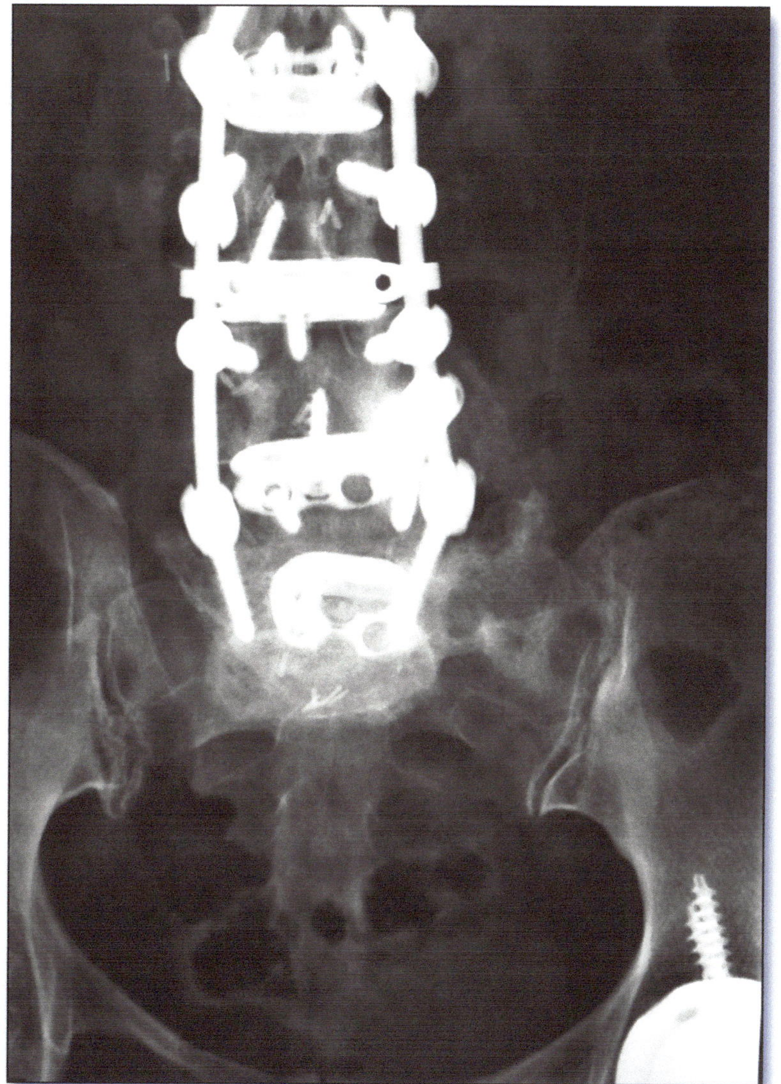

FIGURE 7-5.

This x-ray shows lumbar spinal surgery with multiple screws and hardware and a hip replacement. Chiropractic care post surgery can be essential to keeping the patient mobile, employed and living independently.

debilitated and it does not occur, can you prove your intervention was the main reason for the change in outcome? I know, and my patients know, that the chiropractic and adjunct care they receive keeps them functional and prolongs their abilities to stay independent.

Balance, weight-bearing activity and conditioning will all improve with correcting, even marginally, the posture, leveling the pelvis and increase mobility. The relevant anatomy of the spine in special needs patients has commonly been altered.

Osteophytes, lost joint space and altered curvatures are not part of the normal anatomy of a healthy human spine. These are common features of the arthritic patient, and some patients will have surgical repairs and hardware installed in their spines as well. *(See Figure 7-5.)*

Spinal surgeries are becoming more common in younger patients, but more in the elderly. I find many of the spinal surgeries, not just in the elderly, did not address the chief complaint. So, if the doctor can actually examine and treat the original complaint, despite the surgery, will have a good outcome.

There are two main approaches to dealing with the arthritic spine. The first is segmental and the second is global.

SEGMENTAL ADJUSTING

Segmental adjusting of the arthritic spine can be done with the drop table or the SLI. The patient with limitations in positioning may need to have adjusting done in the seated position or while lying on their side. The palpation of the spine is critical in determining individual vertebral subluxation patterns. Contacting the spinous processes and transverse processes of a particular vertebra to gently drop or tap it, repetitively, into place is the protocol. Even if the patient can be put in a prone position, this is still the protocol.

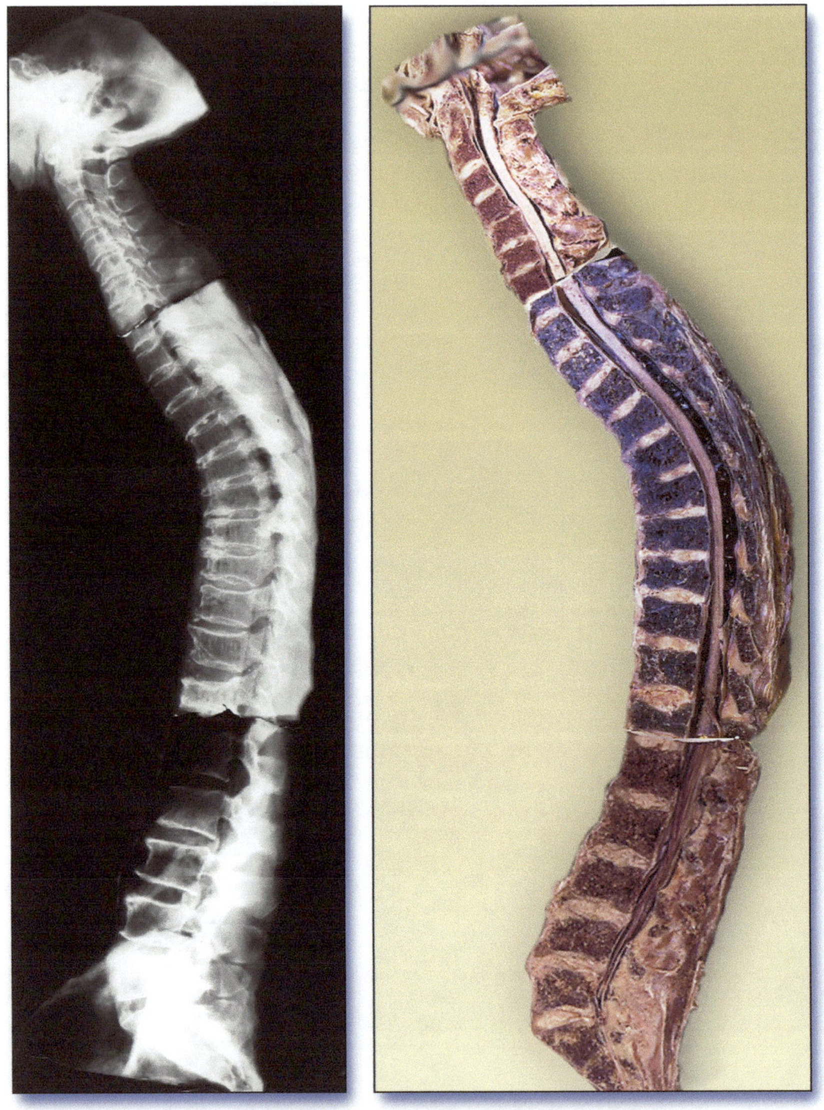

FIGURE 7-6A & B. POSTURAL CHANGES OF THE VERTEBRAL COLUMN CAN DISTRESS THE SPINAL CORD.

Persistent deformation of the Vertebral Column changes the shape and possibly the conductivity of the Spinal Cord.

GLOBAL ADJUSTING

Global adjusting is done to create a change in the shape of each region of the spine. This approach uses postural analysis and X-ray analysis to determine how to do the adjusting. For example, if someone has a hyperkyphosis of the thoracic spine, then putting their thoracic spine in extension would help reduce the kyphosis.

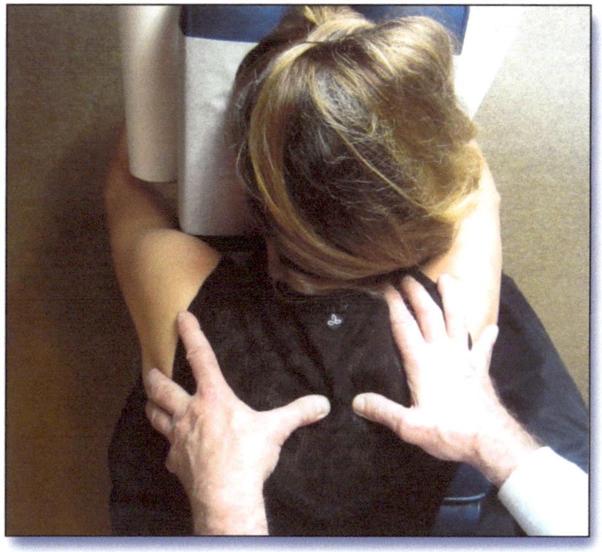

FIGURE 7-7 . PRONE DROP TABLE ADJUSTING OF A SPECIFIC THORACIC VERTEBRA.

Note the specific contact: the left hand is contacting a Transverse Process and the right hand is contacting the Spinous Process

THORACIC SPINE ADJUSTING

Contacting the spinous processes and transverse processes of the vertebrae of the arthritic spine for adjusting can be used to keep the joints mobile. The following figures are typical in patients with advanced arthritis. It is my hope that gentle chiropractic care for our younger patients will help keep these advanced conditions from developing.

In Figures 7-1 through 7-6 arthritic conditions are shown, some whom have and do benefit from Chiropractic care. Keeping patients mobile, active and in their own homes is a very important goal.

In Figure 7 – 7 we demonstrate prone drop table adjusting of specific thoracic vertebra. Note the specific contact, the left-hand is contacting the transverse process and the right hand contacts the spinous process. This would be a set up for a spinous right subluxation for a thoracic vertebra. Figure 7 – 8 a and b show specific contact of a vertebral transverse process for the spring-loaded adjusting instrument (SLI). "a" shows the set up on a plastic spine and

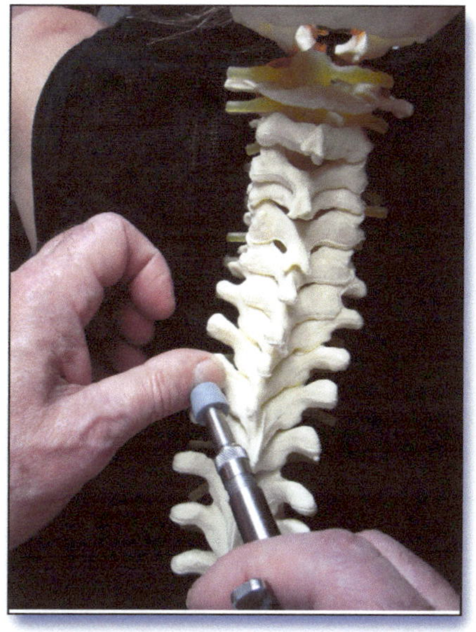

FIGURE 7-8A. DEMONSTRATION OF SLI ADJUSTING OF THE THORACIC SPINE.

The Doctor's fingers can push the Vertebra into the direction of correction, and then the SLI repeated tapping will complete the adjustment.

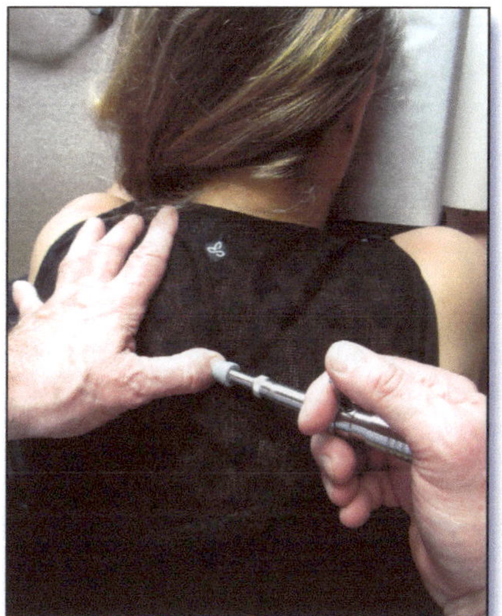

FIGURE 7-8 B. PRONE SLI ADJUSTING OF THE THORACIC SPINE.

Note the specific contact of the Spinous Process.

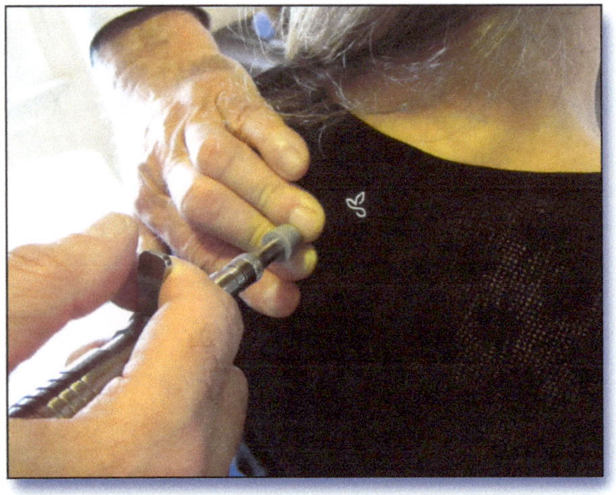

FIGURE 7-9. SEATED SLI ADJUSTING OF THE THORACIC SPINE.

This shows specific, broad contact of a Transverse Process.

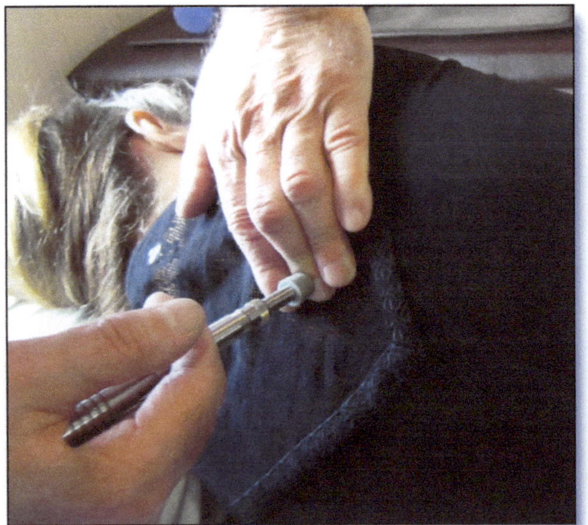

FIGURE 7-10. SLI SIDE POSITION ADJUSTING OF THE THORACIC SPINE.

Note the contact of specific Vertebral segments with the Doctor's hand

"b" is the SLI setup on a patient's thoracic spine. As mentioned before the needs of the patient might eliminate prone adjusting. The SLI allows for different positions that the patient might be more comfortable in. In Figure 7 -9 and 10 we demonstrate SLI adjusting of the thoracic spine in the seated and recumbent positions.

LUMBAR SPINE ADJUSTING

The lumbar spine of arthritic patients can be asymptomatic. The nerves of the degenerated joints are no longer there to transmit pain signals. The musculature of the lumbar region will be hard and rigid from pelvic girdle injury. The work to level the pelvis is covered in Chapter 2. The following figures demonstrate the use of the drop table and SLI to keep the lumbar spine mobile despite impairments. In Figure 7-11a we demonstrate with the plastic spine the specific contacts to reduce lumbar vertebrae rotation. Thumbs are contacting spinous and transverse processes with the drop table *(see Figure 7-11b)*. Use of the doctor's thigh or knee to assist the drop piece to drop is recommended with certain frail or highly distressed patients. In Figures 7-12 a and b we demonstrate the use of the SLI on the plastic spine and then on the patient. Some patients will not be able to tolerate the drop table. The SLI is a lighter use of force and gentler approach. In Figure 7-13 the SLI is being used on lumbar spine on a seated patient and in Figure 7-14 the patient is laying on their side.

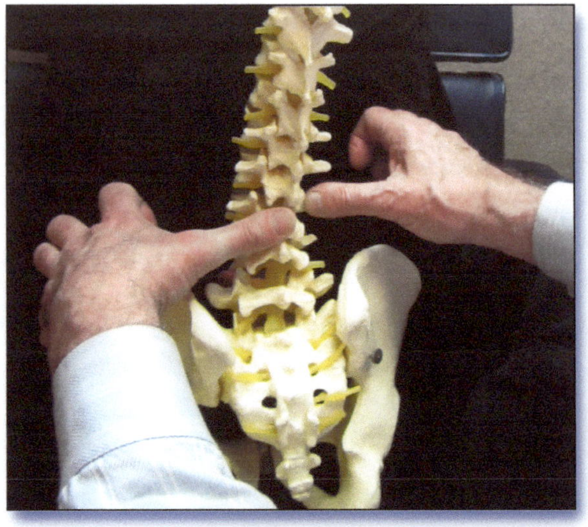

FIGURE 7-11A. DEMONSTRATION OF PRONE DROP TABLE ADJUSTING OF SPECIFIC LUMBAR VERTEBRA.

Note the contact of both the Transverse Process and the Spinous Process.

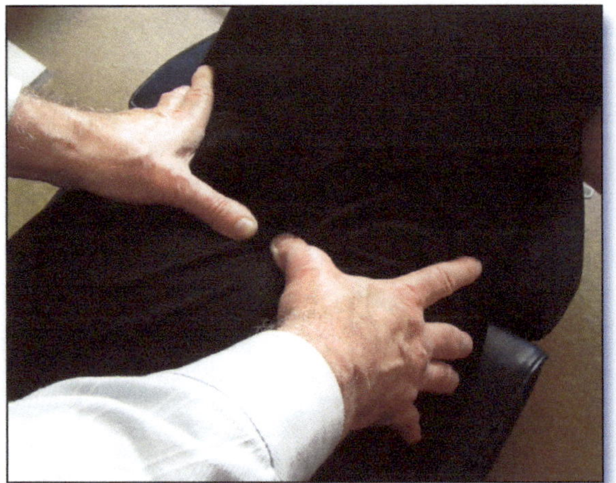

FIGURE 7-11B. PRONE DROP TABLE ADJUSTING A SPECIFIC LUMBAR VERTEBRA.

Note the specific contact, the left hand is contacting a Transverse Process and the right hand is contacting the Spinous Process.

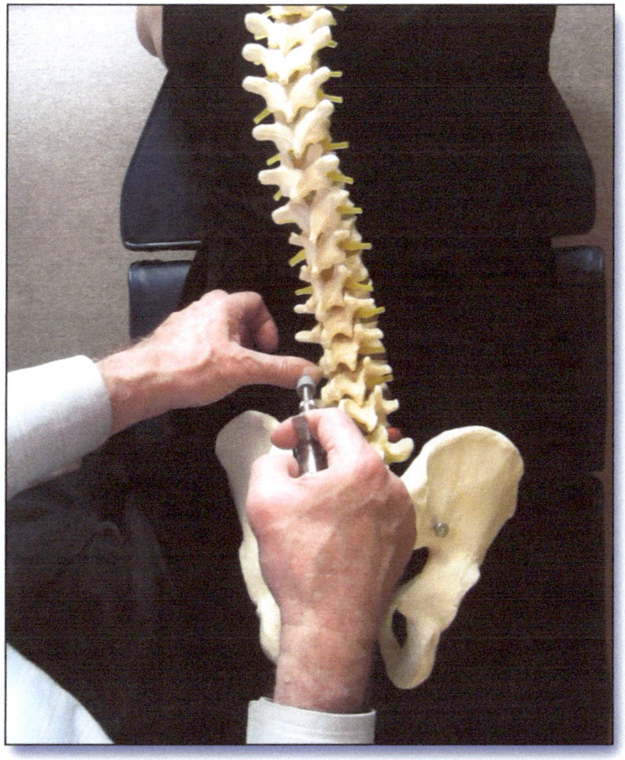

FIGURE 7-12A. DEMONSTRATION OF SLI ADJUSTING OF THE LUMBAR SPINE.

The Doctor's thumb contacts and presses a Transverse Process and the SLI adjusting completes the adjustment.

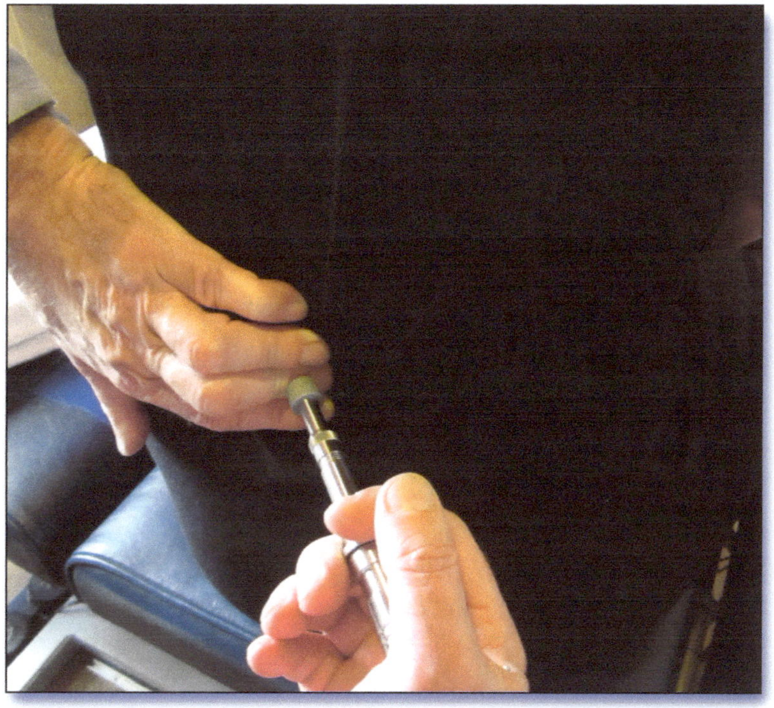

FIGURE 7-13. SEATED SLI ADJUSTING OF THE LUMBAR SPINE.

This procedure can be very helpful to the patient with multiple complications.

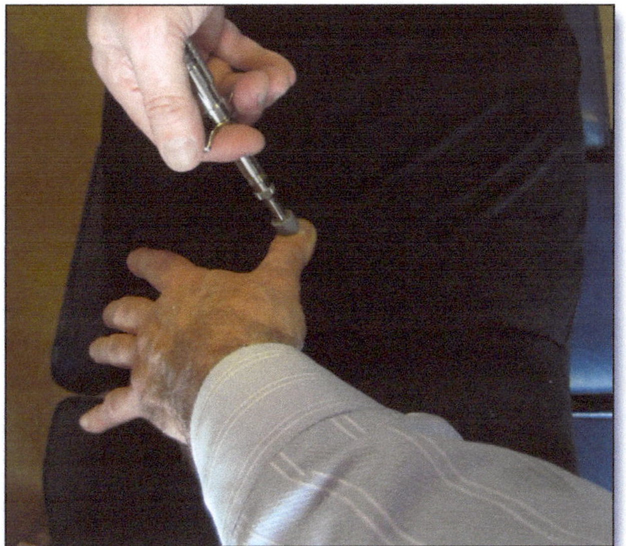

FIGURE 7-12B. PRONE SLI ADJUSTING OF THE LUMBAR SPINE.

Note the specific contact of a Transverse Process.

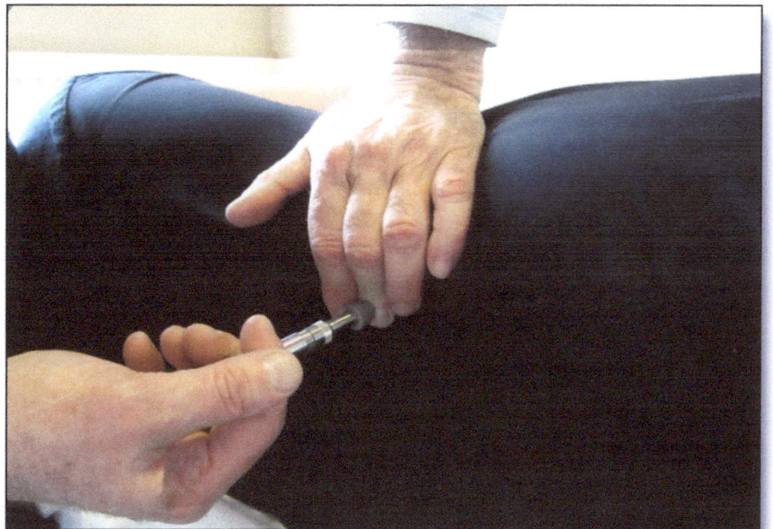

FIGURE 7-14. SLI ADJUSTING OF THE LUMBAR SPINE IN A SIDE POSITION.

This procedure can be used on the patient who will not tolerate prone positions.

GLOBAL ADJUSTING OF THE THORACIC SPINE

Global adjusting of the thoracic spine is done to reduce the kyphosis of the thoracic spine. This is necessary for patients who have acquired a significant anterior weight-bearing deformation of their posture. A large portion of this population will also have a compromised rib cage. This makes the adjusting of the thoracic spine more challenging. Prone adjusting on a patient with rib cage instability is contraindicated. A forceful, posterior to anterior (PA) thrust can add to the patient's rib cage distress pattern. If prone work can be tolerated with hyperkyphosis, generally the doctor can initiate the drop piece with the thigh or knee. This allows the doctor to do multiple, gentle drops without adding to the injury of the anterior joints of the chest, and using a broad contact with the hands to cover as much of the thoracic spine as possible. *(See Figure 7-15.)*

If the patient cannot tolerate prone adjusting, seated postural adjusting can be done. This allows the patient to lean back and put their thoracic spine in as much extension as they can manage. To adjust, the doctor will make a broad contact with the hand and use the SLI, tapping through the fingers if necessary. *(See Figure 7-16.)*

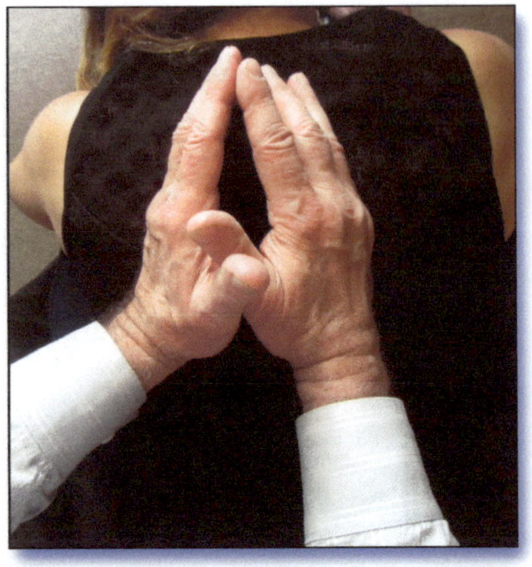

FIGURE 7-15. THE GLOBAL DROP TABLE ADJUSTING OF THE THORACIC SPINE.

Note the broad contact, this is performed in a very gentle manner with the drop piece being activated by the thigh or knee of the Doctor.

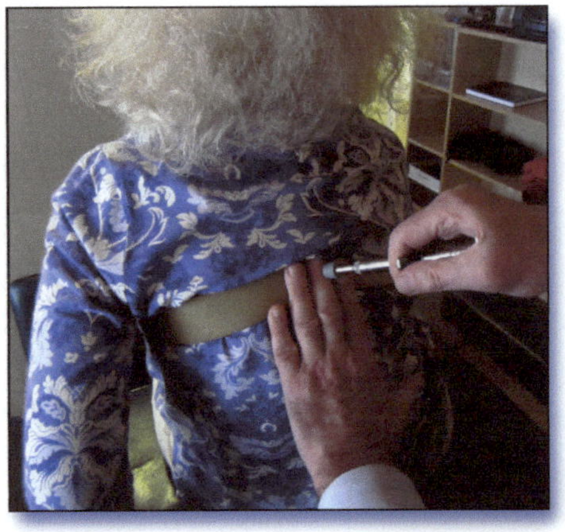

FIGURE 7-16. POSTURAL OR GLOBAL ADJUSTING OF THE THORACIC SPINE TO REDUCE HYPERKYPHOSIS.

This procedure employs a broad contact with the patient leaning back against the Doctor's hand. The broader the contact the more comfortable for the patient.

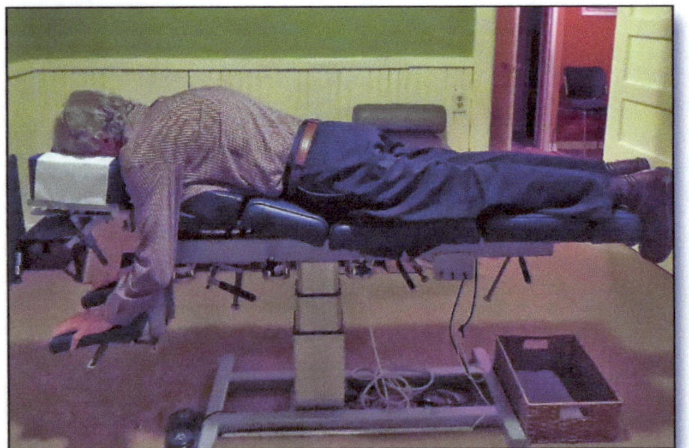

FIGURE 7-16. PRONE EXTENSION OF THORACIC AND LUMBAR FOR ANTERIOR HEAD AND ANTALGIC POSTURES

Drop table or SLI adjusting in this position can give postural relief. Rib cage injury might limit or eliminate this procedure.

MANAGING THE INJURED THORACIC AND LUMBAR SPINES

Managing chronically inflamed and degenerating spines is very challenging. Most patients who have these conditions are older, but not necessarily. We are having more spinal surgeries and joint replacement surgeries on younger members of our society. Generally speaking, the older the patient, the more difficult it is to get them to change their behavior to benefit their health.

The general approach is to inspire your patients to move. This goal is undermined by the older patient becoming more sedentary. Sedentary behavior does not benefit any of the conditions we are treating, but slowing down is generally what happens to us as we get older. There is a coaching aspect to getting people to move more. Motivational talks and even recruiting the patient's family members to become involved with keeping the older patient active is necessary. I consult with every patient about their daily activity levels and their time spent sitting. Every patient that is still working that comes into our office is encouraged to get a sit/stand workstation. Reviewing with the patient the ergonomics of their furniture in their homes and offices becomes necessary. I find quite a few patients have personal habits that bring on their spinal deformities and impede their recovery. Osteoporosis is a common condition in our patients who are 50 years and older, male and female. So everybody should be on their feet as much as possible during the course of their day. Even people in their 20s and 30s should be encouraged to reduce their sitting as much as possible. It would be nice that someday the norm would be good bone density at age 80 for the general population. This change would require an alteration in our collective behavior.

NOTES:

• • •

Online lessons at:
https://youtu.be/B_rIn0x36RI
https://youtu.be/ebgYtH2ShLU

CHAPTER EIGHT

Evaluating, Adjusting and Managing the Knee

The knee is a critical structure in the human being. I've had more than one patient contemplating suicide because of knee pain and dysfunction. The mobility of a patient can be intimately tied to knee function. This is not fully appreciated by anyone until a knee is injured. I feel lower extremity function is critical to managing the injured pelvis and low back and general health of any individual. For a patient whose primary complaint is low back pain and who has a pelvic girdle injury, I always examine the knees, lower leg, feet and ankles. Any of these components that have subluxations and dysfunctional motion patterns can interfere with stabilizing the pelvis. This approach to evaluating and adjusting is not typical and will require some new thinking to fully understand it.

In my opinion, knee arthritis is the result of a subluxated tibia. I have never found a case of an arthritic knee that had the tibia aligned with the femur. *(See Figures 8-1 A and 8-1B.)* I've had discussions with chiropractors about managing their own knee injuries and they will resist care because they have a partially torn anterior cruciate ligament (ACL) or meniscus. They think these injuries doom them to dysfunction. This is not the case. Even with terrible degenerative changes and a complete loss of joint space, realigning the tibia to the femur can improve function and greatly reduce pain.

In one special case, I have treated a knee injury that occurred in the patient 57 years earlier. He had medical care at the time of the injury and had access to orthopedic care for the entire period of time. Not one provider ever realigned the tibia to the femur. He walked with an obvious limp, used a cane, and had no joint space between the two bones. It was obviously arthritic and inflamed. On the first office visit, he had a persistent 15-degree angle in flexion of the knee and he could not fully extend his knee. This was because the tibia was about a half-inch anterior to the femur. The neuromuscular guarding reflex caused his gastrocnemius to tighten, and this left his knee in slight flexion, causing a permanent limp. Realigning the knee on the first office visit changed his gait, and he was able to straighten his leg. At the sixth visit, he came in complaining he'd left his very fancy cane at the gas station and lost it. He said it was all my fault

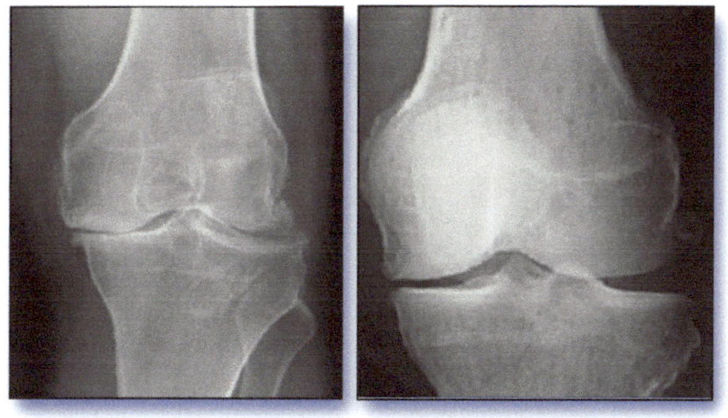

FIGURE 8-1A. SUBLUXATION OF THE TIBIA AND ARTHRITIS

Misaligned tibias are seen with the resulting of joint height.

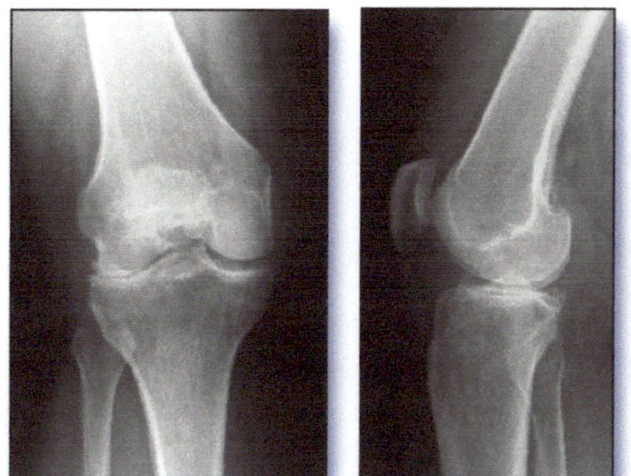

FIGURE 8-1B. TIBIAL SUBLUXATION AND KNEE ARTHRITIS

Misaligned tibia causes erosion of the joint structures

and he actually wasn't happy. I felt funny apologizing for something that was my therapeutic goal. Realigning the knee bones can drastically change someone's mobility, conditioning and prognosis for continued independent living.

The anatomy of the knee is fairly straightforward. The femur and tibia have an articulation that is classified as a hinge joint. In every case that I've seen involving knee arthritis, whether on a radiograph or in an actual examination: the tibia is misaligned with the femur. This results in altered weight bearing, which will deform all the soft tissue components including the capsule, cruciate ligaments and meniscus. *(See Figure 8-2.)* Over time, with a persistent subluxation, these deformed tissues will undergo degenerative changes.

RELEVANT ANATOMY FOR THIS CHAPTER

The femur and tibia:

> *Alignment is critical; all arthritis is related to altered weight bearing.*
> *The cruciate ligaments*
> *These structures are damaged with subluxation.*

The meniscus:

> *This is stressed and eroded with persistent subluxation.*
> *The musculature: all involved muscles will be exhibiting a neuromuscular guarding reflex with subluxation of the tibia.*

The cruciate ligaments are arranged from the attachments in the middle of the joints going medial or laterally in the various directions. *(See Figure 8-3.)* A cruciate ligament injury has to involve a displacement of the tibia relative to the femur. There is no other way for tearing or injury to the cruciate ligaments to occur. Even if it's just instantaneous, and the alignment post-injury is not affected, there is some translation of the tibial plateau away from its normal position with the femur. Cruciate ligament health can only be maintained by realigning the tibia to the femur.

The meniscus is a tough cartilaginous plate with grooves and contours to accommodate the knobs or condyles of the femur. Misalignment of the tibia will cause the condyles to not be in their proper grooves on the meniscus. Persistent displacement in the tibia will cause the meniscus to erode, usually asymmetrically, over time. We label this condition osteoarthritis.

The musculature that moves the knee comes from the pelvis and the lower leg. (See Figures 8-4 and 8-5.) Misalignment of any of these superior or inferior components will cause stress on the knee and make the musculature tight with a neuromuscular guarding reflex. The quadriceps, the biceps femoris, vastus medialis, sartorius, gracilis, vastus lateralis all attach to the innominate. Subluxation of the sacroiliac joints and pubic symphysis will cause all these muscles to tighten.

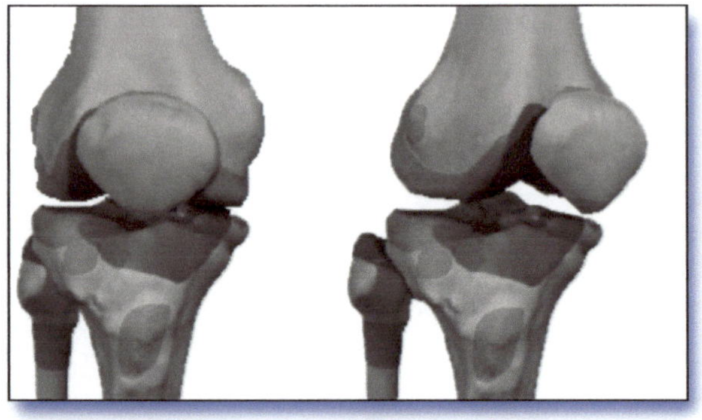

FIGURE 8-2. THE SUBLUXATED KNEE.

The Tibia has a proper position under the Femur. Any change in this relationship will affect the soft tissue and will result in generative changes. Loss of joint space and changing the shape of the Distal Femur and Proximal Tibia due to Wolf's Law is the expected outcome.

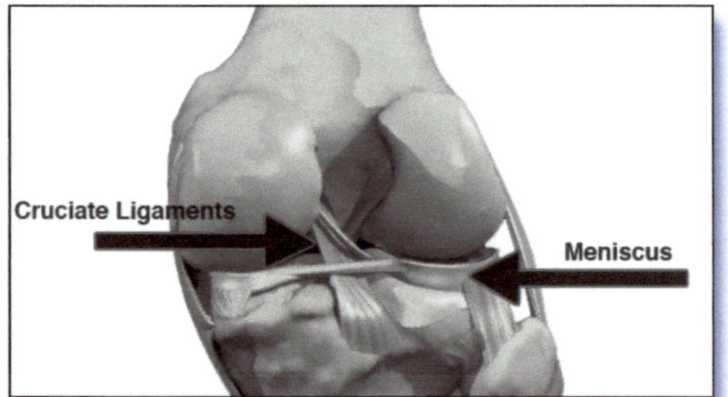

FIGURE 8-3. THE STRESSED INTRINSIC STRUCTURES

The intrinsic joint structures of the knee have to be damaged when translation of the tibia occurs. Optimal recovery is only possible when a realignment has occurred.

The gastrocnemius attaches to the inferior or distal femur, crossing the knee joint and going to the calcaneus. Calcaneal subluxation will cause the gastrocnemius to tighten, interfering with the function of the knee. Any displacement of the tibia

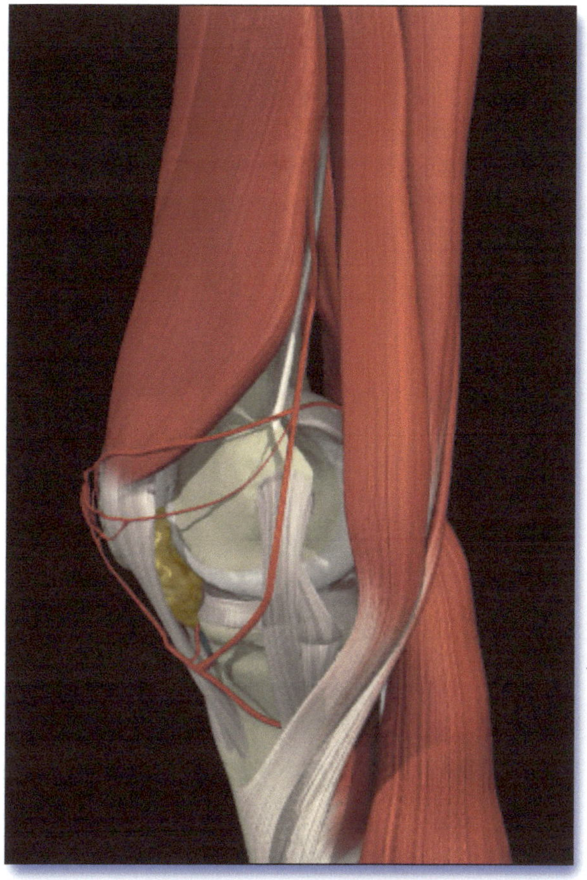

FIGURE 8-4. THE MEDIAL VIEW OF THE KNEE.

All these muscles guard to prevent misalignment. Trigger points, contracture and distortion of the leg are the result of chronic subluxation of the Tibia.

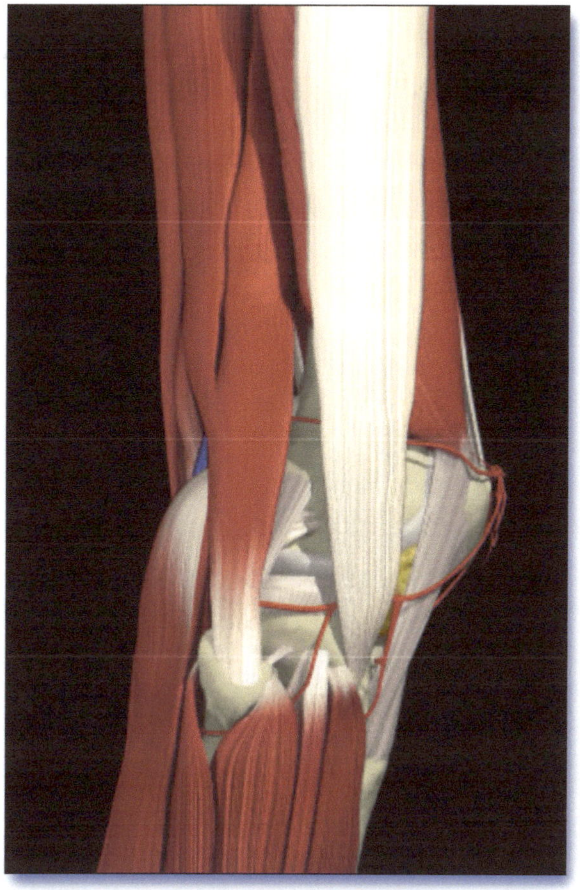

FIGURE 8-5. THE LATERAL VIEW OF THE KNEE

These muscular structures can be affected by other joint dysfunction patterns in the mechanical chain.

will cause all these muscles to tighten. These are all neuromuscular guarding reflexes that are evoked by peripheral joint subluxation patterns.

The knee is not a separate and distinct structure, it is an integrated part of the lower extremity. Any component of the lower extremity in dysfunction will affect some aspect of the whole chain. This opinion is not shared by the knee orthopedists I have encountered over the years. The thinking in that community is that the knee is a separate structure and has nothing to do with the hip or the ankle. Gait analysis before knee surgery is not the protocol of care. I feel this puts patients at risk. I had a patient who had two arthroscopic knee surgeries with no relief of her knee pain. I did a gait analysis on her and saw her ankle was collapsing on one side. I adjusted her ankle and put a small brace on it and her gait analysis changed and her knee pain was gone. She wanted me to help her sue her knee orthopedist. I told her that he had not deviated from the practices of his community, and therefore no malpractice had taken place (from a legal point of view that is). Logical thought processes in the application of medicine do not always take place. But if the procedures in question are standard in the medical community, no laws have been violated – except maybe the laws of common sense and good judgment.

EVALUATING THE KNEE

> ***Palpate the knee, in extension, looking for femoral condyles. Palpation of the condyles indicates tibial displacement.***

> ***Palpate for the tibial plateau, with knee in extension. Finding the plateau indicates tibial displacement.***

> ***Orthopedic testing, takes seconds to perform, and is usually negative. (Adjust even if tests are positive.)***

> *"Structural Testing": press the tibia in the direction of correction to see if the muscles soften and reduce the tenderness.*

> *Assess any patterns of knee subluxation: anterior tibia, posterior tibia, external rotation, internal rotation, lateral tibia and medial tibia. Most common in MVAs and falls: posterior, externally rotated and lateral tibia.*

Evaluating the knee is complicated by the acuteness of the injury. Very acutely injured or swollen knees can be difficult to palpate. My approach is pretty straightforward: where are the condyles and where is the tibial plateau? With the knee extended, the tibia should be lined up with the femur. I should not be able to feel the underside or inferior aspect of the condyles. I should not be able to feel the top of the tibia when the knee is extended. Sometimes, fully extending the patient's knee is not possible because the gastrocnemius will be so tight. It's tight for a reason and the doctor must find out why – it is not misbehaving. This muscular rigidity is from a distressed joint structure's nerve endings feeding its distress back to the spinal cord, and the spinal cord's response is to make everything tight to keep the joint as stable as possible – a neuromuscular guarding reflex.

Orthopedic testing can be done in just a few seconds: anterior draw, posterior draw, knee drop, lateral and medial stress tests. But there will be some knees that can't do the testing. So, in these cases, you do the best you can, finding where the parts are. Again, where are the condyles and where is the tibial plateau?

Structural testing is a technique which involves pushing a bone back towards its alignment and evaluating the muscular response. I will start to push the tibia back towards my notion of alignment for that knee and note the response. I'm looking for relief: "Does this feel better?" Rigid muscles going soft is the positive testing result we are looking for. Muscle guarding should be involuntary. The patient cannot relax these types of guarding patterns. Deep breathing and massage do not get these muscles to soften, and will not overcome the guarding reflex the injured joint has provoked from the spinal cord. The only things that will make the muscles relax are: adjusting the joint, general anesthesia and death. We always prefer the first option!

These patterns of knee subluxation are directly related to the mechanism of injury. Sometimes you know what happened because the patient's reporting is precise and sometimes you're dealing with someone who says, "I didn't do anything." I really like a clear description of the injury. It helps me visualize what happened, and what I need to do is usually the opposite of what occurred.

An anterior tibia is a hyperextension injury of the knee. *(See Figure 8-6.)* The gastrocnemius will tighten with an anterior tibia and it can be characterized by a slightly flexed knee. Five to fifteen degrees of flexion without the ability to fully extend the knee will be common. Going downstairs or downhill can be very painful.

The posterior tibia is common with falls and foot on the brake at impact in a motor vehicle accident. *(See Figure 8-7.)*

Rotational injuries to the knee will occur with falls and poor positioning of the legs while seated. *(See Figure 8-8.)* On palpation, just the medial plateau on the medial side of the patella will be prominent. If both the lateral and medial plateau can be felt on either side of the patella, the tibia has translated anteriorly. But if only the medial plateau is palpable, then that's an external rotation of the tibia. If the lateral tibial plateau is prominent on the lateral side of the patella, there is an internal rotation of the tibia. *(See Figure 8-9.)* In any of these cases, you find the tibial tuberosity is not lined up with the femur.

With the translation of the tibia laterally, the inferior medial femoral condyle will feel like a lump and be very tender to the touch, especially on the inferior aspect. (*See Figure 8-10.*) Drawing the tibia laterally should give relief when tested.

Medial translation of the tibia is not that common, but the tibial plateau will be prominent on the medial side of the knee. *(See Figure 8-11.)*

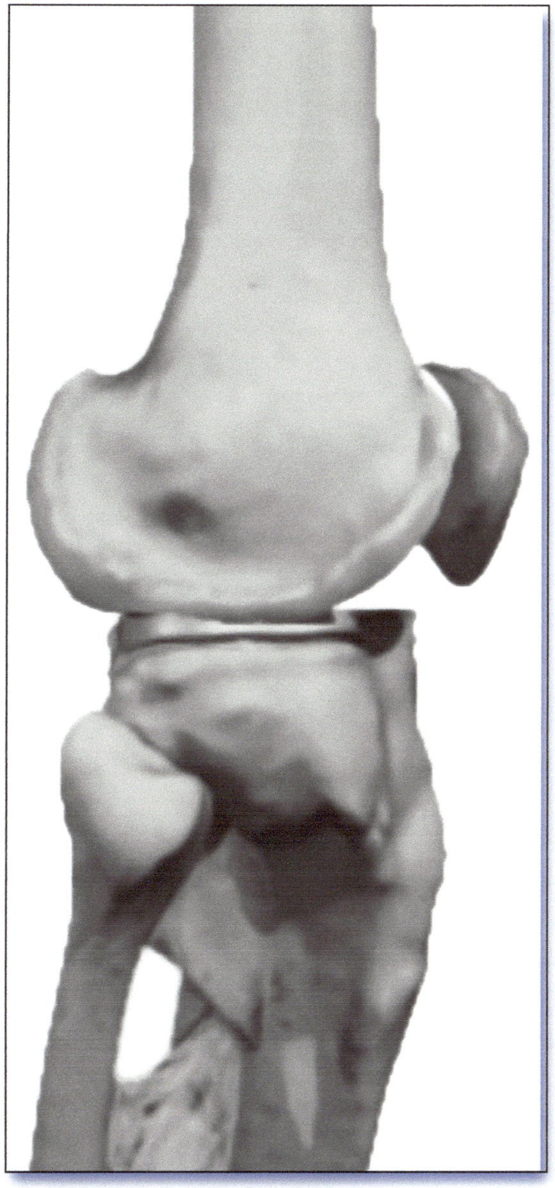

FIGURE 8-6. THE ANTERIOR TIBIA

The anterior tibia is characterized by the edges of the tibial plateau that are prominent relative to the femur.

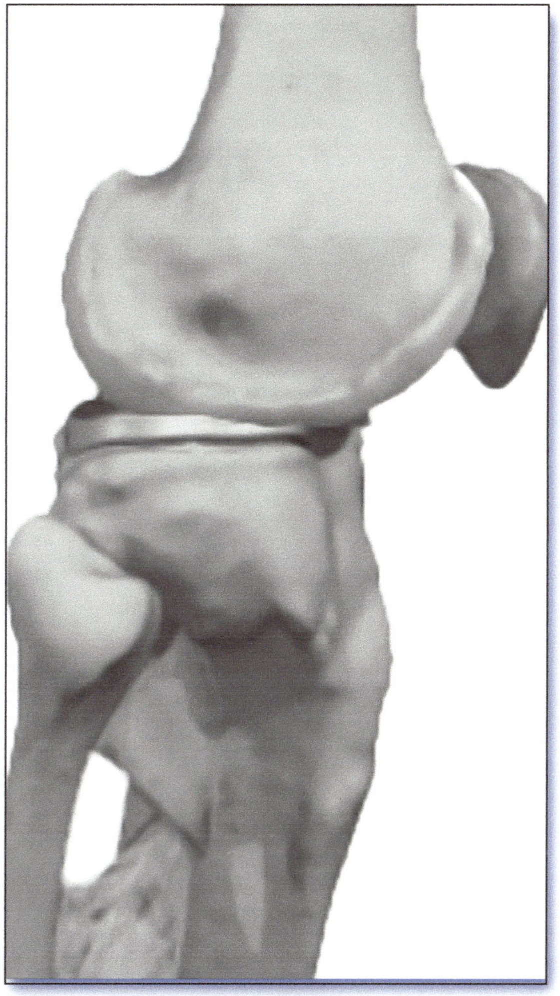

FIGURE 8-7. THE POSTERIOR TIBIA

The Posterior Tibia has as its main features the palpable inferior Femoral Condyles. The capsule and the ligaments can all be very sore and tender to the touch. Gently draw the tibia forward and see if there is any relief. A posterior draw test would aggravate this injury.

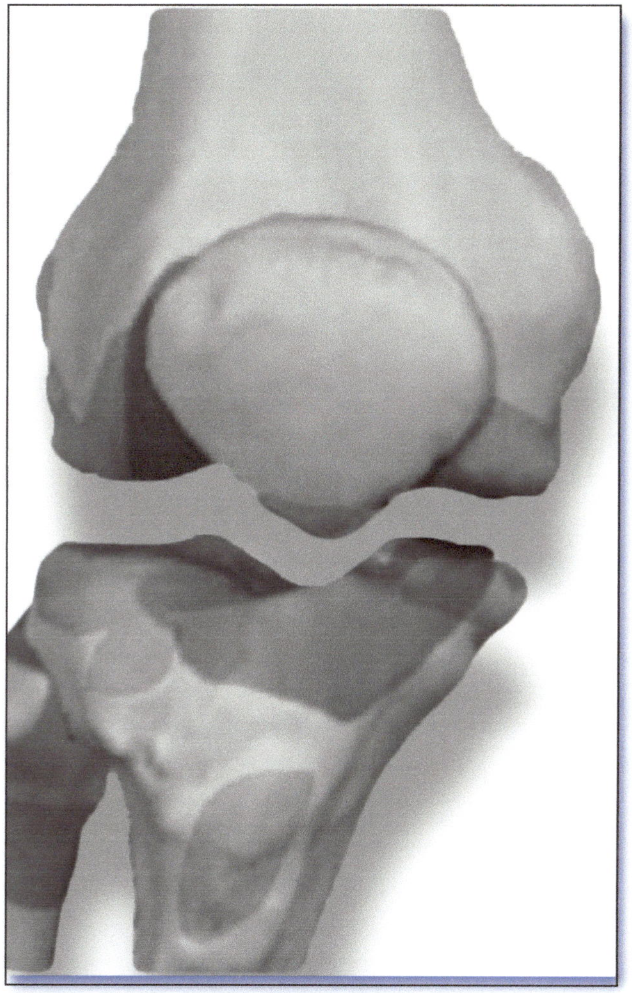

FIGURE 8-8. THE EXTERNAL ROTATION OF THE TIBIA

External rotation of the Tibia characterized by the Medial Tibial Plateau being anterior to the Femur's Medial Condyle.

ADJUSTING THE KNEE WITH A DROP PIECE

1. The tools:

> *A portable drop piece*
>
> *A firm cervical roll*

2. The knee is placed over the roll which is on top of the drop piece

3. All adjusting is done gently with a firm grip and simultaneous distraction, if possible.

Adjusting the knee with a drop piece or a small portable device is a really useful approach to reducing the subluxations of the knee. Use a cervical roll of four inches in diameter, placed underneath the knee. The position of the roll will become more specific with each subluxation pattern that we will discuss.

I have had many patients appear to be terrified of chiropractic care, and using the small drop piece on their extremity problems has been acceptable to them. They are grateful for a non-manipulative approach. I show them how the drop piece works and say, "Your knee does not make this noise." That gets them to relax a bit. Sometimes, I'll do a few mock drops just to get them a little more relaxed. It helps, with the apprehensive patients, to bring up some distraction. You might have some questions from the examination or their intake chart that can get them talking and take their attention away from your adjusting. I've had many patients say, "But it doesn't feel like you're doing anything!" And I say, "You're welcome."

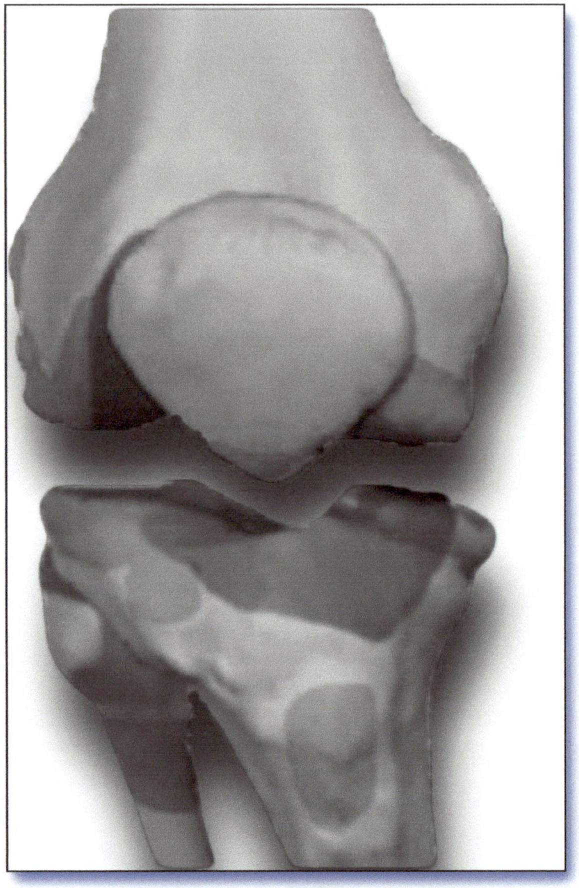

FIGURE 8-9. THE INTERNAL ROTATION OF THE TIBIA

The internal rotation of the Tibia will be characterized by the lateral portion of the Tibial Plateau being prominently anterior to the Femoral Condyle. Again, only the lateral Tibial Plateau is prominent, not both sides.

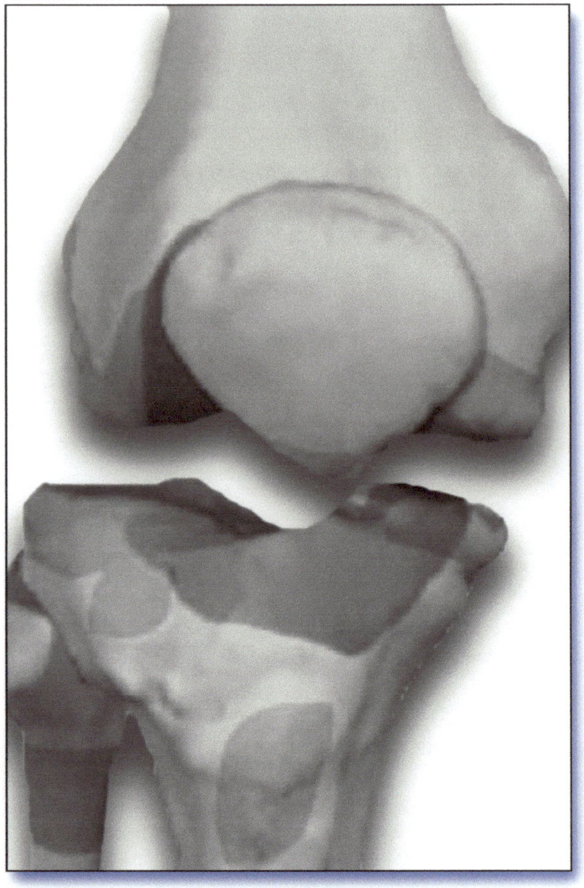

FIGURE 8-10. THE LATERAL TIBIA

The features of the Lateral Tibia is the medial; inferior Femoral Condyle will be palpable. It also should be very tender to the touch.

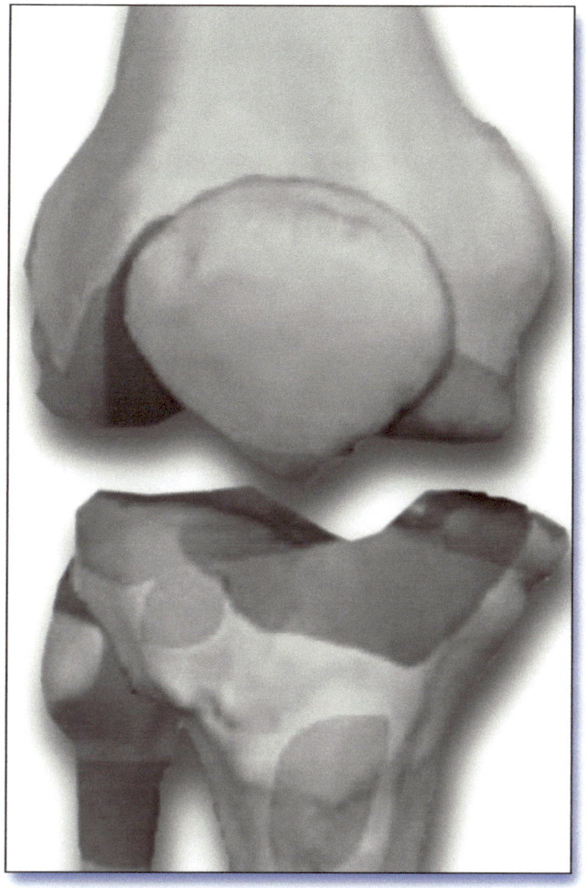

FIGURE 8-11. MEDIAL TIBIA

The main characteristic of a medial Tibia is the medial Tibial Plateau is palpable on the medial side of the knee.

Finding an innocuous way to intervene in someone's health problem should be one of our therapeutic goals, as chiropractors.

ADJUSTING THE POSTERIOR TIBIA

The posterior tibia has as its main features the palpable inferior femoral condyles. The capsule and the ligaments can all be very sore and tender to the touch. Gently draw the tibia forward and see if there is any relief. A posterior draw test should aggravate this injury.

Like many of the maneuvers we have previously discussed, this follows the same pattern: be very careful and perform multiple, gentle drops. If possible, use a slight distraction. Firmly grip the tibia, simultaneously pull inferiorly as you perform the drop. This distraction should be done only in patients that do not have joint replacement surgery of the hip or the knee. It is not uncommon for me to have to drop 25-30 times in the first session. The firm roll is placed under the tibia, inferior to the knee joint. *(See Figure 8-12).* The drop is on the femur (not the patella). Proceed until a correction is accomplished.

ADJUSTING THE ANTERIOR TIBIA

The anterior tibia is characterized by the edges of the tibial plateau prominent relative to the femur. The gastrocnemius doesn't like this, and so a chronic anterior tibia can be characterized by a slightly flexed knee. The correction for this is to put the cushion underneath the femur and drop on the tibia. *See Figure 8-13.*

ADJUSTING THE ROTATED TIBIA

External rotation of the tibia will be characterized by the medial tibial plateau being anterior to the femur. Just the medial plateau will be prominent on the medial side of the patella. If both the lateral and medial plateau can be felt on either side of the patella, the tibia has translated anteriorly. But if only the medial tibial plateau is palpable, then that's an external rotation of the tibia. An additional sign of this is if the tibial tuberosity is not lined up with the femur. To correct, place the firm roll under the knee and internally rotate the tibia if it is externally rotated and drop. *(See Figure 8-14).* Rarely does the tibia rotate medially, but the setup for correction would be the same, except rotate the tibia externally and drop.

ADJUSTING THE LATERAL TIBIA

The features of the lateral tibia is the medial, inferior femoral condyle will be palpable. It also should be very tender to the touch.

The set up is to have one hand on the medial femur and the other hand on the lateral part of the tibia. A thrust with the hand on the Tibia lateral to medial. The upper hand, on the femur can stabilize or performing a thrust medial to lateral. This depends on the health and level of injury. Both hands moving is for a less inflamed knee. *See Figure 8-15.* The lateral subluxation of the tibia can be the most painful displacement pattern.

FIGURE 8-12. SET UP FOR A POSTERIOR TIBIA.

Note the roll is under the Tibia, and the drop is on the Femur.

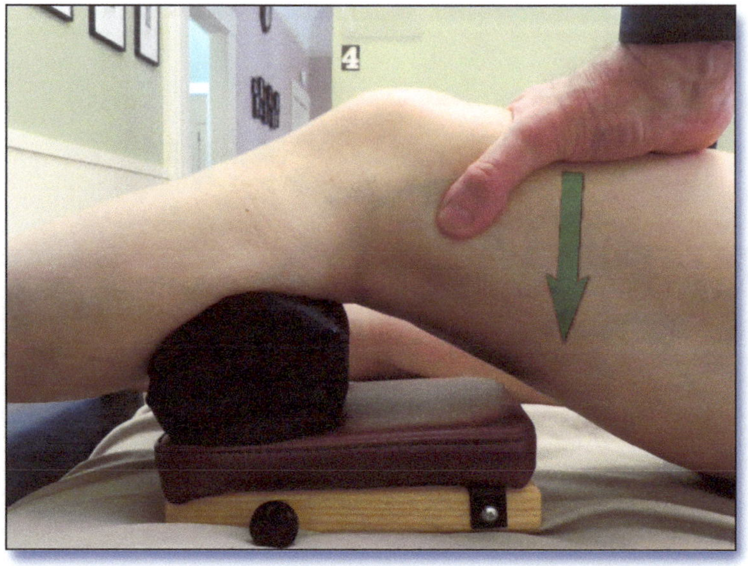

ADJUSTING THE KNEE REPLACEMENT

Knee replacements are done primarily to remove damaged cartilage and remodeled cortical bone and put new surfaces on the tibia and sometimes the femur (see Figures 8-16a and 8-16b). If it's just one, usually the tibia, it's called partial replacement. If it's both the femur and the tibia, it's a full replacement. These replaced services don't change the dynamics of the subluxation complex of the knee. Even with new surfaces, the tibia can still be misaligned to the femur, giving the same neuromuscular guarding reflex. The damaged bone and the degenerated meniscus do not give off pain signals. The muscular efforts to hold an unstable and misaligned knee together with weight-bearing activities will still be painful and limit motion.

FIGURE 8-13. SET UP FOR AN ANTERIOR TIBIA.

Note the firm roll is under the Femur, superior to the Knee joint. The drop is on the Tibia.

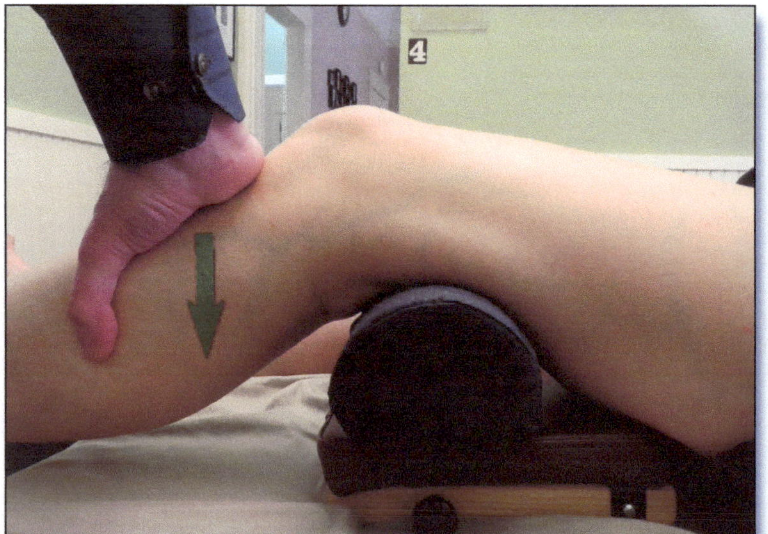

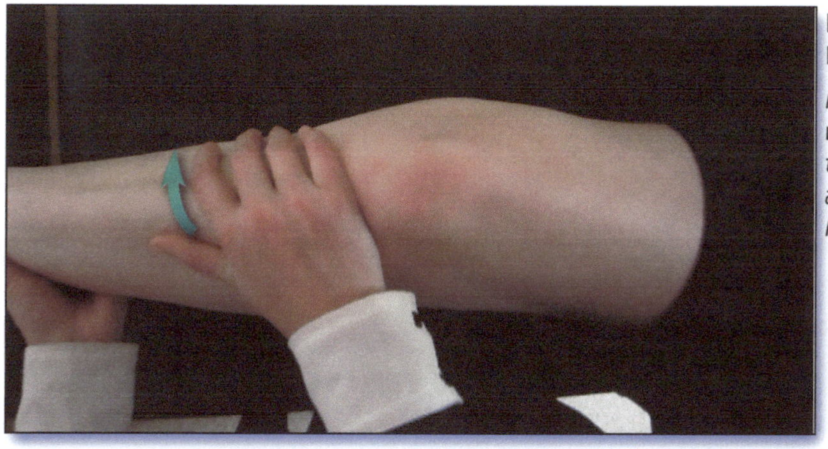

FIGURE 8-14. SET UP FOR ADJUSTING A ROTATED TIBIA.

Note the inferior hand of the Doctor, as well as the superior hand, is contacting the lower portion of the leg to affect a rotation of the Tibia relative to the Femur.

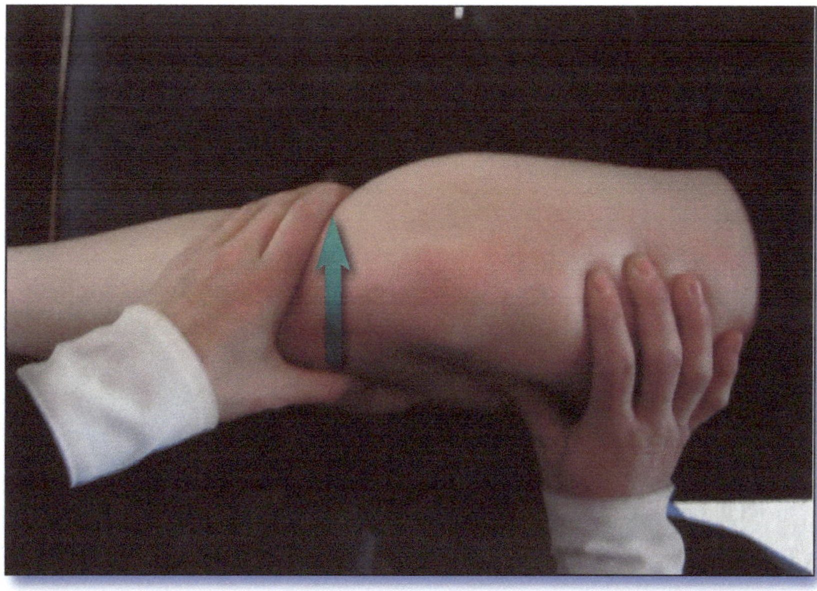

FIGURE 8-15. ADJUSTING THE LATERAL TIBIA.

The superior hand is stabilizing the Femur and the inferior hand is thrusting lateral to medial.

Realigning the bones with replaced surfaces is essentially the same protocols as the 'normal' knee. The gentleness of the procedure is essential. The repetitiveness of it is the source of the force. The deformation of the joint capsule weakens its ability to keep the alignment with twisting, bending and pivoting of normal activity. Realigning joints is the only hope that the joint capsules have in regaining full integrity and strength.

MANAGING THE INJURED KNEE

> *Review personal habits; knee crossing, leg sitting*

> *Review employment issues*

> *Review activities: gardening, yoga*

Managing a knee injury can be more difficult than adjusting the knee. Reviewing personal habits with the patient is very important. Most personal habits will have developed before a specific injury. In the case of the knee, this is really important because we as Americans and in Western society sit for prolonged periods of time and deform our legs. This is normal behavior in our population. People sit on their legs, crossed their knees, twist them around chair legs and generally don't think about them if they are not standing on them. All these habits I characterize as 'non-weight bearing postures'. Non-weight bearing postures that deform an injured knee can be painless at the time. But when the patient becomes weight-bearing, then the pain can suddenly strike them from "out of nowhere". There is a remoteness in time from the exacerbation while seated and the pain or feeling the knee is coming-out from underneath them later when they are weight bearing.

Therefore, it is necessary to review all personal habits involving leg crossing, leg sitting and leg tucking. Frequently patients will deny they do this, but their persistent subluxation patterns will give them away. Sometimes weeks after denying that they cross their legs they come in and say "Oh my gosh, I'm doing it all the time, it's driving me crazy."

People that are employed using a computer have well-established habits with their legs underneath the desk. Their legs are out of view and they are focused on the computer screen and their tasks. So it is necessary to review all employment issues. How often are they at the computer, what other tasks do they have as part of their job description? People in the trades have usually challenging issues. This is where work limitation orders and letters to the employer have been helpful. Can some tasks be brought up off the floor and put on a bench or table to keep from being on the knees? There are many issues the doctor can be helpful with looking at well-established job description from a fresh point of view. I'm the advocate for the injured knee, not the completion of their job description.

All other activities have to be reviewed including gardening, yoga and other exercise, and resting postures. This is where crossing the legs as patients watch TV or read are critical factors because of the time frames. Reading or watching TV for three or four hours is completely normal at night or on the weekends.

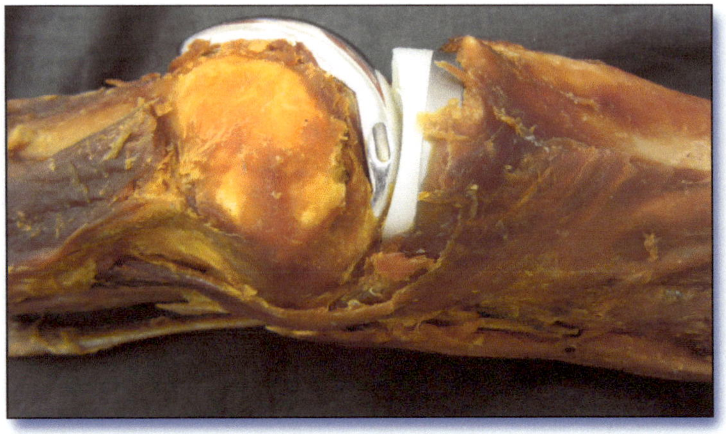

FIGURE 8-16 A. A TOTAL KNEE REPLACEMENT

Note that the surfaces have been replaced with steel and plastic. The knee cap is removed in some procedures. There is a wide range of prosthetic devices. Despite the new surfaces, the soft tissues surrounding them are all still embedded with sensitive neurological structures keyed to altered biomechanics. These altered biomechanics result in splinting and rigidity of the tissues, which cause complaints of pain, stiffness and lack of mobility.

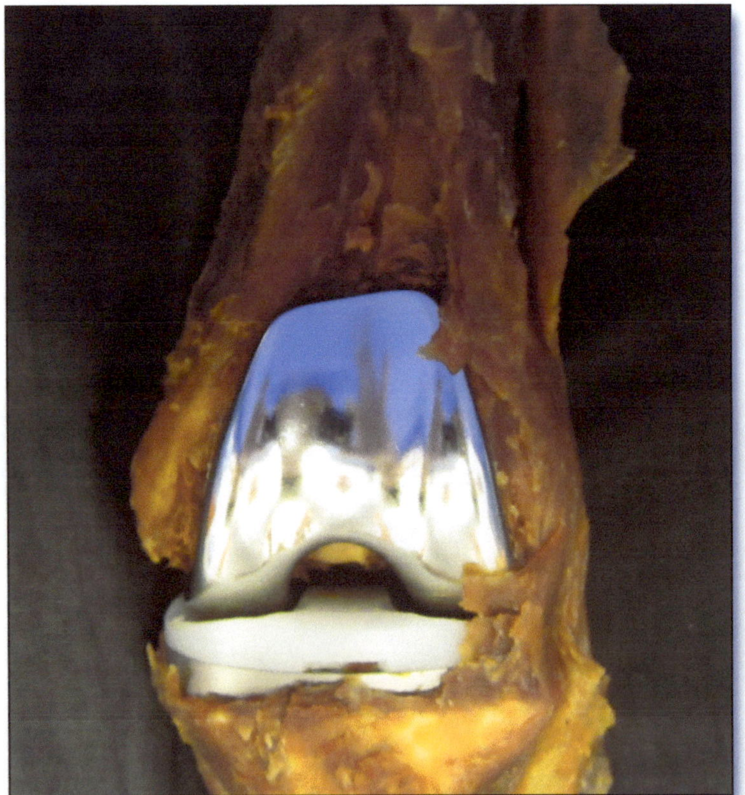

FIGURE 8- 16B. ANTERIOR VIEW OF A TOTAL KNEE REPLACEMENT

You would hope that after the pain and trouble of knee replacement surgery, you would have everything lined up. But some people have such rigid tissues from the chronic nature of the condition that a few weeks or months of rehab cannot reverse all the structural remodeling. You also must review their personal habits.

Three or four hours of deforming an injured knee can be disastrous for the inflamed injured tissues of the knee. Extending one leg from the sofa to an ottoman with a hyperextension injury to the knee will irritate and will cause continued instability of the ligaments. Then, put the other ankle on top of that extended knee pushing it into hyperextension. You start to get the picture. Non-weight bearing postures can push a minor injury into a debilitating condition.

Any yoga postures or exercises that put the patient on their knees must be evaluated. Also, the knee crossing in meditation or other similar type activities has to be evaluated. Sometimes I will have the patient assume a certain position of the knee and palpate it in that position. If it is really tender to the touch, (more than when in a neutral position) this shows the patient the inadvisability of that posture. Kneeling while gardening or doing yard work needs to be reviewed. Can any of those tasks be done on their feet? How about a low seat (they make these) for the garden?

Years ago, I had a 66-year-old obese female patient present with terribly swollen knees. I couldn't even assess them via palpation, as they were so swollen and painful to the touch with +3 flinch responses. We did a full 360° ice wrap on both knees for 20 minutes. I needed the tissue to be as numb as possible for evaluation. On evaluation, I found both tibias to be posterior. I asked her if she had a history of falls. She said no. I asked her if she had a history of motor vehicle accident with her knees impacting the dashboards. She said no. I asked her if she did any kneeling, and she said she was a Catholic nun. And I said, "Well, I'm not a theologian but I don't think kneeling is required, Sister." So she started praying in the seated position. With our care and her cessation of irritating activities, she had normal appearing knees and no pain within two weeks.

NOTES:

• • •

Online lessons at:
https://youtu.be/rXvqfcNluf4

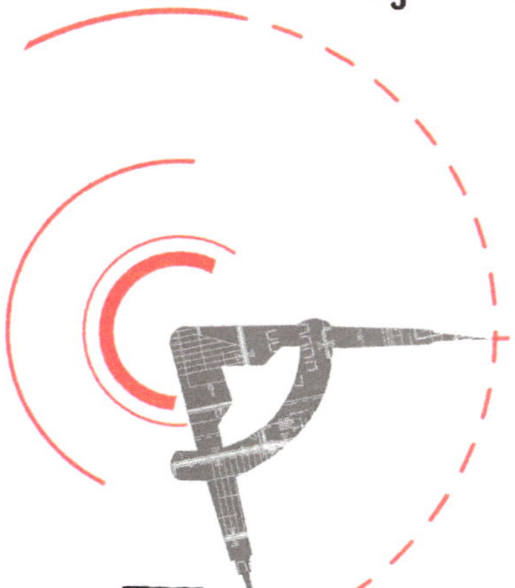

CHAPTER NINE

Evaluating, Adjusting and Managing the Lower Leg

This chapter is about evaluating, adjusting and managing the injured lower leg. I find this topic to be extremely important for many reasons. Most significantly is the fact that most leg pain is generated by an injury to the leg itself. JMPT published a study a few years ago stating that 80 percent of the people with radiating leg pain had confusing and confounding symptoms. The symptoms did not match any dermatomal or nerve root patterns. Evaluating the legs of these individuals was limited to pulses, reflexes and the pinwheel test. This is not a thorough evaluation of the leg. So it seems likely to me that the 80 percent with the confusing and confounding symptoms in that study actually had injured legs. The minimal evaluation process did not bring to light the joint dysfunction and guarding patterns characteristic of an injured leg.

Leg, foot and ankle dysfunctions are a leading cause of disability, the need for assisted living, a gradually declining loss of independence and a reduced quality of life. Few providers actually restore normal architectural features of the injured leg, foot or ankle. Even if manipulative care is used often, these procedures do not leave the joints realigned. Subluxation and ligament injury is the basis for the injuries that the lower extremity experiences. Not only do these joints get subluxated, the ligaments that hold these joints together are injured and chronic instability patterns develop. Once the injuries have occurred, the neuromuscular guarding reflex comes into play and makes muscles and tendons tight – and leads to contractures and the permanent loss of motion, and entraps neurological and vascular structures causing deficits in nerve function and vascular perfusion.

Leg and foot injuries change someone's interaction with their environment, alter their occupational opportunities, and lead to sedentary behavior and deconditioning. I cannot even list all of the adverse effects of the loss of a graceful, easy gait, but I will mention again a study from a few years ago that showed in a long-term study that a slow awkward gait is a 100 percent predictor of measurable cognitive decline within ten years. That should be a big wake-up call to get our patients to be more aggressive in getting gait abnormalities addressed. Also, chiropractors should be getting lots of referrals from the mental health care community, but this is not the case. Since 85 percent of the U.S. population has arthritis now, our future will have debilitating or reduced functional capacities issues, as well as a diminished quality of life.

As a new chiropractor more than a quarter-century ago, I had constant leg pain. Everyone at the college I went to assumed it was my L5-S1 disc that was the source of my leg pain. I had the signs of loss of disc height on an x-ray and was tender at the L5-S1 joint. So I embarked on a course of daily decompression therapy with a backswing or inversion table, and my leg pain got worse. Now I should add some details about my medical history: I was a long-distance runner in high school and college and had continued to run for another 15 years. My running had become difficult and painful from the leg pain and cramping of my hamstrings and calf muscles. I went on a final run with my classmates at the chiropractic college, but my legs finally seized up on me and cramped in such a severe manner that I was on my tip toes with knees bent, staggering and finally falling over. Teachers and students alike thought this was a blown disk. No one ever examined my legs. Decompression therapy added to the instability of the injured ligaments of my lower legs, ankles and feet. I was mystified, as were my colleagues, by my lack of response to the decompression therapy. My leg pain got worse and my running days were over.

I started my practice with constant leg pain and when it was slow in the office, I would get on the back swing and do more decompression therapy. The stretching of my legs and low back on the backswing felt good while I was on the swing. The relief was very transitory. I was fortunate enough to be a dissection instructor at the college I attended. My time in the lab investigating pain patterns led me to the conclusion that my legs were injured. I also started to evaluate and assess the legs, feet, and ankles of my patients and found that almost everyone had signs of joint dysfunction and pain patterns that were actually emanating from the injured leg and ankle structures themselves. The spine might be involved, but it wasn't to be the major source of relief. So, the treatment and care of my injured legs has allowed me to remain in practice all these years. I have to do daily things to manage my chronic leg, foot and ankle injuries, but this protocol resulted in my being fully active and still seeing around 100 patients a week. I have a walking regimen, and I believe my managing my injuries will keep me functional for years to come.

RELEVANT ANATOMY FOR THIS CHAPTER

- *The proximal and distal tibiofibular joints*
- *The musculature of the region: tensor fascia latae (TFL), iliotibial band (ITB), all the muscles of the leg (most go to the foot)*
- *The subluxation of the fibula can cause: "hip" pain (ITB Syndrome), "shin splint" pain, "Charlie Horse" cramping, Restless Leg Syndrome, heel pain, big toe pain, arch pain and pain on the top of the foot.*

I have treated 16 people over the years that have had back surgery performed for relief of leg pain. They came to me with the continued leg pain post-surgery. They all had injured legs and reported to me that no one had ever examined their legs! I've also had hundreds of cases of chiropractic patients with a history of leg pain whose previous chiropractors ignored their injured legs and focused on their spines.

I don't think there's any surgical or chiropractic procedure that could be performed on the spine that would realign the fibula or the calcaneus. I have a construction background and I must say, fuzzy thinking doesn't get the job done in that field either. The lights don't come on just because you're a nice guy. All your connections have to be right. There is no forgiveness for poor performance on the job site; you're gone. So I say this to my students, and many of them don't listen to me because they refer patients to me and they haven't done this: *if someone comes into your office complaining of leg pain please, please examine the leg.*

It seems so basic, but in our age of advanced imaging and the mistaken notion that the disc is the source of all pain, we have forgotten basic protocols. Rule number one in examination procedures is *examine the patient's complaint*. Don't read the radiographic report and make assumptions. I recently saw a TV commercial for USC Medical Center where they claim they have a new minimally invasive micro-discectomy to relieve leg pain. So the ad says, if you have leg pain, give us a call and schedule one of our minimally invasive procedures today. It doesn't mention examining a leg, so I believe this approach puts patients at risk. The studies I've read how a patient has a greater chance of being worse after back surgery for relief of radiating symptoms than being helped. (There is a 65 percent failure rate on these procedures!) The literature discusses what a failure is: the patient is worse after the surgery than before. So this is what I found with those 16 patients: they still have their injured legs after the surgery and now they have a wound on their spine. They classify themselves as being worse than before the surgery.

I feel the quality of medicine has declined by the emphasis on the radiographic findings and neglecting completely to physically examine the patient. This is a source of billions of dollars a year in lost productivity and unnecessary medical procedures and hospitalizations. This chapter covers how to evaluate, adjust and manage an injured lower leg. If successful, you will be able to restore someone's mobility, dramatically improve their quality of life and possibly save them unnecessary surgical procedures.

The following explanation of relationships between the joints and distant symptoms and complaints cannot be verified in any of the textbooks or scientific literature that I've encountered. These observations are mine and in part based on the principles established by the assumption that the human body is an exquisitely designed piece of equipment. Therefore, the body's components don't randomly misbehave. In my clinical experience, muscle tightness, rigidity and pain when palpating the structures of the lower leg indicate injuries to the lower leg.

I was blessed for a number of years to be a dissection instructor at the local chiropractic college while I was in a full-time practice. Questions that developed in my mind about a patient's condition would lead me to investigate these complaints in the anatomy lab. Among the observations that I made is that joint dysfunction causes neuromuscular guarding reflex patterns initiated by the spinal cord when this joint dysfunction is perceived. Commonly, the pain pattern develops at the opposite end of the muscle's distressed joint structure. I call it "remote but related pain" – origins and insertions. The muscle that is distressed has Sharpey's Fibers that insert into the cortex of the bone at its insertion. The constant guarding pattern will cause these Sharpey's Fibers to become inflamed which will be the conscious source of pain for a lot of patients.

On evaluation, the doctor may find the entire muscle group is distressed, possibly with trigger points and other problems like contractures, congestion and signs of poor circulation, as it is difficult for a muscle that is clenched all the time to have proper circulation. So in my view, tight muscles don't necessarily need to be stretched. They need to be relieved of the neurological messages to tighten. I need to find the joint or joints that are distressed and relieve the guarding pattern. So according to this view, there are a lot of therapeutic interventions that are trying to fight the central nervous system's protective mechanisms. Tight muscles that are painful to the touch give me information about the condition of the joints they are associated with. They don't mislead me. My perspective is a different type of approach to evaluating and managing injuries.

The proximal and distal joints of the fibula are different. The proximal tibiofibular joint is a tough synovial joint. Sometimes people hear and feel a "pop" when this joint subluxates and they think it is the knee they have injured. The distal joint is "syndesmosis" or a fibrous joint. And there is the interosseous ligament that runs between the two holding it all together. I feel the failure or injury to these three structures is responsible for most leg pain. Instability in these three structures is not in the International Code of Diagnosis book. Injuries to the proximal and distal joints are listed, but not the whole unit. I have found many people with this type of instability, including almost all the patients that had back surgery for relief of leg pain.

The top of the fibula has the iliotibial band and the long head of the biceps femoris attached to it. I will not name all the muscles of the lower leg, but most of them attach to the foot in some manner. They also have some relationship, directly and indirectly to the alignment and proximity of the tibia and fibula. A separation of the two bones would involve a neuromuscular guarding reflex from almost all of the muscular structures of the lower leg. Some of these guarding patterns would be felt in the foot, the thigh or the hip, as well as the leg.

According to this perspective, certain pain patterns and syndromes are actually unrecognized injuries to the lower leg. The Ilio-Tibial Band Syndrome is almost invariably a separated proximal tibiofibular joint. "Shin Splints" is a separation of the fibula from the tibia, usually from running and jumping activities. A "Charlie Horse" or calf cramping is usually a combination of dehydration (with possible magnesium depletion) and distress to the lower leg via this separation of the two bones.

I have found Restless Leg Syndrome or Jumpy Leg Syndrome to be a product of the separation of the two bones. My explanation of this condition is that the muscles are being recruited by the central nervous system to hold the lower leg together once the separation has occurred. All through a day of weight-bearing activity, the muscles are required to hold the lower leg together and move the patient. The rigid nature of the muscular tissues does not allow for a normal capillary blood flow. Once the daily activities have ceased and the patient is in bed or off their feet, the muscles of the lower leg will start to fasciculate or twitch to facilitate capillary blood flow. The muscles of the lower leg are oxygen deprived, and the muscular activity is to restore as much circulation as possible. So the condition that keeps people awake at night is part of a defensive mechanism. Medicine's approach to this problem is to suppress the central nervous system with pharmacology. So the complaint of feeling dopey and tired after using these medications would be prevalent.

I found a number of cases of heel pain being primarily caused by the separating of the proximal tibiofibular joint. Soleus and gastrocnemius can both become distressed by the separation of the bones proximally, and the pain will be felt distally at the heel. Big toe pain, pain at the first metatarsal-phalangeal joint (MP Joint) and arch pain can all be because of a distressed hallucis tendon. Hallucis longus and brevis muscles are deep and become distressed when the fibula and tibia separate. The pain is usually not consciously felt in the belly of the muscles. The pain is felt at the terminus of the tendons in the foot. The same thing is true for the peroneus muscles: when proximal tibiofibular joint subluxation occurs, the pain is usually felt in the terminus of peroneus longus in the lateral part of the foot.

The proximal tibiofibular joint is very close to the knee and can "pop," becoming sore and inflamed when certain types of twisting or pivoting activities take place. *(See Figure 9-1.)* I've had many patients come in and put their hand right on that joint and call that knee pain. This injury occurs frequently in tennis players and skiers. This injury is tough to manage with such athletes because they want to get back on the court or the slopes quickly. The ligaments of this joint complex can take months to heal. I found many patients that have permanent injury to these ligaments require reduced activities and bracing to manage the instability and pain. Of course, some of the patients will injure both the knee and the tibiofibular joints. Both need to be adjusted to regain a normal functioning of the leg.

Figures 9-2 and 9-3 show a view of the lower leg in which the displacement or subluxation of the fibula would distress all the muscles of the lower leg. The muscles of the lower leg are recruited in a neuromuscular guarding reflex pattern to hold this structure together. Most people I have examined have some degree of this injury. Palpate the peroneus longus muscle on yourself and your patients. Note how hard and tight this muscle is on most people. This is a sign of lower leg injury.

THE ILIOTIBIAL BAND

In my opinion, the Iliotibial Band (ITB) Syndrome is caused by subluxation of the proximal tibiofibular joint. *(See Figure 9-4.)* Pain at the top of the crest where the ITB inserts on the upper part of the iliac crest is caused by the subluxation of that joint at the other end of its origin. Pain at the trochanter can be caused by the iliotibial band being so taut that motion or laying on that side at night can become very painful.

The lateral view of the lower leg shows the relationship of the lower leg to the foot and ankle. The dysfunction of the proximal tibiofibular joint can cause peroneus and tibialis anterior distress in the foot and ankle region. I consider the foot and ankle in the lower leg to be a functional unit, although each of these require separate adjusting protocols and management protocols.

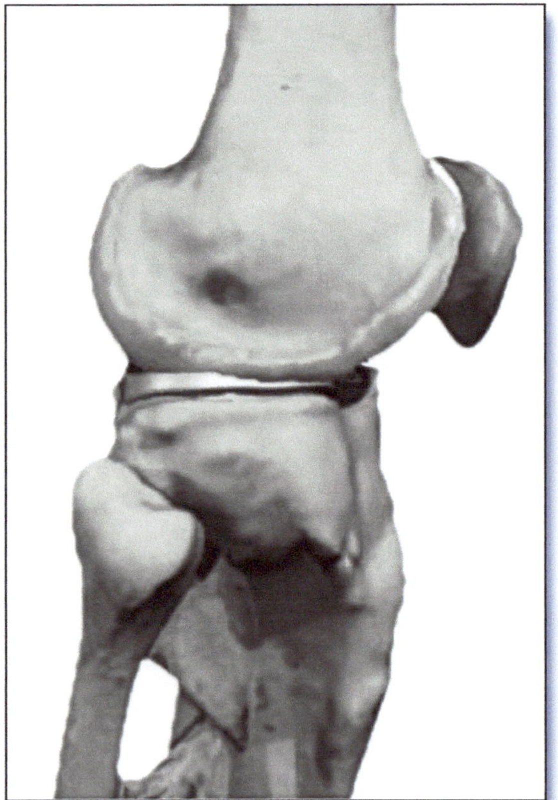

FIGURE 9-1. THE PROXIMAL FIBULA TIBIAL JOINT AND THE KNEE

Note the proximity of the Fibula Joint with the Tibia and the knee. Injury at the fibula joint can be felt to be knee pain by the patient. A careful examination is required to distinguish the two.

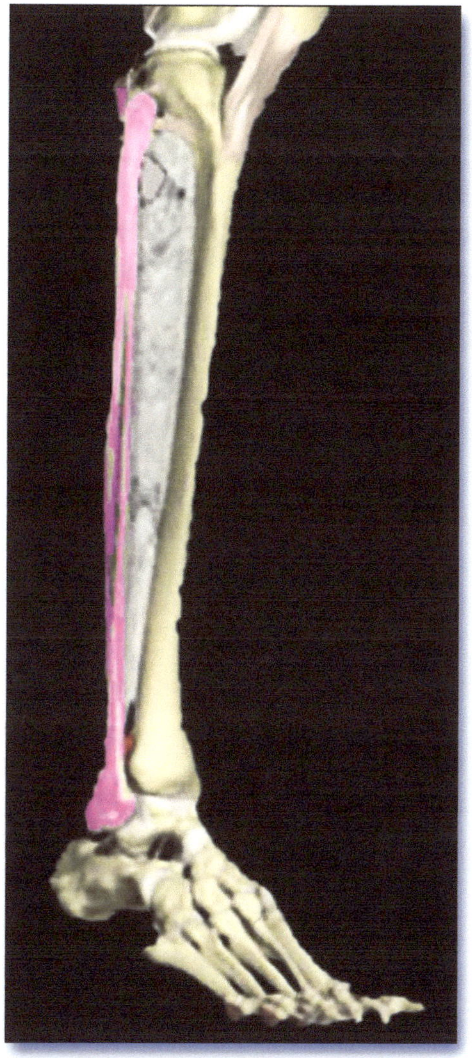

FIGURE 9-2. THE LOWER LEG WITH THE INTEROSSEOUS LIGAMENT

Note the Interosseous Ligament would have to be injured for this kind of subluxation to occur.

EVALUATING THE LOWER LEG INJURIES

- *The palpation of the proximal "tibiofibular" joint*
- *The palpation of the TFL (looking for "hip" pain)*
- *The tibiofibular SQUEEZE TEST: squeeze the proximal tibiofibular joint while provoking the tender TFL, and look for change*
- *The palpation of the distal tibiofibular joint, squeeze for signs of relief of tenderness*

In evaluating the lower leg injuries, it can be simple on one level, but the range of symptoms and complaints can be quite varied and complex. Palpating all of the muscles of the lower leg is a necessary part of assessing an injury of the lower leg. This should be done with the leg at rest. The doctor must actually touch the joint at the top, front and back. It's be common that when there is a separation, it can especially be felt in the posterior aspect of the joint. I explore around behind the fibular head with an index finger, and if there is a gap there, I consider it a sign of lower leg injury. Also, that's frequently a very painful place to palpate and it evokes +3 flinch response on some patients.

If there is a hip pain complaint, I want to palpate the iliotibial band or the tensor fascia latae (TFL). Rigidity and pain on palpation are the things I'm looking for. So with this condition, I would introduce what I call the "Tib-Fib Squeeze Test." *(See Figure 9-6.)* The test is performed while provoking the painful complaint by squeezing the proximal fibula and tibia together. The complaints could be iliac crest pain or pain in the lateral digits of the foot. I have the patient or myself poke or palpate the distressed area of the complaint. While maintaining this irritating touch, I then squeeze the fibula to the tibia and maintain it for 15 to 20 seconds. I'm still surprised sometimes at how the responses occur with this test. I recently had a patient come in with a complaint of left iliac crest pain and right third, fourth and fifth toe pain. On the

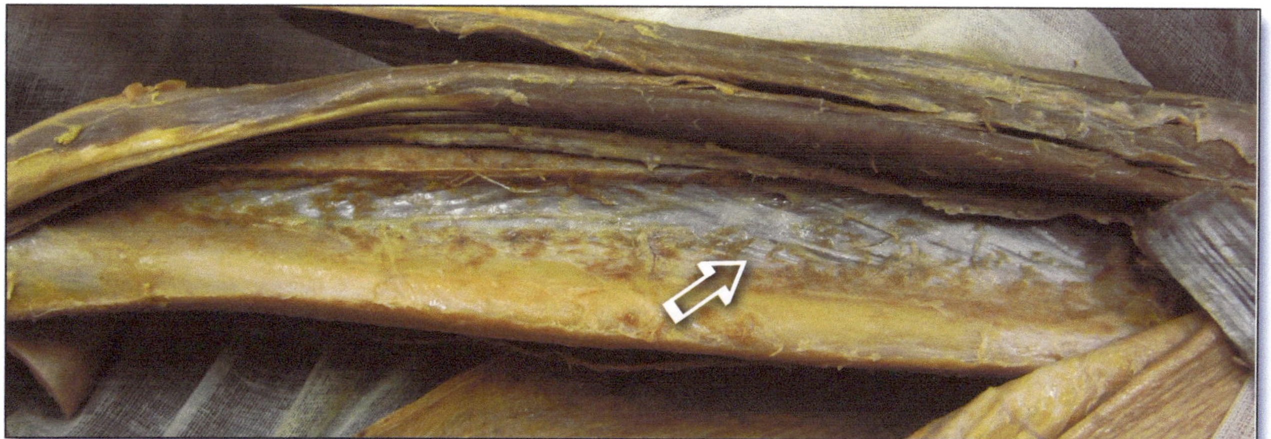

FIGURE 9-3. THE INTEROSSEOUS LIGAMENT OF THE LOWER LEG.

This is a tough fibrous tissue that has to be strong and flexible

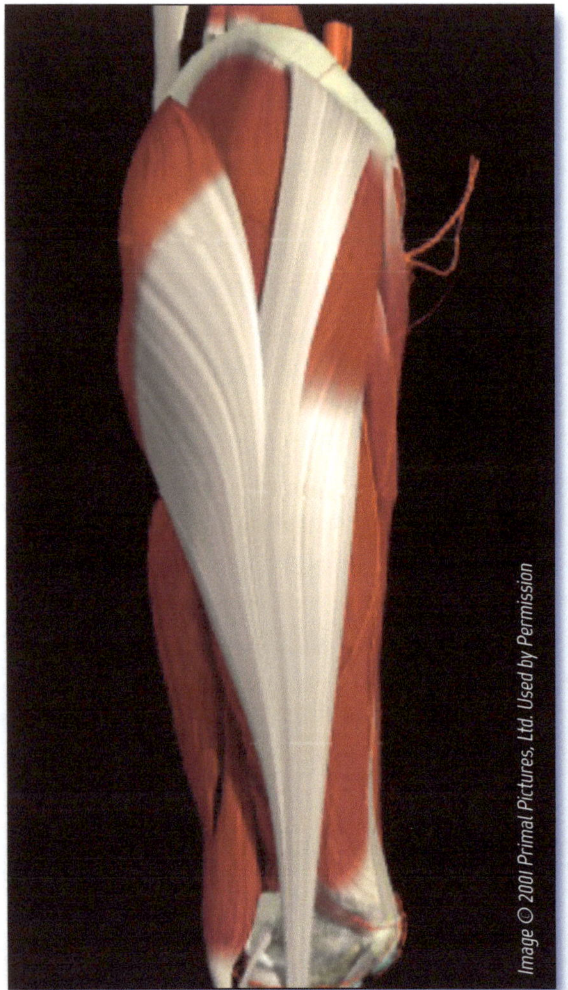

FIGURE 9-4. LATERAL VIEW OF THE THIGH.

Note the ITB is attached to the Fibular Head and inserts at the Iliac Crest.

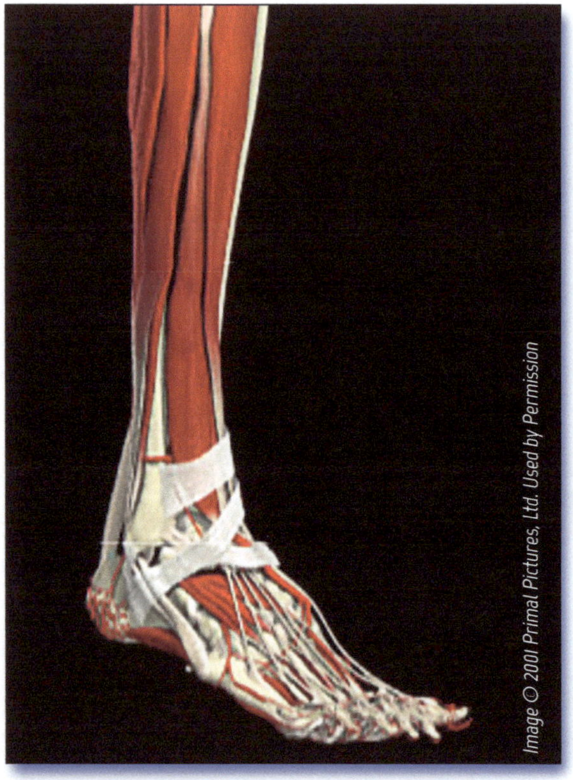

FIGURE 9-5. LATERAL VIEW OF THE LOWER LEG

Note the musculature of the lower leg goes to the foot.

left side, I palpated her in the area of the iliac crest and produced the pain that she was complaining about. I then squeezed her left fibula to the tibia and the pain slowly faded away as my pressure continued. I then went to the right foot and squeezed the toes, provoking the pain, and then I performed the tib-fib squeeze test and the pain slowly faded away.

This particular patient had the most proximal and distal complaints I find associated with the subluxation of the fibula from the tibia, as well as a history of marathon running and a current occupation as a dog agility trainer – two activities that can certainly produce a leg injury. A very common pain pattern is that the distressed joint will provoke a neuromuscular guarding reflex, and the pain pattern is felt where the guarding muscle inserts at the opposite end from the distressed joint. The iliotibial band originates on the top of the fibular head and inserts on the edge of the iliac crest. *(See Figure 9-3.)* So it makes sense to me that hip pain or pain in the trochanteric region can be produced by a subluxation of the proximal tibiofibular joint. The same thing applies to peroneus, thus the toe pain from a proximal tibiofibular joint subluxation.

My approach is to evaluate the complaints from the extremities first and in the spine later. I find many more lower extremity injuries than I do herniated discs. I do the same procedure with toe pain, heel pain, arch pain and pain on the top of the foot. If the tibialis anterior is extremely unhappy with a proximal tibiofibular subluxation, the pain will be felt across the top of the foot where the tibialis anterior's tendons splay out across the top of the foot going to the toes. In fact, I believe "hammertoe" is at least in part caused by the tibiofibular separation and the rigidity of the muscle passing down through its tendons, (which will curl or hammer the toes, a very tough condition to reverse).

It is also important to palpate the distal tibiofibular joint, which is part of the ankle complex. If there is pain at the inferior aspect of the fibula, I will draw the proximal fibula inferiorly to see if it relieves the pain at the ankle. This is a common injury from jumping or landing on the feet with a lot of force. The fibula will be knocked superiorly from the force of the contact with, usually, concrete or asphalt. With the tib-fib squeeze test, I can access all the muscles of the lower leg to see if there's a change in tone or reduction in pain as the compressive test is maintained.

A few years ago, I had a 38-year-old patient present with severe right hip pain. He was antalgic with a cane and severe limp. He said he couldn't put any weight on his right leg without severe hip pain. He said he'd had an injury to his right hip when he was eight and had a hip replacement. Then he had another when he was older, and it had failed, breaking his femur. He spent two years in a wheelchair recovering so they could do yet another hip replacement. He presented ten years later. He said he had been fine for a while, and then the pain in his hip had started to become worse and it gradually had gotten to the point where he could not put any weight on his leg. He had had six epidurals in the last month before he came into our office.

I started his assessment by taking hold of his right lower leg and foot. I wanted to start with the talocalcaneal (subtalar) joint and I found his heel bone was grossly out of place. There was a +3 flinch response and he arched his back in pain. Then I went up to his proximal tibiofibular joint, and he had the same severe response. I asked him to stick his thumb in the worst part of his hip pain and he did. I then pulled inferiorly and medially on his fibula head. I counted to ten and he said the pain was going away. I maintained my pressure to a count of 30, and he said the pain was completely gone.

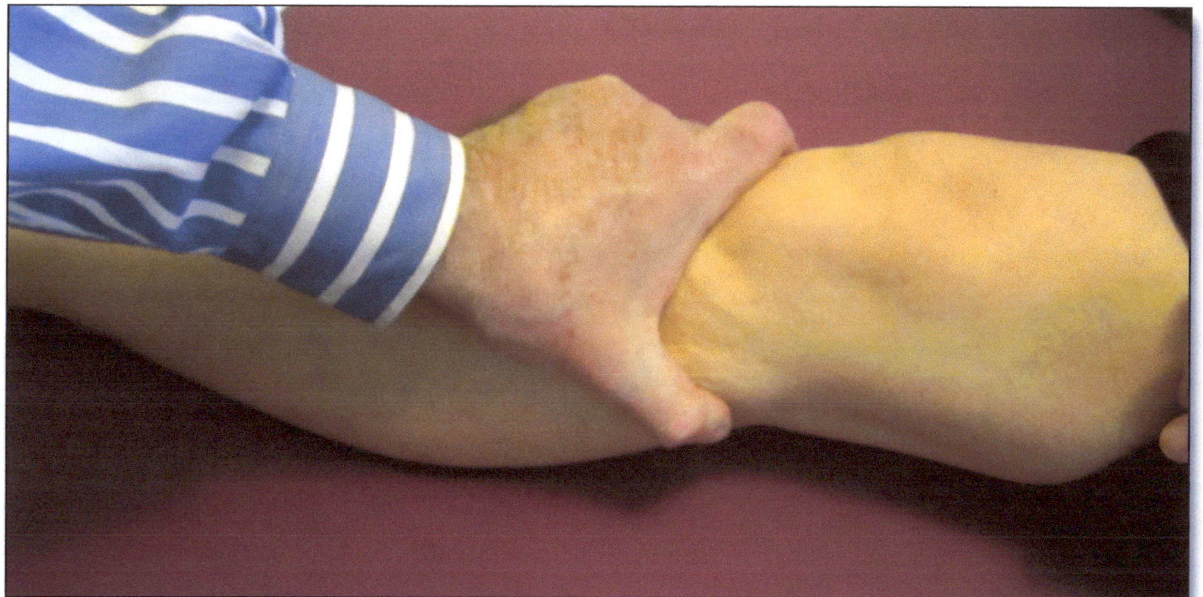

FIGURE 9-6. THE FIB-TIB SQUEEZE TEST.
Note the Doctor's hand is squeezing the Fibula to the Tibia

I also evaluated his spine and pelvis. He had a significant subluxation of the right innominate, including the pubic symphysis. We then proceeded to the treatment area and I put him on a tilted up drop table. [In Chapter 2 in this book, I discuss how to adjust someone's pelvis with a hip replacement, someone who is in severe pain and cannot be put in the prone position. I start with the pelvis because there is so much muscle mass attached to the pelvic girdle that once guarding responses are modified, it's easier to deal with the lower extremities.] Then I went to the lower leg and adjusted his fibula, and then his foot and ankle. I had also found he had a posterior talus.

After all the adjusting, I put a tibiofibular belt on his proximal tibiofibular joint and taped his ankle and foot. I then had him stand up. He did so, and put all his weight on his right leg. He rejoiced and started to walk around with his cane over his head. At one point, he said he was speechless and one of my staff members said, "He doesn't sound speechless to me!" I said to her, "Tell me, do we need drugs in this clinic?" She said "No!," and gave me a high-five.

Figures 9-7 and 9-8 are an X-ray study of the lower leg. Figure 9-7 shows the normal appearance of the fibula's relationship with the tibia. The right photo shows someone who is injured, and was having right leg pain and an inability to put her full weight

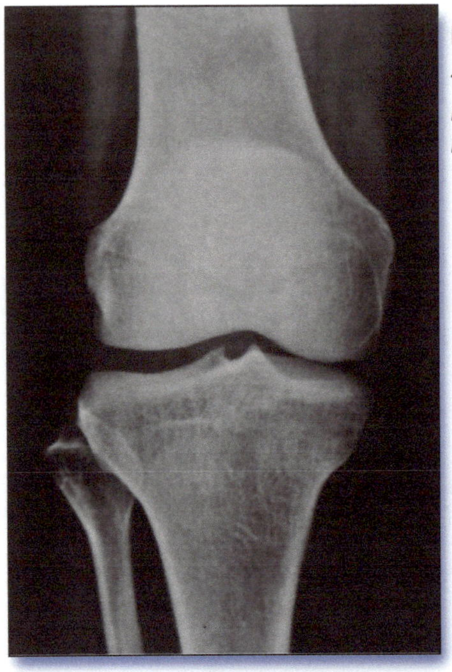

FIGURE 9-7. THE NORMAL FIB-TIB JOINT, ANTERIOR VIEW

Note the overlap that the Fibular head has with the Tibia.

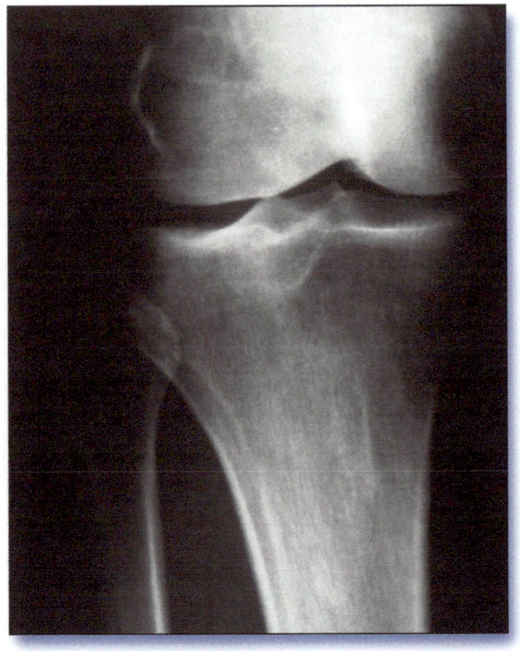

FIGURE 9-8. THE SUBLUXATION OF FIBULA, ANTERIOR VIEW

Note the reduced overlap of the Fibular head and the bigger gap between the two bones.

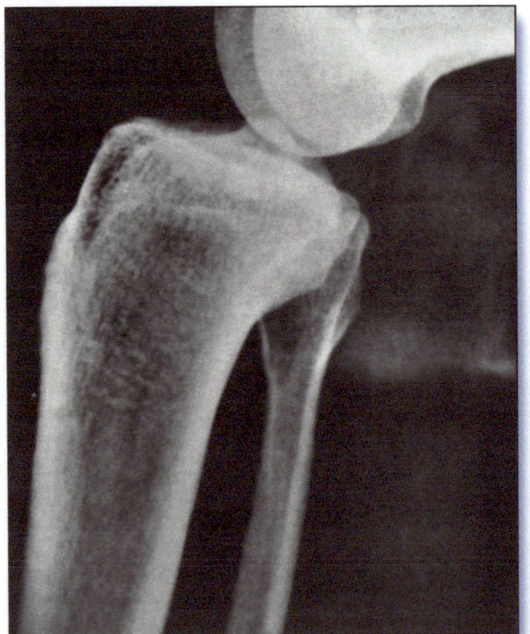

FIGURE 9-9. THE NORMAL LATERAL VIEW OF THE TOP OF THE LOWER LEG

Note the close relationship between the Fibular Head and the Tibial Plateau.

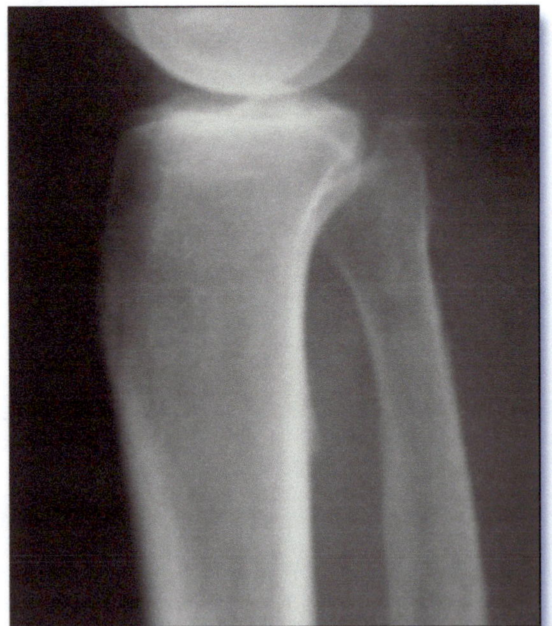

FIGURE 9-10. THE LATERAL VIEW OF A SUBLUXATED FIBULA

Note the Fibular Head is separated from the Tibia and the larger space between the two bones.

on her leg. You can see how much bigger the space is between the two bones and how the top of the fibula is closer to the top of the tibia in the right hand picture.

Figure 9-9 is an X-ray of a lateral view of the normal leg. Figure 9-10 is the same injured person as in Figure 9-8. Note the difference in space between the two and that Figure 9-9 has the fibula closer to the tibia. Figure 9-10 shows the signs of a separation of the fibular head from the tibia. This is the most common subluxation pattern of the fibula, it being superior and lateral to the tibia. This patient's X-ray report had the word "normal" appear four times. The patient wanted to know why a radiologist would call her films "normal." I said that there were no fractures, tumors or infections, so he was trained to call that "normal." An orthopedist usually doesn't look at the films, just the report, and that's how patients end up with drugs and exercise as the only intervention. I asked my patient, "What drugs would put those two bones back together?" She said "None," and I said, "Now you know more than your orthopedist."

ADJUSTING THE FIBULA WITH THE SPRING LOADED INSTRUMENT (SLI)

Contact the proximal fibula and squeeze it to the tibia and tap the fingers that lie above and around the fibula head, medially and inferiorly

> ***Supine: The Doctor's thumb is pulling the Fibula in the direction of correction and then the SLI is used on the thumb repetitively. See Figure 9-11.***

FIGURE 9-11. THE SLI ADJUSTING OF THE FIBULA SUPINE POSITION

The Doctor's thumb is pulling the Fibula in the direction of correction and then the SLI is used on the thumb repeatedly..

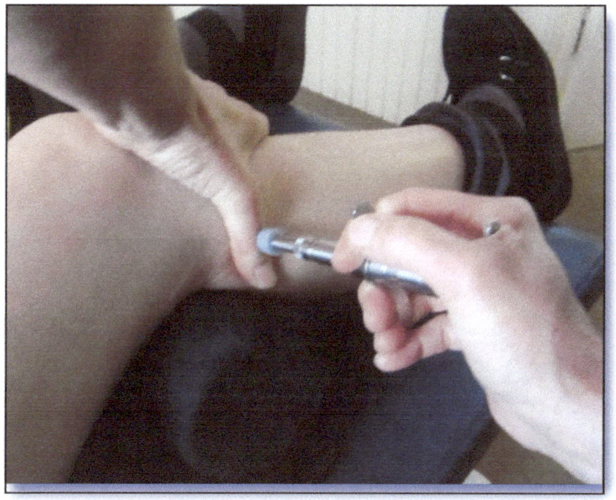

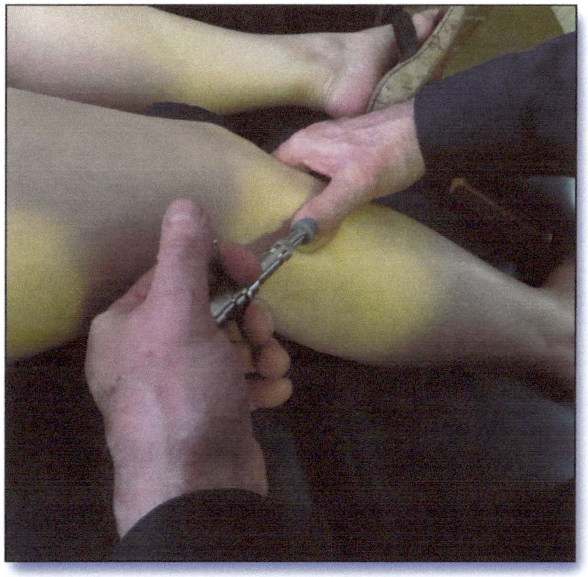

FIGURE 9-12: SLI ADJUSTING OF THE FIBULA LATERAL POSITION

The doctor's thumb is pulling on the fibular head in the inferior and medial direction. The SLI is used on the doctor's thumb, repeatedly.

FIGURE 9-13: SLI ADJUSTING OF THE FIBULA PRONE POSITION

The doctor's thumb is pulling the fibula inferiorly and medially while the SLI is used repeatedly

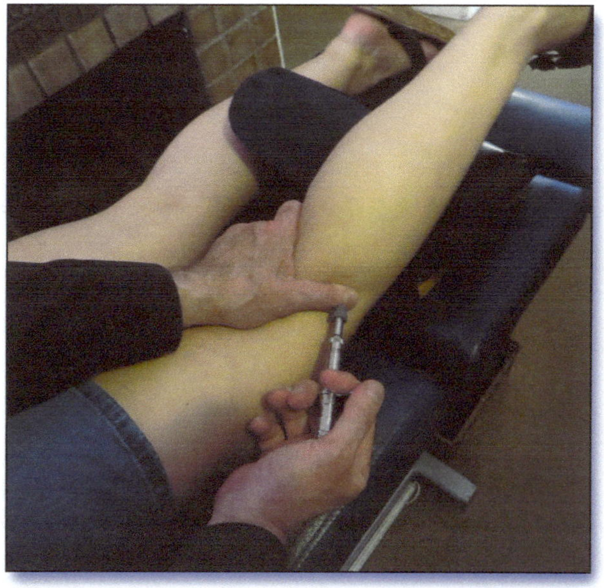

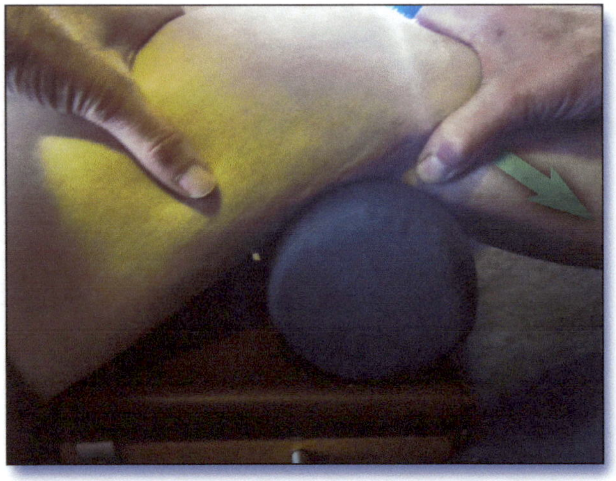

FIGURE 9-14. USING A THE DROP PIECE ADJUSTING OF THE SUPERIOR FIBULA

The knee is placed over the drop piece with a firm roll. The Doctor's thumb firmly contacts the top of the Fibula, squeezing the Fibula to the Tibia and then drop several times.

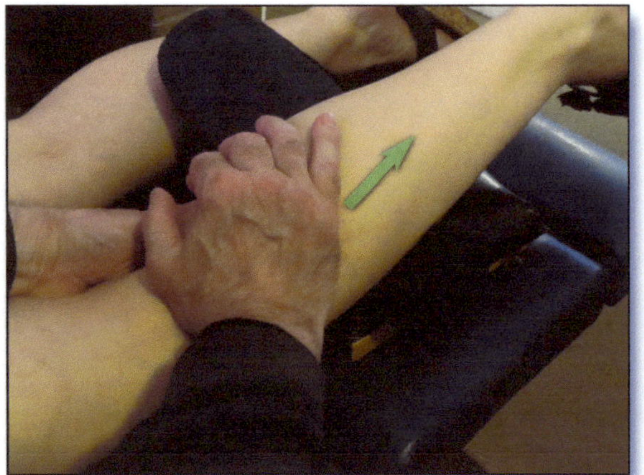

FIGURE 9-15. USING A THE DROP PIECE ADJUSTING OF THE SUPERIOR FIBULA PRONE POSITION

The doctor's hand has thenar contact on the fibula head. The line of thrust is superior to inferior, and lateral to medial. (Down and in)

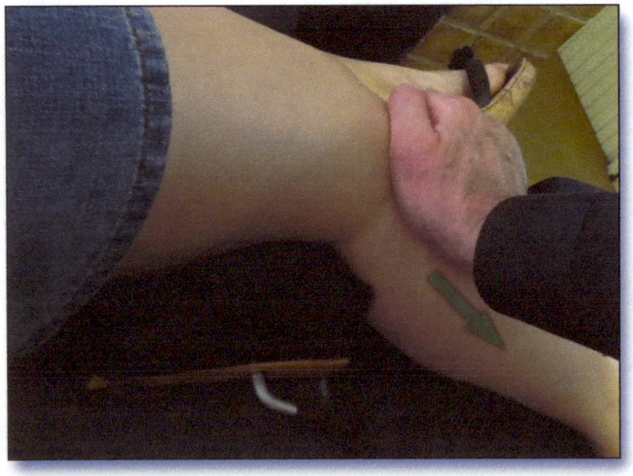

FIGURE 9-16: DROP TABLE ADJUSTING OF THE FIBULA LATERAL POSITION

Fibula adjusting from a lateral position is done with the doctor's hand with thenar contact on the fibula head. The line of drive is superior to inferior, and lateral to medial. (Down and in)

> ***Lateral:** The doctor's thumb is pulling on the fibular head in the inferior and medial direction. The SLI is used on the doctor's thumb, repeatedly. See Figure 9-12.*

> ***Prone:** The doctor's thumb is pulling the fibula inferiorly and medially when the SLI is used repeatedly. See Figure 9-13*

ADJUSTING THE FIBULA WITH THE DROP PIECE

Put the drop piece with a roll under the knee. The Doctor's thumb firmly contacts the top of the Fibula, squeezing the Fibula to the Tibia and then drop several times.

Please note all procedures are gentle and firm, don't expect the first drop to complete the correction.

> ***Supine:** Squeeze the fibula to the tibia and drop (sometimes the fibula needs to be moved inferiorly, so an inferior component to the thrust is needed). See Figure 9-14.*

> ***Lateral:** The doctor's hand has thenar contact on the fibula head. The line of drive is superior to inferior, and lateral to medial. (Down and in) This position gives the mechanical advantage to the doctor, especially if there are big displacement patterns, or if the doctor is smaller than the patient. See Figure 9-15*

> ***Prone:** The doctor contacts the fibular head with thenar contact. The thrust is inferior and medial. See Figure 9-16.*

Different subluxation patterns,i.e. superior and inferior, might make the best mechanical position for the doctor with the patient in a different position than prone. Also the size of the patient relative to the size of the doctor might be a factor in choosing which position to use.

MANAGING THE LOWER LEG INJURY

Managing the lower leg injury can be difficult. In listing the degree of difficulty, I think that adjusting the joints is the easy part. It's more difficult to evaluate and make the correct diagnosis.

FIGURE 9-17
DIFFERENT TYPES OF BRACES

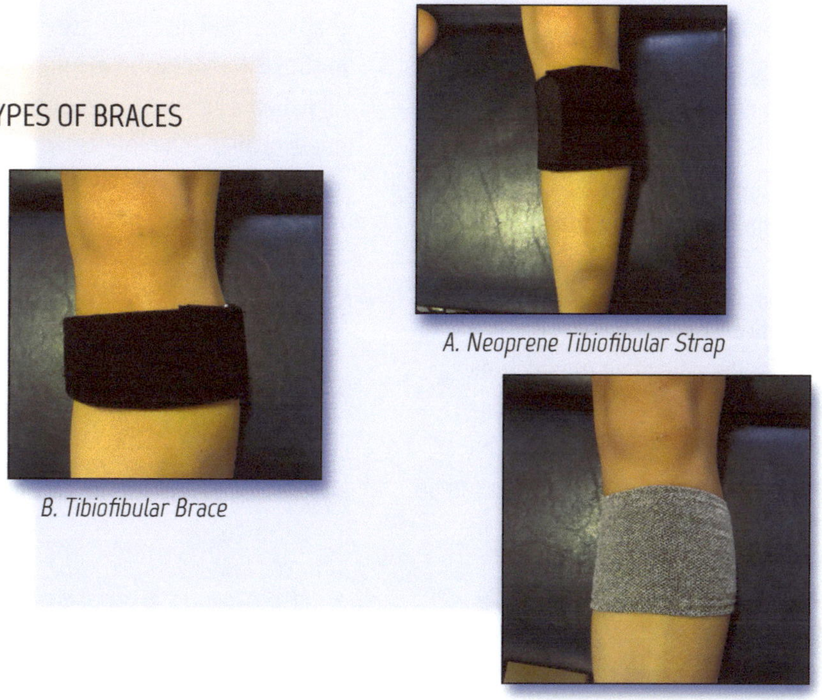

A. Neoprene Tibiofibular Strap

B. Tibiofibular Brace

C. Compressive Sleeve - There are a variety of these braces on the market.

BRACING

- *A compressive brace can be very helpful.*
- *Evaluate the types of compressive braces and sleeves.*
- *Circulation issues can develop with braces in this region.*
- *This is a difficult injury to manage for active patients*
- *Supportive footwear is important.*

If you have read the previous chapters in this book, you know I'm in favor of bracing.

If I can get a brace to help restore normal function, weight-bearing activity and conditioning, I will use it. Some injuries in the categories of modern injuries we have described will result in permanent impairment. Some injuries will not allow a full recovery. So managing the injury, in some cases, on a daily basis, is necessary.

I ran on pavement for 25 years. I have permanent impairment to my lower legs and feet. As I said earlier, at the time of this writing, I am in full-time practice seeing on average 100 patient visits a week. I am past the usual retirement age. I have no intention of letting my age or my injuries impair my ability to work, however I need braces to be able to continue. Driving my car and being stuck in traffic is more painful than being on my feet working all day. But that's how it will be for some patients with these types of injuries. Managing the dysfunction and pain with braces is so much more efficacious than taking drugs and restricting or limiting my activities because of the pain, which is what the majority of suffering patients do.

The compressive strap is the most helpful for an injured lower leg. I frequently use what I call a tibiofibular strap, which is a neoprene strap with a bit of Velcro *(see Figure 9-17a),* or a tibiofibular brace which is a canvas strap with a buckle. *(see Figure 9-17b)* The latter is more durable, and I use it on folks who are very physically active. The neoprene strap is usually recommended for people that are having trouble moving around. We vary the size from 2-inch to 4-inch. I find the larger folks with a lot of tissue on the lower leg to respond to the 4-inch strap better than the 2-inch strap. There are also endless choices of compressive sleeves on the market. They vary widely in material, cost, size and shape. *See Figure 9-17c.* Your choice in braces should depend on your patient's individual needs.

Circulation issues can develop for people in this region, including varicose veins. The use of the braces or straps should be selective. By that, I mean that the patient wears the braces when they are active and they take the braces off when they are off their feet. The exceptions are when the pain keeps the patient awake at night, especially if ITB syndrome keeps them from laying on their side in bed. The strap can be very helpful in this situation. Selective use has a disadvantage: without conscious pain, patients forget to put it on. The pain developing in the activity of the day will remind them to put the brace on, but they've usually left it at home. Some people will be better at managing these injuries than others. Patient compliance is an important part of resolving the problem.

People that insist on continuing to run marathons or have a high level of activity despite a lower leg injury are difficult to manage. Supporting and adjusting the leg, as well as consulting with the patient on proper footwear and possibly modifying some of their activity is essential. A main chiropractic principle is that a body wants to heal. So I'm amazed at how some patients recover despite their lack of compliance and refusal to reasonably restrict or modify their behavior. Getting a patient to acknowledge that there is an actual injury to manage can be a challenge.

Again, I want to mention the number of times I've seen patients that are post spinal surgery for relief of leg pain that still have injured legs. It is a very sad comment on our quality of medical care, that palpatory examination procedures are considered passé by a lot of our healthcare community. So when evaluating someone who has suffered any injuries, please be thorough about examining the lower leg and foot. I've seen patients diagnosed with diabetic neuropathy as an explanation for their leg and foot dysfunction, but by restoring the normal alignment and instituting supportive devices including proper footwear, the 'diabetic neuropathy' resolves.

Please don't assume that injury to the spine is always the cause of lower leg pain and dysfunction. In later chapters, I will discuss these same issues as they relate to stroke, traumatic brain injury and spinal cord injury. All patients deserve to have a thorough evaluation made of all of their injuries instead of assumptions about their condition.

THE ERGONOMICS OF THE LOWER LEG INJURY

- *Review personal habits (e.g., leg crossing, sitting, kneeling activities).*
- *Walking and running on asphalt and concrete are to be avoided.*
- *Hydrotherapy is recommended, especially if knee, lower back and other injuries are present.*

The ergonomics of the lower leg injury is a complex subject. Patients invariably have personal habits that relate to their legs, knees and feet. Some of these personal habits will interfere with the recovery of more recent injuries. Patients with desk jobs are usually not aware of what they do with her feet, legs and knees while seated at the desk, as they are focused on their tasks. Patients curl their legs around the legs of the chair, they sit on one leg or they cross their knees and their ankles without ill effect for years. Normal legs, knees and ankles can probably take quite a bit of distortion without becoming injured. But after a car accident or a fall, these habits can make the leg injury worse or keep it from resolving.

The challenging part for the doctor is to get the patient to become aware of these habits and change them. Sometimes I've recruited a spouse to help manage a change in behavior regarding the legs. I routinely have patients deny they sit on their legs or cross their legs for weeks before they discover that they are doing it all the time. I will have been suspicious of the habits the whole time because I'm expecting better results from the care and it's not happening. I feel when I restore normal joint alignment and function that there should be some improvement at the next office visit. When this has not happened, I want to know what forces have intervened to stop the healing processes.

We live in a paved environment. Walking and running on asphalt and concrete will not help any of the injuries to the lower leg. Reducing contact with asphalt and concrete can be next to impossible for the urban dweller. Footwear is a way to modify that contact. So paying attention to the patient's footwear is important when dealing with a leg injury or a foot injury. Supportive footwear is available, but it's usually a bit more expensive. I advocate the use of boots, as lace- up six or eight inch boots can really help stabilize leg, ankle and foot injuries. I will discuss this in greater detail in the chapter on foot injury.

Hydrotherapy can be very helpful to a patient who has the entire lower kinetic chain injured. Ensuring patient mobility and weight-bearing is of the utmost importance after these types of injuries. This can be difficult when the pelvis, knees, lower leg, ankle and foot are all injured and the joints are unstable. Getting into a pool and engaging in normal motion patterns can be essential for establishing ligament stability and maintaining or reestablishing the health of the muscles, vascular structures and neurological structures that have suffered injuries.

NOTES:

• • •

Lower Leg videos:
https://youtu.be/2q-kDcW5_Vc
https://youtu.be/rbEjBnDfFns
https://youtu.be/kxiuozSKuvI
https://youtu.be/q5EWZy7yEBO
https://youtu.be/MLSQFvnuWJ4

CHAPTER TEN

Evaluating, Adjusting And Managing The Foot And Ankle

Evaluating, adjusting and managing the injured foot and ankle properly can improve someone's mobility and quality of life. The modern injuries that are occurring in our population include injuries to feet and ankles. Asphalt and concrete are not kind to the human foot. During a car accident, a foot on the brake at the moment of impact can cause permanent injuries. When treating traumatic brain injury patients, as well as motor vehicle accident victims, earlier providers assumed foot and ankle dysfunctions were caused by disc or spinal injuries or brain injuries

Evaluating the foot and ankle properly can reveal joint problems that cause dysfunction. Rehabilitation of any of these types of injuries should be focused on improved mobility. Foot and ankle function would be critical for the rehabilitation of the spine and pelvis and many other conditions, including cardiovascular problems. An inability to walk or walk without pain and with stability could keep rehabilitation limited in scope, and reduced outcomes could be anticipated.

The foot and ankle, like every other structure in the human body, has a "building code." If you alter the architecture of the structure and violate the building code, dysfunction must be expected.

With this chapter, I intend to show how to assess the foot and ankle area, and adjust it in a gentle manner. As with all the adjusting protocols I teach, I isolate the forces of intervention to the targeted area. I do not want to do anything to the probably injured leg, knee, hip or pelvis. I will describe and depict specific adjusting maneuvers for the foot and ankle using the portable drop piece, as well as taping and bracing methods to help maintain the alignment and holding adjustments.

I have been able to successfully change the shape and shoe size of quite a few feet over the years. The first example is myself: I am currently wearing a size 10 ½ shoe. A few years ago, I was wearing a size 12 shoe. This change in shoe size came from putting the heel bone back in place and realigning my metatarsals with the mid-foot. I use tape to support the changes I'm making with the adjusting protocols. In this manner, I very quickly went from a 12 to 11 ½. It took about a year to go from 11½ to the 11. In the following months, the size 11 shoes became too big! I also see this happen with many patients. When the heel bone is brought back into its normal position, it is closer to the toes. When the arch is raised, it shortens the foot as well. These two main approaches can change the shape and therefore the function of the foot.

One of my patients began treatment with me as a 74-year-old obese bookkeeper who hadn't liked to walk since age 14 because of foot pain. By the time she was 78, she was walking regularly, including taking her new dog to the dog park. She lost 38 pounds and looked much younger. I've had patients as children with deformed feet that cause their shoes to be deformed as well. Sometimes, the shoes look like someone's taken a belt sander to one side of them. With children, it can take six to eight weeks to change the shape of their feet. Some adults, if they are compliant, can have the same results as quickly.

Plantar fasciitis, if it really is plantar fasciitis, is almost invariably a subluxated calcaneus. Sometimes, people call any pain on the underside of the foot "plantar fasciitis." So you have to do a thorough assessment of the complaint.

There is a reoccurring theme through these chapters: if someone comes into your office complaining of foot pain, please examine their feet and lower legs! As you'll see in the next section, the muscles that operate the toes and ankle arise from the lower leg. Lower leg injury can cause foot pain, which needs to be recognized. Also, footwear is a big factor in foot pain. Most women's shoes do not do an adequate job of protecting their feet from the harsh environment of asphalt and concrete. I find almost everybody in a paved environment has calcaneal subluxations. The heel striking on asphalt and concrete is the only thing I can contribute to this finding. Mother Earth absorbs your heel strike, while asphalt and concrete send the force into your spine.

I have a study from the early 1990s that shows that a heel striking on asphalt or concrete is a micro-trauma to the L4 and L5 discs. The study didn't mention the adverse effects of a heel strike on any of the joints from the heel to the L5 joint. However, I figured that if there is micro-trauma to the lower lumbar spine, it cannot be good for the intervening joints – the foot and ankle especially. So when I'm advocating a walking regimen for my patients, I discuss the need to walk on natural surfaces. I ran on pavement for 25 years and altered the shape of my feet. I had quite a bit of foot and ankle dysfunction from my athletic activities. But as a high school and college athlete, I didn't pay attention to or worry about the long-term consequences of my activities. This was the primary reason my feet got bigger over the years: they were collapsing. Even after I stopped running, walking on unnatural surfaces did not help my situation. So this minor change of walking on Mother Earth can have a significant positive impact on foot and ankle injury resolution, especially for younger patients.

RELEVANT ANATOMY FOR THIS CHAPTER

- *The talocalcaneal/subtalar joint, talocrural/talar mortise joint, tarso-metatarsal (mid-foot) joints, inferior tibiofibular joint*
- *The muscular structures of the region: gastrocnemius, peroneus, the hallucis group and plantar fascia — most of the muscles of the lower leg go to the foot*

In reviewing the relevant anatomy, I don't want to bore readers with a whole lot of anatomical names. I feel the need to keep it simple. A lot of times, I find the explanation I give to patients is not much different from what I would say to a class of doctors!

The relevant parts of the foot for the purposes of this discussion are the joints between the heel bone and the ankle bone. The talocalcaneal joint is a complex, tough joint that is actually made up of three components, all with different angles. I consider the heel bone to be the keystone to the foot. The big toe tendons, the flexors of the little toes, the Achilles tendon and the plantar fascia, among other structures, are attached to the calcaneus, so subluxation of the calcaneus can cause problems and pain in these structures.

The foot has multiple complex joints. The architecture of their shapes imply that this complexity is essential to the foot's function. *(See Figures 10-1 and 10-2.)* Change the architecture, or allow "building code violations" into the structure, and you have to expect a change in function. Altered weight bearing, as with any other part of the body, will cause bones to remodel and joints to erode.

The underappreciated part of this fundamental change in shape is that it also alters the length of the nerves, as well as the arteries and veins. They will also suffer from persistent deformation, resulting in poor circulation and impaired neurological function. In studying the nerves of a frog in a biology lab, it was discovered that the nerves have decreased conductivity when they are stretched. So as the foot subluxates and becomes longer, expect decreased sensation and motor function from the stretched and distressed nerves. The stretching of the arteries will cause the lumens to narrow, delivering a reduced blood supply. The deformation of the veins will cause them to collapse, and swelling and edema can be expected. (*See Figure 10-5.*)

Figure 10-3 depicts the anatomy of the lateral leg and foot, showing that most of the muscle tissue is shared between the lower leg and foot. So I consider the lower leg and foot to be a functional unit. Injuries

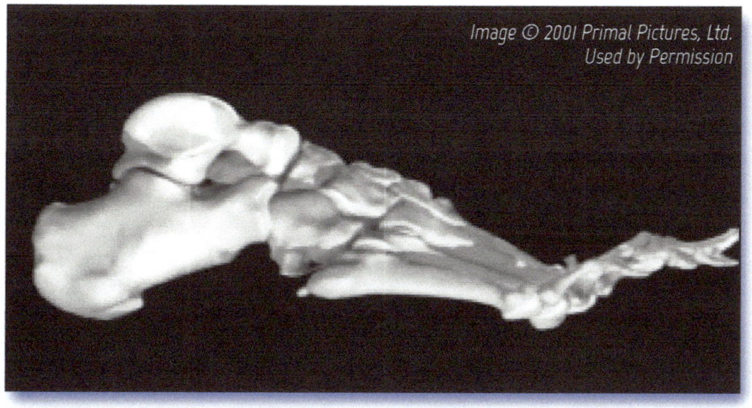

FIGURE 10-1. THE LATERAL VIEW OF THE FOOT.

Note the smooth top to the foot and that the calcaneus and talus are aligned

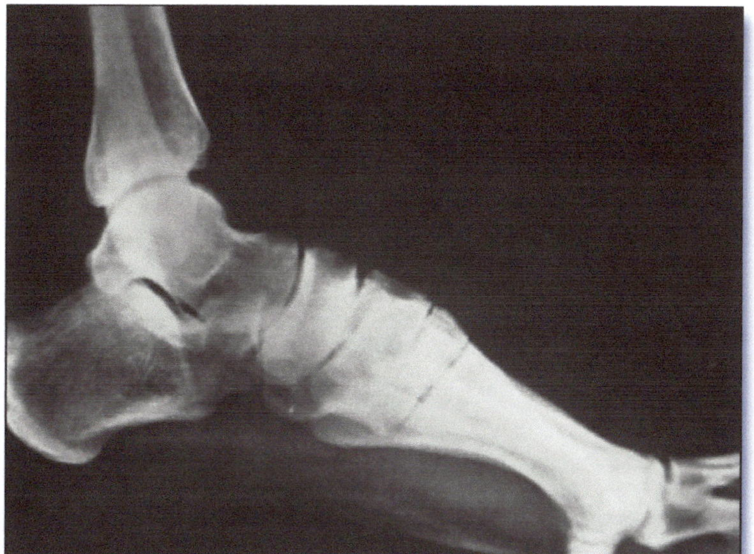

FIGURE 10-2. LATERAL VIEW OF THE FOOT ON X-RAY

Note the top of the foot has smooth curved arch, as well as the inferior arch.

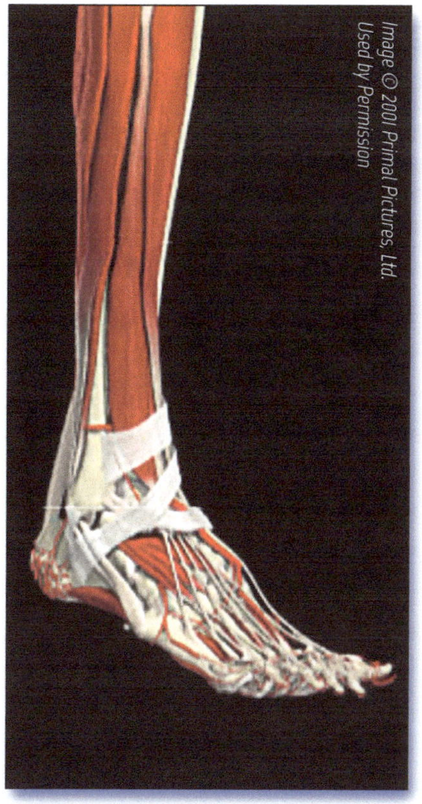

FIGURE 10-3. THE LATERAL VIEW OF THE LOWER LEG AND FOOT

Note the muscular structures that go from lower leg to the foot. Lower leg dysfunction is often felt in the foot.

to the lower leg almost invariably have adverse consequences for the foot. Most pain patterns in the foot have some relationship, if not their origin, in the lower leg.

Podiatry looks at the foot as a separate structure from the leg. I have an article written by a podiatrist about bunions. The first line of the article says, "Bunions of the first metatarsal-phalangeal joint are caused by a misalignment of the base of the first metatarsal with its joint at the cuneiform." The article then proceeds to describe the surgical procedure of taking a wedged piece of bone out of first metacarpal and using pins to hold this new shape until it heals. The podiatrist author never mentions realigning the misaligned joint. I consider podiatric care to be based on an incomplete understanding of the anatomy of the region and very often podiatrists' interventions lack logic and comprehensive understanding. Therefore, I consider most people under podiatric care to be at risk for further injury and unnecessary surgical procedures. I'm sorry to make such a harsh judgment about a profession, but I've had many patients over the years that had podiatric interventions that didn't really solve the problem, or worsened it. (I got a dozen roses from a patient when I saved her daughter from foot surgery. The surgeon had performed many surgeries on the patient's mother and she was confined to a wheelchair from foot pain).

The entire structure of the lower leg and foot must be evaluated to create a more rational intervention that deals with the full scope of the injuries. Figure 10-4 is the medial view of the lower leg and foot. Note how the big toe tendons come down behind the medial malleolus and attach to the heel bone. Separation of the proximal fibula and tibia combined with a subluxated calcaneus can produce severe arch pain, metatarsal-phalangeal (MP) joint pain and big toe pain. Any one of those, or all in combination, would be caused by these "remote" subluxation patterns. Hopefully, I am making a good case for why a foot and ankle complaint should have an evaluation of the lower leg included. This is especially true when so many people come into chiropractic offices complaining of sciatica, when in fact, it's an injured leg that's the cause of the complaint.

As I was preparing this chapter, I had another new patient yesterday with over 30 years of left leg sciatica, with tingling and numbness of the foot. He had lumbar surgery for this complaint 30 years earlier. This pain pattern affected his sleep and his ability to stand and change positions. He had subluxations of the pelvis, tibia, fibula, calcaneus, talus and metatarsals. He left our office with a fib-tib brace and his calcaneus and talus taped. He said he could put all of his weight on his left leg for the first time in 30 years. He said, "As I stand here I'm out of pain right now, but I've got two miles of fence post holes to dig this weekend." (The patients will drive you crazy. Someday, I would like to write a book called "You Did What?") You could try to talk to him about being reasonable about his injured leg and low back. But he is 68-years-old, and the best thing I could say was, "We should see you on Monday."

The talocalcaneal joint is extremely important to the integrity and function of the foot. Not only is the plantar fascia attached to the calcaneus, but the neurovascular bundles that proliferate out to the plantar surface of the foot are also bound to the calcaneus. (*See Figure 10-5.*) Calcaneal subluxation can result in neurological and vascular deficit as well as musculoskeletal distress patterns.

EVALUATING FOOT AND ANKLE PROBLEMS

> *The calcaneus should be under the talus (Calcaneus Draw Test).*

> *The talus should be under the mortise/ talocrural joint (Talus Draw Test).*

> *The metatarsals should be lined up with the cuneiforms.*

> *Determine the lower leg involvement in the complaints (Fib-Tib Squeeze Test).*

I have gone through a number of textbooks on this subject and I feel that there is a simplified version of evaluating the foot and ankle. However, I'm going to add the complication of including the lower leg in assessing foot and ankle problems – because when considering the foot and ankle only, the main points are: Where is the heel bone? Where is the ankle bone? Are the metatarsals aligned with the mid-foot? I know that there can be lots of other problems with the foot and ankle, but those three points are critical to getting a foot functioning properly again.

In evaluating the talocalcaneal joint, find the lateral malleolus and place a thumb underneath it, palpating

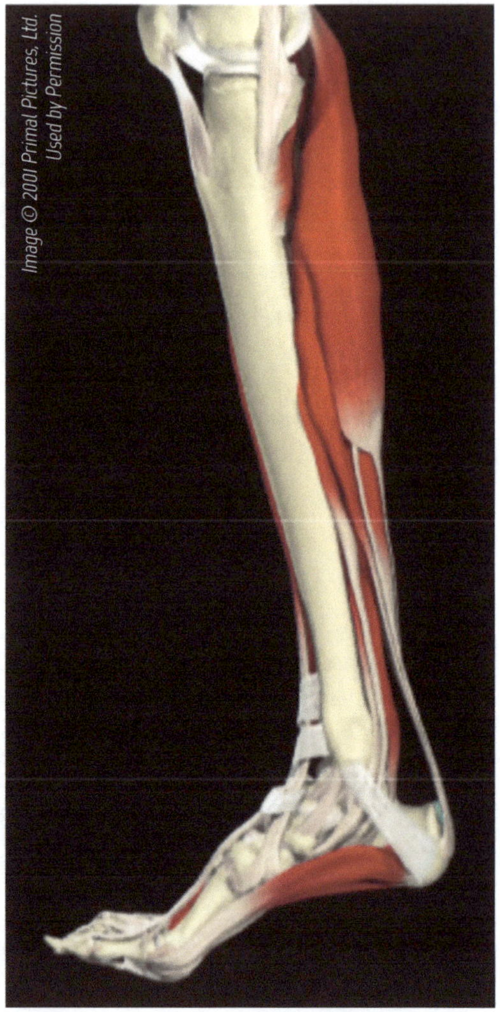

FIGURE 10-4. THE MEDIAL VIEW OF THE LOWER LEG AND FOOT

This view of the lower leg shows the large muscles that move the foot.

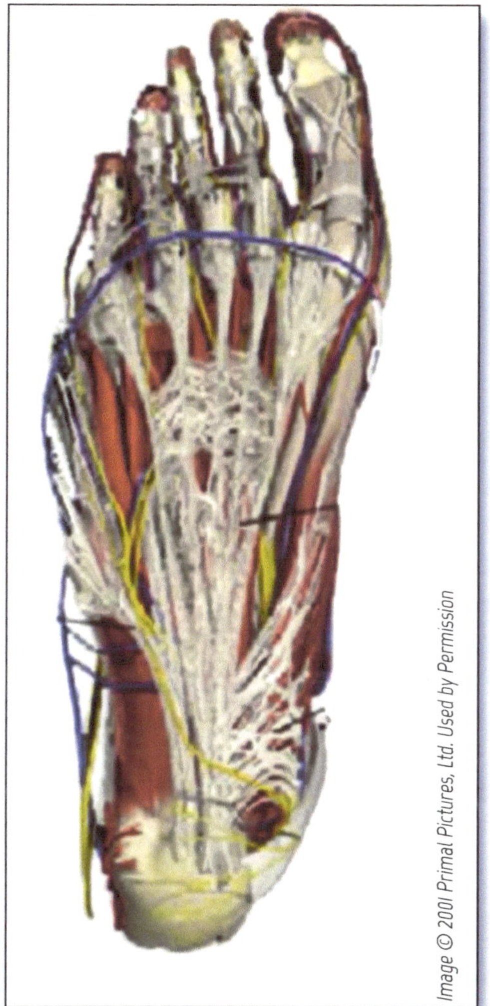

FIGURE 10-5. THE UNDERSIDE OF THE FOOT

The tendons, arteries, veins and the plantar fascia will stretch and deform with subluxation of the calcaneus.

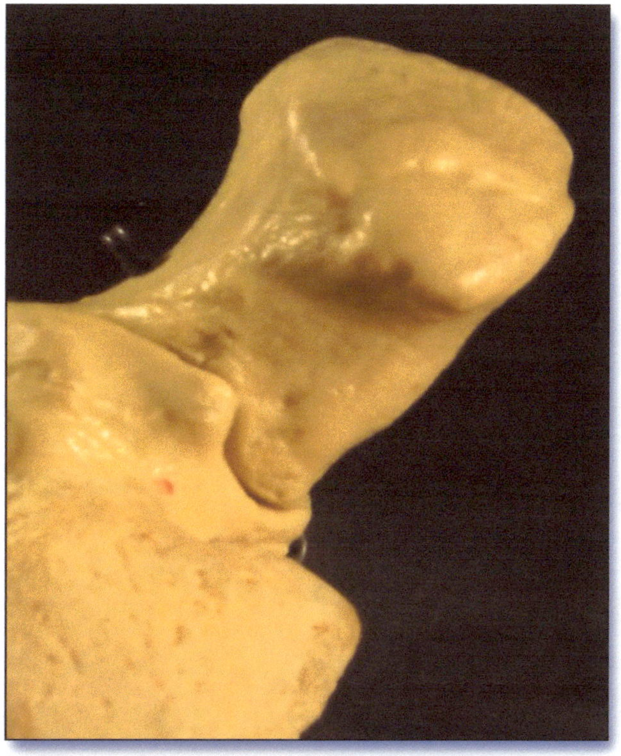

FIGURE 10-6A THE NORMAL CALCANEAL/TALOR JOINT

Viewed from above and behind. The joint should be smooth when aligned and non tender.

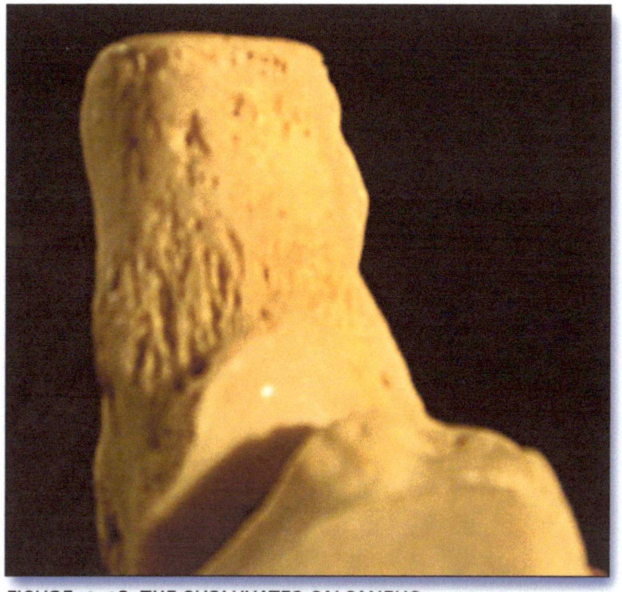

FIGURE 10-6B. THE SUBLUXATED CALCANEUS

Viewed from above and behind. The ridge of the top of the calcaneus is protruding and will often be very tender to the touch.

for a shelf or ridge. *(See Figures 10-6a and b. Figure 10-6a is the aligned talocalcaneal joint. Figure 10-6b shows the subluxated calcaneus with the talus.)* The lateral side shows the calcaneus having subluxated posteriorly and laterally relative to the talus. This ridge is likely to be very painful to the touch. *(See Figures 10-7a and b).* Most of the time, this is a complete surprise to the patient.

The ankle bone or talus should be properly positioned underneath the mortise joint. If it's not aligned, then the words "instability" or "unstable" will commonly be used by the patient. This is also the case with heel bone displacement. But in combination, the two displaced joint complexes can be a real functional problem for the patient. Chronically, these folks will complain of always recovering from one ankle sprain or the other. As soon as one ankle starts to feel less painful, they sprain the other one. The metatarsals are very commonly out of place, and getting them lined up with the cuneiforms is essential to getting the foot to function properly.

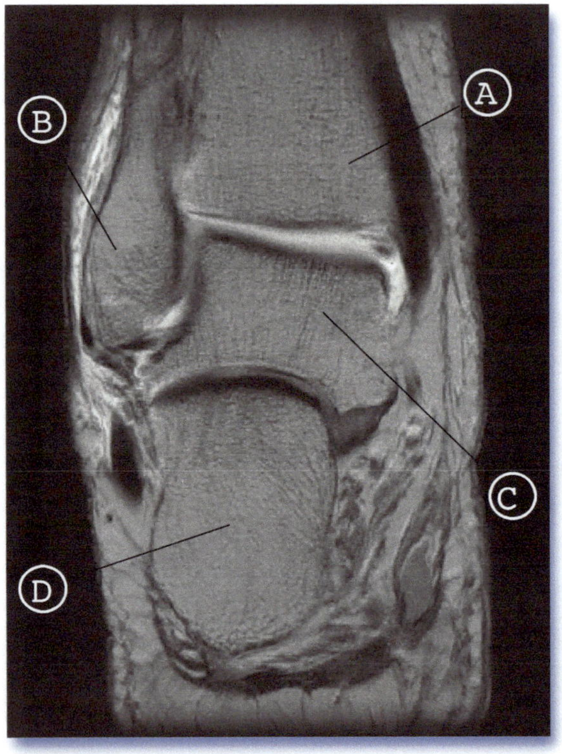

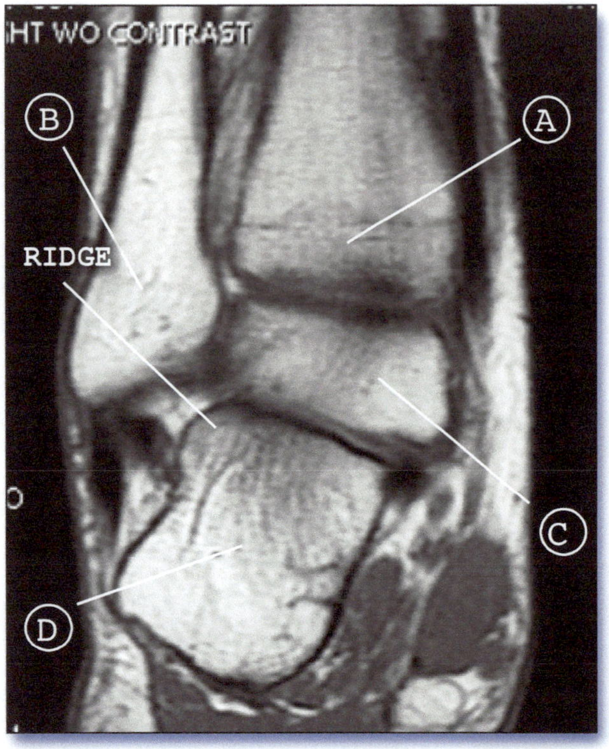

FIGURES 10-7A&B. MRI IMAGES OF NORMAL AND SUBLUXATED CALCANEUS

Figure 10-7a is an MRI of a normal Tibia, Talus and Calcaneus alignment.

10-7b is an MRI of a lateral subluxation of the Calcaneus, patients chief complaint is the medial side of the Calcaneus.

A. Tibia *C. Talus*

B. Fibula *D. Calcaneus*

THE CALCANEAL DRAW TEST

To test the involvement of the subluxation, I provoke the patient's complaint: big toe pain, tingling and numbness of the foot, plantar fasciitis or arch pain, whatever it is. Either the patient or I will provoke the complaint and then I will pull or push the calcaneus back into place, and count to 30. Over ninety percent of the time, the symptoms start to fade with the maintained pressure of holding the calcaneus in place. (*See Figure 10-8.*) This is important for two reasons: one, it is a diagnostic for me and, two, it illustrates to the patient the heel's involvement in their complaints. The more the patient understands and appreciates the full extent of their injuries, the more they tend to be compliant with your care and requests for changes in their behavior and footwear.

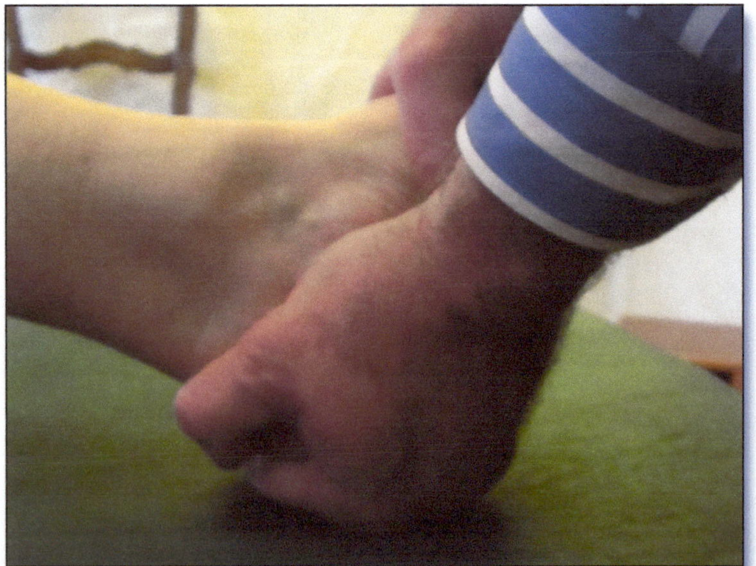

FIGURE 10-8. THE CALCANEUS DRAW TEST

The doctor grasps the posterior aspect of the heel bone and, while stabilizing the mid-foot with the other hand, pulls or draws the heel bone forward or anterior and medial.

TALUS DRAW TEST

The talus or ankle bone has a distinct and important relationship with the lower leg. I have had so many patients over the years complain of unstable ankles. They have been all making accurate architectural statements about the subluxation patterns they suffered. If the ankle bone is not properly aligned underneath the mortise/talocrural joint, the whole foot is misaligned under the leg. Certain positions and activities would make that worse. Also, "feeling like the foot is going to come out from underneath the leg" is actually an accurate statement. The body will respond appropriately and tighten up all the involved muscular structures to create a semblance of stability in the misaligned joint. Ligaments will become inflamed and arteries, veins and nerves will become entrapped when we have this important joint lose its alignment and stability.

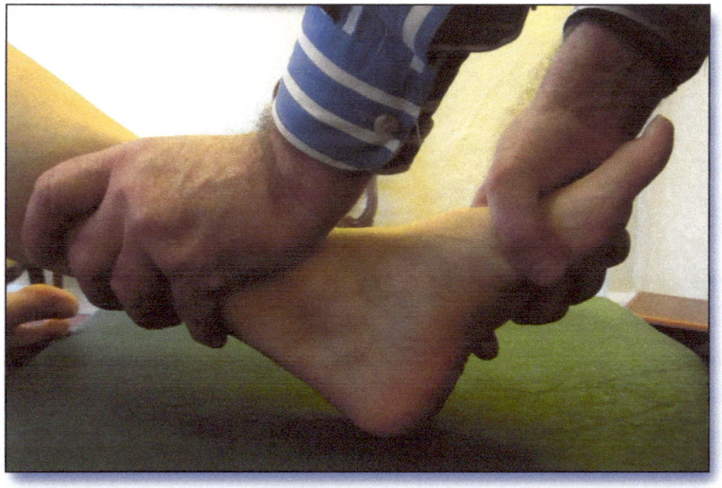

FIGURE 10-9. THE TALUS DRAW TEST

The foot is in a neural position and the doctor's hands grip the foot and the lower leg. The leg is pressed or drawn posteriorly or anteriorly. Note the position of relief.

The talus can slip posteriorly and the underside of the mortise/talocrural joint can be felt on palpation. This is a critically important joint when inability to walk is a chief complaint. Additionally, the talus can be forward or anterior to the mortise joint and the dome of the talus is prominent in the neutral position. These are subtle changes, but important ones, and I am going to repeat that *if you do not look for it, you will not find it.* So when I'm evaluating the foot and ankle, I'm looking for specific subluxation patterns that are very common. I will then test my findings by pulling or pushing the bones or joints back into place and waiting for 20 to 30 seconds to see if there is a change in the tone of the muscles or tendons or other symptoms. (*See Figure 10-9.*)

When assessing the lower leg involvement in foot and ankle problems, ask if any of these tests are positive, which manifests as lessened pain.

- *Big toe pain: squeeze the proximal tibiofibular joint, assess the big toe pain while maintaining the squeeze. (If positive, see Chapter 9).*
- *Big toe pain: pull the calcaneus anteriorly and medially and assess the big toe pain while maintaining the pulling.*
- *Heel pain: Squeeze test, Squeeze the proximal tibiofibular joint while provoking the heel pain. (If positive, see Chapter 9).*
- *Heel pain: Pull the calcaneus anteriorly while provoking the heel pain.*
- *Plantar Fasciitis: Pull the calcaneus anteriorly while provoking the plantar pain.*
- *Arch pain: Pull the calcaneus anteriorly and medially while provoking the arch pain. Repeat while performing the Fib-Tib Squeeze test.*

The Fib-Tib Squeeze Test is used to distinguish the involvement of the lower leg from any of the symptoms of the foot. *(See Chapter 9.)* One extra thing to note is that pain across the top of the foot is commonly tibialis anterior tendon tension from a separation of the fibula to the tibia at the proximal joint where the origin of the tibialis anterior muscle inserts to both bones. It's a simple test and can be done in just moments.

This evaluation protocol can be done in less than three minutes once it has been well-practiced. This takes far less time than it takes to fill out the paperwork to get an MRI of the lumbar spine. Testing for sciatic pain can be done very simply by putting a thumb into the sciatic notch of the patient's symptomatic side and pressing firmly. Press firmly on the lumbar spinal vertebra and have the patient take a deep breath and cough simultaneously. If neither of these tests is positive, then taking an additional three minutes to evaluate the leg can be extremely important.

Again, there is nothing I can do to the lumbar spine with chiropractic care or surgery that would actually fix the lower leg or foot injuries that are so common in our population. In promoting the idea of rational care, properly identifying and treating the injuries is essential.

ADJUSTING THE TALUS WITH THE DROP PIECE

Posterior talus: *place the foot with the back of the heel in contact with the drop piece, drop posteriorly on the lower leg. This is best with the knee bent and supported. Repeat. (See Figure 10-11a.)*

Anterior talus: *place the end of the lower leg on the edge of the drop piece, with the foot hanging off the drop piece. Drop on the foot with it in a neutral position to the leg. This is best with the knee bent and supported. Repeat. (See Figure 10-11b)*

ADJUSTING THE CALCANEUS WITH THE DROP PIECE

Posterior Calcaneus: *Set the back of the calcaneus on the drop piece, best with knee bent and supported. Grip the talus and mid-foot and drop towards the back of the calcaneus. Repeat. (See Figure 10-11.)*

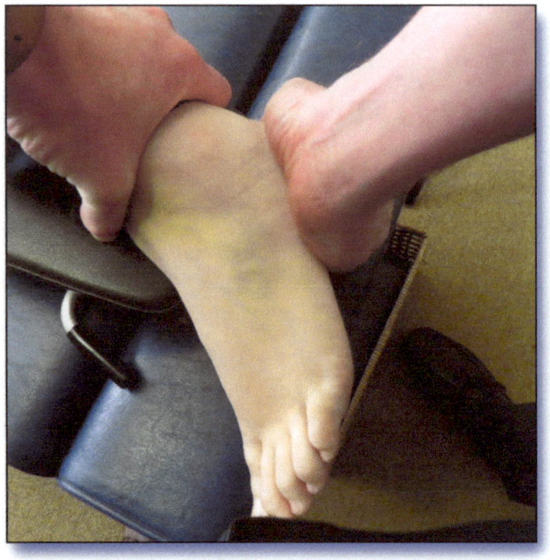

FIGURE 10-10. ADJUSTMENT FOR A LATERAL CALCANEUS

The medial side of the foot is placed on the drop piece with the calcaneus off the edge. Drop lateral to medial.

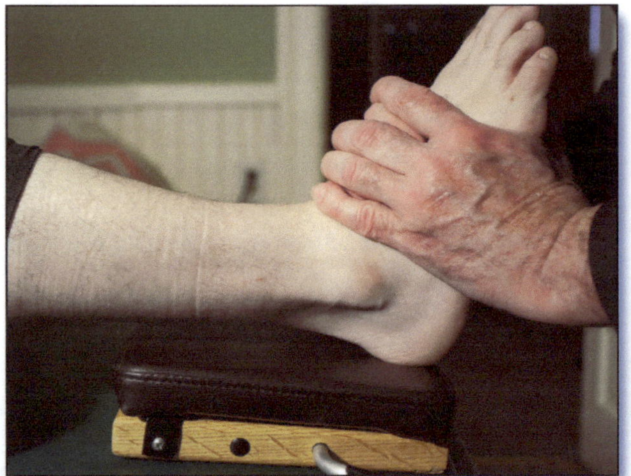

FIG. 10-11A. ADJUSTING THE POSTERIOR CALCANEUS OR ANTERIOR TALUS ON THE DROP PIECE.

The calcaneus is placed on the adjusting piece with the hand on the foot; the thrust is down into the drop piece. This setup can be used on an anterior talus or a posterior calcaneus.

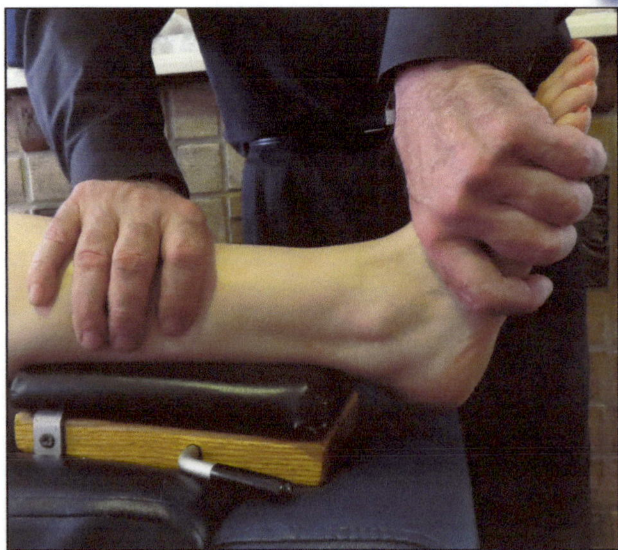

FIGURE 10-11B ADJUSTING THE ANTERIOR TALUS ON THE DROP PIECE

Place the end of the lower leg on the edge of the drop piece, with the foot hanging off the drop piece. Drop on the foot with it in a neutral position to the leg.

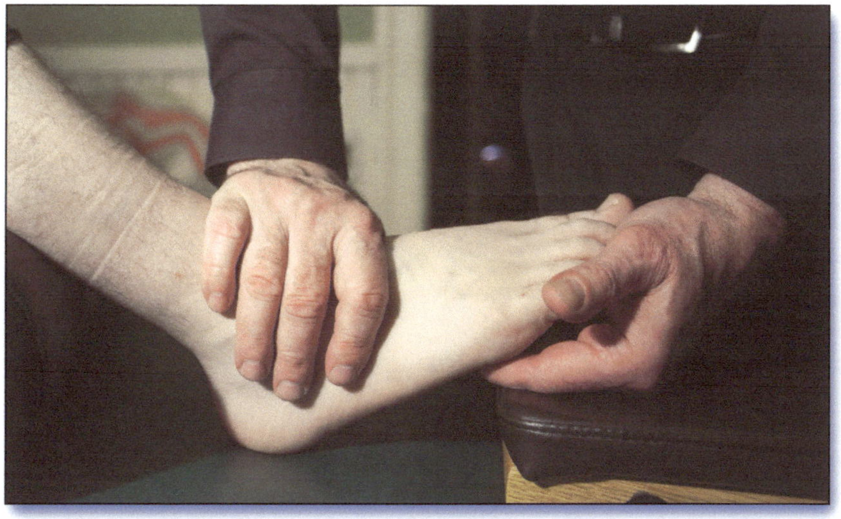

FIGURE 10-12. THE SUPINE ADJUSTING OF THE MID-FOOT

The Doctor's fingers are held in a rigid curled position contacting the inferior part of the base of the metatarsals, while the other hand contacts the top of the cuneiform and drops.

Posterior and Lateral Calcaneus: *Set the back of the heel on the drop piece and roll the foot externally ten to 15 degrees. Grip the talus and mid-foot and drop towards the drop piece. Repeat. (See Figure 10-10.)*

ADJUSTING THE MID-FOOT PRONE POSITION

Inferior metacarpals: *place the top of the foot on the drop piece, with the cuneiforms at the edge and the foot hanging off the drop piece. Contact the base of metatarsals, on the plantar surface, just distal to the cuneiforms. Drop. Repeat. (See Figures 10-12 and 10-13.)*

Inferior cuboid or navicular: *place the foot and ankle on the drop piece with the cuboid or navicular just off the edge. Contact the plantar surface each and drop.*

Please note all the procedures should be gentle and firm. Don't expect the first drop to complete the correction.

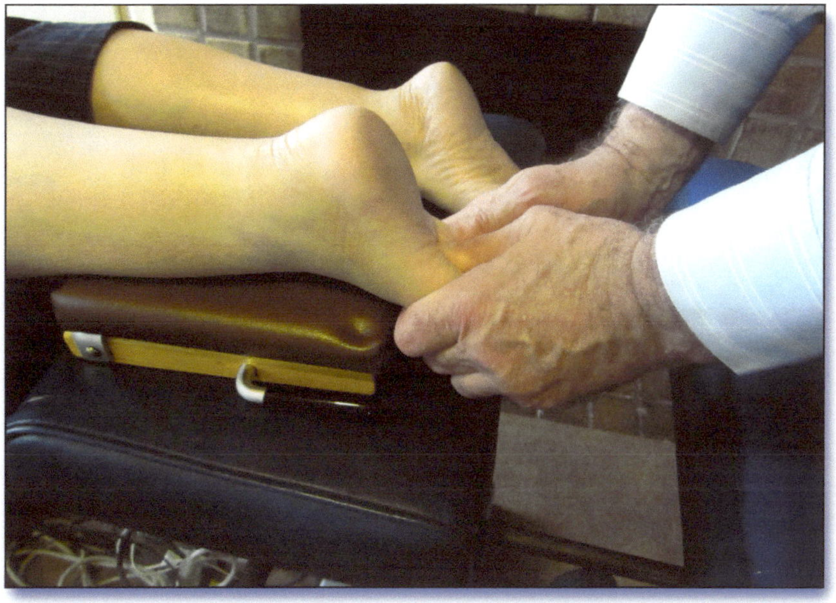

FIGURE 10-13. PRONE ADJUSTING OF THE MID-FOOT

Note the foot is placed with the superior cuneiforms on the top edge of the adjusting piece, while the doctor's thumbs are on the proximal metatarsals. Thrust is down toward the drop piece.

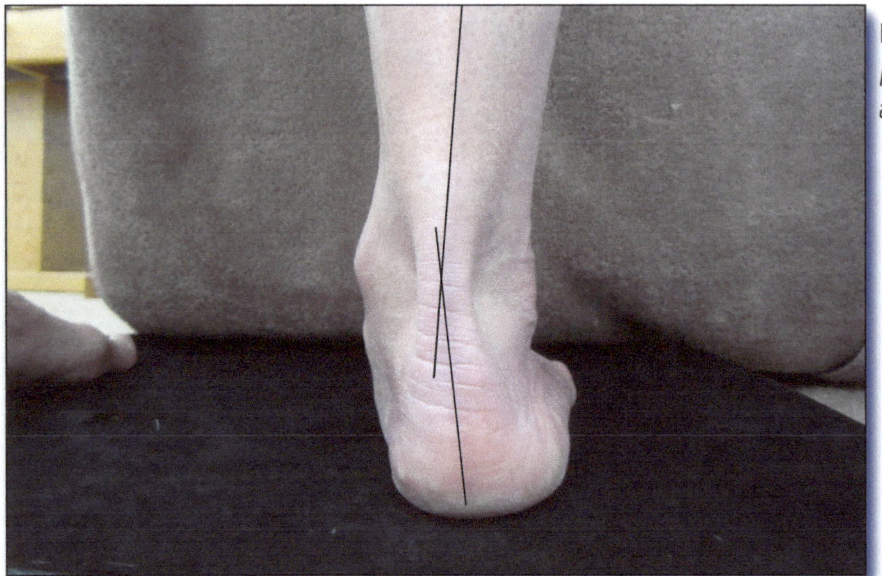

FIGURE 10-14 THE LATERAL AND POSTERIOR CALCANEUS

Note the lateral displacement of the heel bone the angle between the medial and lateral malleolus

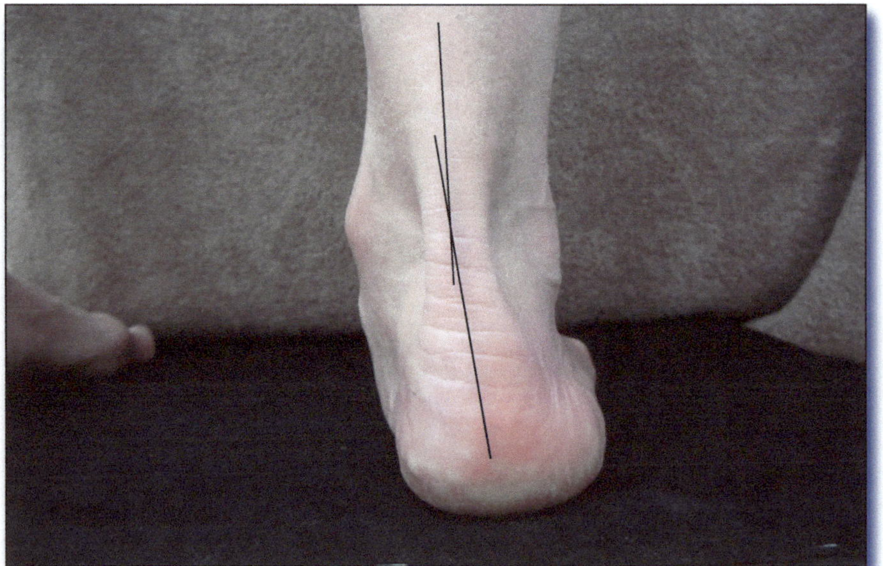

FIGURE 10-15 THE ADJUSTED CALCANEUS

Note the slight decrease in angle of the Achilles Tendon

Foot and Ankle videos:
https://youtu.be/GIhtj-7ViV4
https://youtu.be/BSiXeZlxnxM
https://youtu.be/eSplLgk_Ne8
https://youtu.be/522bz1mI-5g
https://youtu.be/kEhpkFUqsYo

TAPING, BRACING, ORTHOTICS AND FOOTWEAR

Any support to provide structural integrity is important.

Taping Protocols

Taping can be very helpful for flare-ups of chronic cases

- *Posterior/lateral calcaneus*
- *Lateral calcaneus*
- *Posterior talus*
- *Anterior talus*

Bracing

- *The Figure-8 brace*
- *So many types available*

Orthotics

- *Make an orthotic for extreme cases.*
- *There are so many types available.*
- *The normal architecture of the foot should be restored before the impression for the orthotic is made*

Footwear: The New Zealand Study

- *An athletic shoe company sponsored seminar on lower extremity problems.*
- *The doctor should be the advocate for the injured foot, not shoe designers.*
- *Good footwear treats the foot like Mother Earth and absorbs the heel strike.*

Taping, bracing, orthotics and good footwear are part of what most people need to recover from a foot injury. At the very least, good footwear must be discussed with patients. A lot of foot problems are a combination of misplaced joints, inflamed soft tissues and an altered gait. Chronic foot problems will usually involve altered or misshapen footwear, which is another indication of the need to have a multifaceted approach to the problem.

To start the intervention, the adjusting is absolutely essential. This is followed by the taping of the foot and ankle. Different subluxation patterns require a different taping pattern. I use a firm tape called "Tensoplast." I had one patient call it "duct tape for the body." I don't use Kinesio or similar tape because it's too stretchy. The Tensoplast is pretty tough and can be kept on for a few days and will survive hot showers, if they are brief. It will come off in a hot bath. I have taught patients to tape themselves. It has been a lifesaver for some who have traveled internationally for weeks and who need that stability the tape gives them.

In all these protocols, the base wrap is not applied tightly. We are not trying to squeeze the foot. The base wrap in all these protocols is just gently placed on the foot and wrapped completely, so the tape has a fair amount of contact with itself.

Bracing the foot and ankle is the next thing I do after taping. Some people can't handle the tape because of dermal responses. The braces last longer and can be self-applied easier than the tape. The most common brace I use is a "figure-8 brace". It is good for most ankle sprains and easy to put on and remove. There are so many other types of braces that I can't stock all of them in my office. We have catalogs full of them, and occasionally there are braces available at Walgreens and Rite Aid that are cheaper than anything I can get in my catalogs. The patient and I will go over the pictures of the braces in the catalog and then they can go out and buy one in ten minutes at the corner drugstore.

Orthotics can be essential for maintaining the proper foot architecture. In extreme cases, I will make an orthotic for the patient and tape it to their foot. By "extreme case," I mean swelling and pitting edema that is so severe the patient can't wear shoes. They usually have a shuffling gait and it will be assumed that this is congestive heart failure or diabetic neuropathy. It is tough to evaluate the completely swollen limb but with care, it can be done. Most the time, there is no arch and the heel bone is out of place, as is the ankle bone. So I will make an orthotic out of orthopedic felt and tape and make an arch support that has an exaggerated appearance and tape it to their bare foot. Of course, adjusting the subluxated joints is essential to this process. But in the cases I've seen that were extreme, within seven to ten days, the patient has had normal appearing feet and the edema has dissipated.

Orthotics for more normal cases are readily available. My concern is that the impression for your orthotic may be made with a subluxated foot. I think the impression for the orthotic should be made with a foot free of subluxation patterns. I will tape the foot after adjusting, then have the taped foot used to make the impression for the orthotic.

Footwear can be a real problem. Most of the time the patients present with footwear that will not help us solve their foot and ankle problems. I have a fair amount of doctors, nurses and therapists as patients and we have to have serious conversations about what they're doing to their feet with their shoes and other forms of footwear.

Because I deal with people with multiple health problems, I am routinely telling people to walk more. This is tough to do with painful feet, injured legs and lousy footwear. I recommend boots, usually lace-up, to protect the ankle and foot. In 1990, New Zealand's National Defense Forces Boot Camp did an experiment with athletic shoes versus boots. Fifteen hundred recruits got the standard issued boots and the other 1500 got athletic shoes. The athletic shoe group was plagued with foot and ankle injuries throughout the three-month boot camp. Hardly any problems occurred with the group wearing boots.

Years ago, I went to a seminar on lower extremity problems sponsored by Nike and Reebok. They were absolutely grilled by the doctors in attendance. They admitted under harsh questioning that athletic shoes lose 50 percent of their original supportive qualities after 800 miles. This is before signs of visual wear. If you are active and either running or walking, as part of your health regimen, 800 miles comes pretty quickly. For most of us, it would be three or four months. They admitted that when the shoes look worn that they are at less than 20 percent of their original supportive qualities. Boots will last a whole lot longer, and are not that much more expensive than your average athletic shoes. Needless to say, I never saw them do this type of seminar again.

I'm often running into the issue of unacceptable footwear for female patients. I always have to say the doctor is the advocate for the injured foot, not your fashion statement. I've had patients come to chiropractic care because the podiatrist was going to make them wear a boot, and it wasn't going to go with any of their outfits. So it was unacceptable.

Good footwear treats your feet like Mother Earth would: absorbing your heel strike. Most of us in this country live in a paved environment. So I recommend walking on earth as part of anyone's health regimen. When you can't do that, the footwear must treat your feet like the Earth does, and absorb your heel strike.

TAPING FOR THE SUBLUXATED HEEL BONE (CALCANEUS)

The calcaneus subluxation can cause plantar fascitis and heel pain, and also knee, hip and groin pain. The lateral and posterior calcaneus, is common and a source of debilitating pain. (*See Figure 10-14.*)

Adjusting the calcaneus is done to correct both the lateral and posterior components of the subluxation pattern. The adjusting of the calcaneus (*see Figure 10-14*) can make only a slight difference in an advanced case. This is why the taping procedures can be helpful. We will have to do two taping procedures, one for the lateral component and one the posterior component. (*See Figures 10-16 and 10-18.*)

Taping for Posterior Calcaneus

We will start with the posterior taping. An anchor is placed around the mid-foot. It is not tight, do not squeeze the foot. (*See Figure 10-16.*) The posterior wrap is started on the lateral side of the foot and brought around the back of the heel and cut short of the anchor. The posterior wrap is pulled firmly towards the toes and secured to the mid-foot with an outer anchor. (*See Figure 10-17*)

Taping for Lateral Calcaneus

The taping for the lateral component of the subluxated heel is started with an anchor at the lower end of the leg (*see Figure 10-18*). The lateral wrap is started on the lateral side of the foot, brought under the heel and is cut short of the anchor. (*See Figure 10-18.*) The lateral wrap is then pulled firmly up the leg towards the hip to the end of the anchor and then secured to the leg with an outer anchor. (*See Figure 10-19.*) These two procedures should help correct the subluxations and improve proper weight bearing and mechanics. (*See Figure 10-20.*) Note the improved alignment of the heel to the leg – please compare Figures 10-22 and 10-15.

This taping can be done over sheer or other thin tight stockings if there is skin sensitivity to the adhesive to the tape. Again, we use Tensoplast tape, which can be kept on for days and worn while showering.

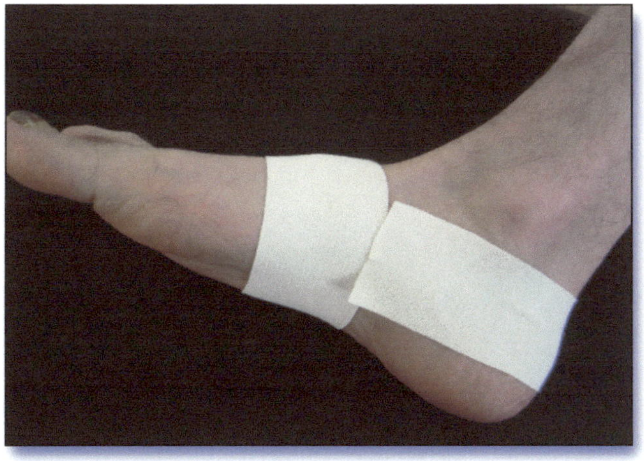

FIGURE 10-16 TAPING FOR A POSTERIOR CALCANEUS

Note the anchor around the mid-foot. The posterior wrap is cut short of the anchor.

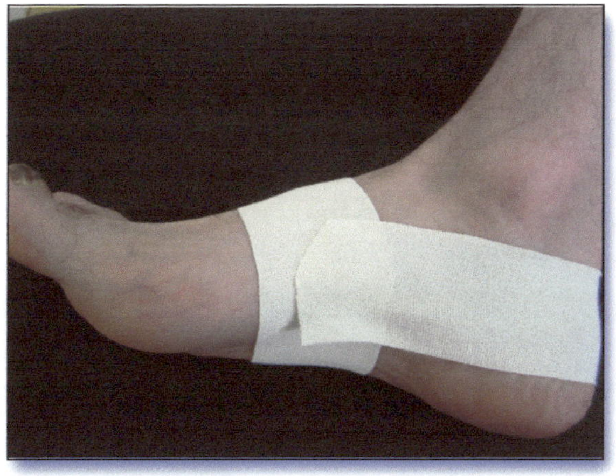

FIGURE 10-17 THE MEDIAL VIEW OF FOOT TAPING FOR A POSTERIOR CALCANEUS

Note the posterior wrap has been pulled forward onto the anchor and another, outer anchor, will be applied

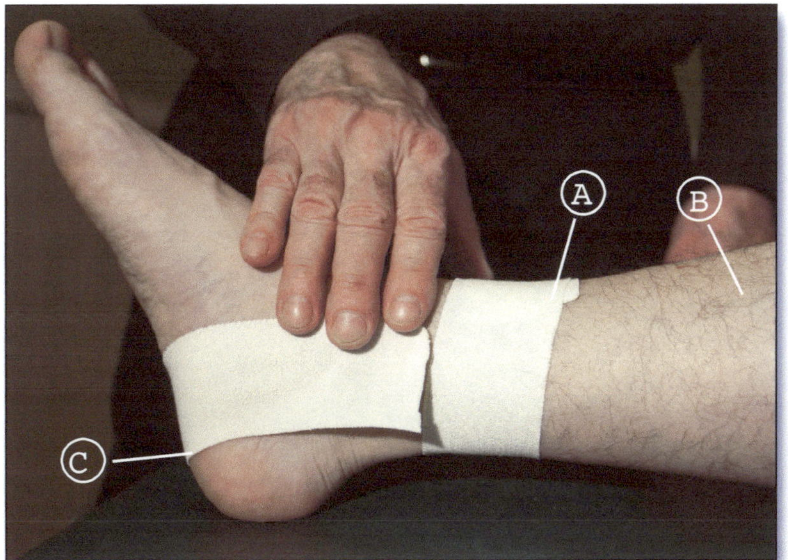

FIGURE 10-18 TAPING FOR A LATERAL CALCANEUS

The posterior wrap is cut short of the anchor.

A. Anchor around lower leg

B. Leg

C. Lateral wrap

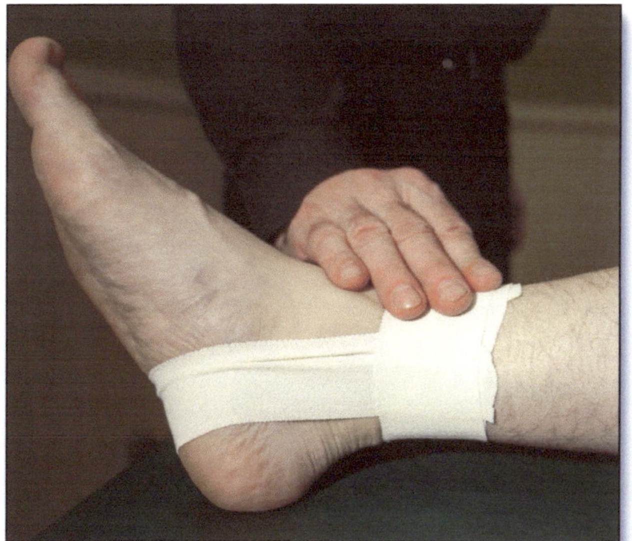

FIGURE 10-19 THE MEDIAL VIEW OF FOOT WITH COMPLETED TAPING FOR A LATERAL CALCANEUS

Note the lateral wrap has been pulled up onto the end of the anchor and another, outer anchor, has been applied

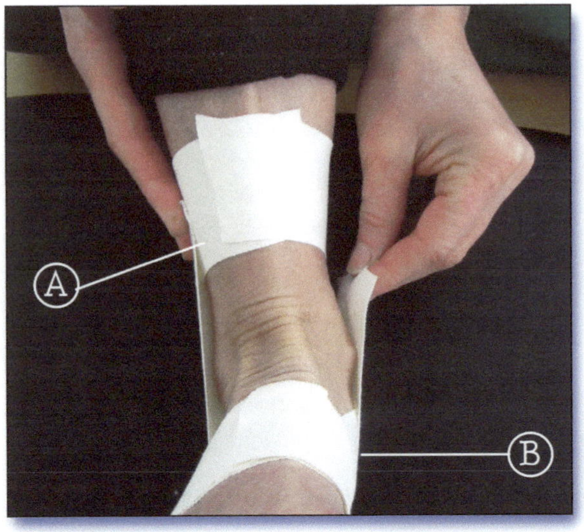

FIGURE 10-20 TAPING FOR A LATERAL CALCANEUS

Note the anchor on the lower leg, 4″ above the ankle, the lateral wrap is applied from lateral to medial, under the calcaneus and cut short of the anchor

A. Anchor on lower leg

B. Lateral wrap starting on the lateral side of the leg

FIGURE 10-21 THE MEDIAL VIEW OF COMPLETED LATERAL AND POSTERIOR CALCANEUS TAPING

The lateral wrap was stretched to cover the inner anchor and another outer anchor has been applied

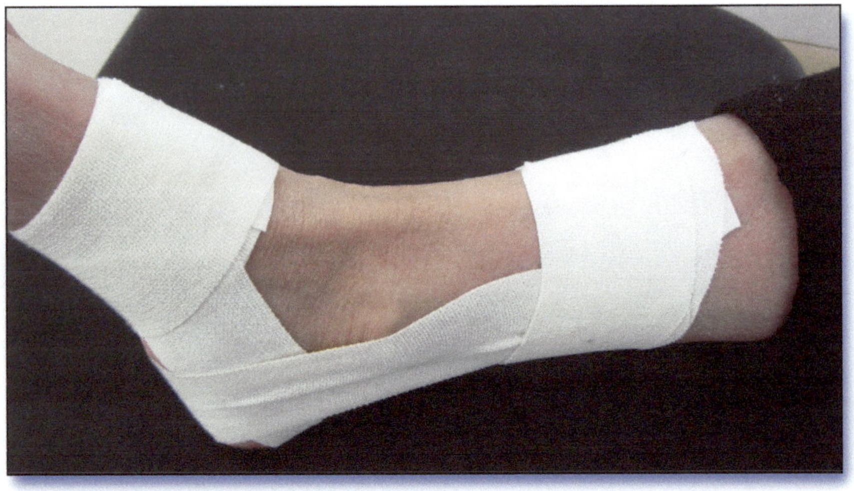

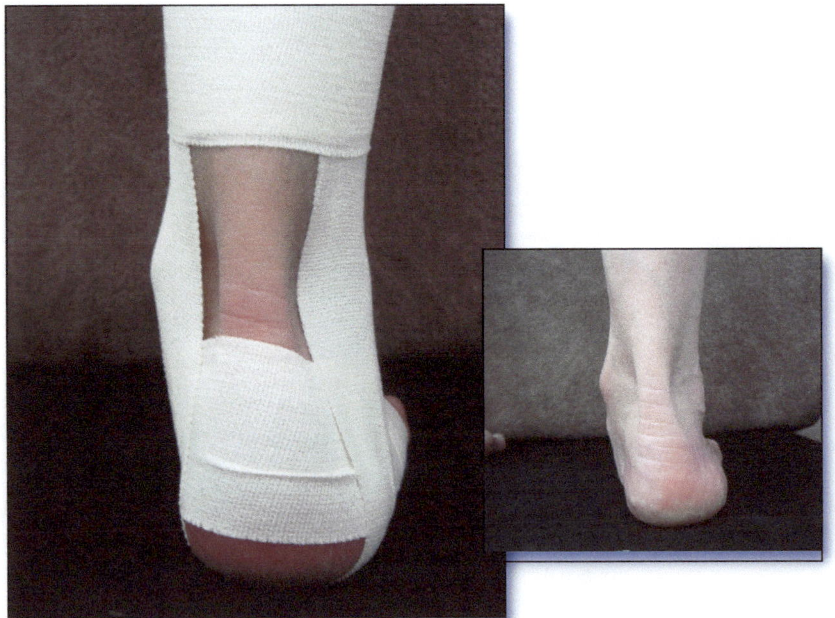

FIGURE 10-22 THE TAPED HEEL WEIGHT BEARING

Note the improved alignment of the heel to the leg and how the maleolei are more level — see (repeated) Figure 10-15 inset at right.

CHAPTER ELEVEN

Evaluating, Adjusting and Managing The Effects of Traumatic Brain Injury and Stroke

This chapter is about the chiropractic care for patients who have suffered traumatic brain injuries and/or strokes. I know there is a branch of chiropractic involving neurological diagnoses and treatments using and focusing on the brain. The protocols discussed here have to do with the additional injuries that are common with traumatic brain injuries and strokes. I am assuming the patient is stable from the events that caused their major health problems. The best way I can illustrate this is by discussing a few case histories.

Case 1 : Childhood Brain Injury (?)

The first case history involves a 26-year-old patient with an obvious gait impairment (*see Figure 11-1*). She had a brace on her left leg, which she used in a swing gait when she walked. She was run over by car when she was four years old, unconscious for five days and then after stabilization was transported to a large rehab facility for a year. She spent the next five years in a wheelchair and after that was fitted for the leg brace. She knows the term "upper motor neuron lesion." She knows the phrase "positive Babinski's." She used both those terms on the intake form and during the examination procedure. She also notes that she has to urinate five to six times an hour, and when she is on public transportation, she has to wear adult diapers

Upon examination, I found that her left pubic bone is so posterior that I could feel the whole inside of her right pubic bone. Her sacrum was significantly rotated to the left. I found her left tibia to be posterior to the femur by more than half an inch. This subluxation pattern caused a permanent bend or angle of her left knee at 15 degrees. She could not extend her knee. She had little ability to further bend her knee but she could only extend it as far as the 15 degrees. Her gastrocnemius and Achilles tendon were extremely rigid and her left foot was in a significant and rigid plantar flexion without the brace. The entire leg musculature was hard. There was no flaccid paralysis about her leg at all. My question was: is this truly paralysis?

I also found that I could put my thumb underneath the mortise joint of the lower leg on the left, which meant her talus or her whole foot had moved posteriorly to the leg. Her left big toe was raised. When you stroked the underside of her raised left big toe, it quivered. This is what is described as a "positive Babinski's." I took her lower leg in one hand and her foot in the other hand and I drew the foot forward relative to the leg. Her big toe dropped to a normal position. Then I stroked the underside of her big toe. There was no quivering. So the question I have is: can peripheral entrapment syndromes mimic upper motor neuron lesions? (The answer is "Yes.")

Her bladder problems were blamed on the brain injury and not the pelvic girdle subluxation pattern. To put her leg brace on every morning, she would sit down in a chair and put the brace on the floor in front of her, place her leg and foot into the brace, lean forward and press her leg and plantar flexed foot into the brace and attach it to herself with Velcro straps. She had welts on her leg and foot from the straps. This does not appear to be your classic "foot drop" case where there is a flaccid paralysis and a floppy foot. Her whole hip, and foot were rigid. I began by adjusting her pelvis, knee, and foot – and she got up off the table and started to walk with hip flexion, knee extension, toe rise and heel strike. It was still an obvious altered gait. But the lateral swing phase of her gait was gone.

She turned to me and said, "I want to talk to Oprah!," and burst into tears and did a face-plant on my chest. Within two weeks, her bladder problem was gone. I later took her to the monthly meeting of the "Brain Injury Support Group of the East Bay." We had her tell her story. Afterwards, I asked the 20 people in the meeting, "How many of you feel you had multiple injuries at the time your head was traumatized?" They all raised their hands. I then asked, "How many of you feel those additional injuries are being written off as manifestations of your head injuries?" They all kept their hands up. I then asked, "How many of you feel you would benefit from evaluations of the additional injuries?" Their hands stayed up.

Next I did a study of the brain-injured group and found that every single one of them had injuries that were interfering with their functioning and quality of life. A neuropsychologist, (like the doctor running the support group), typically will not evaluate all of the additional injuries.

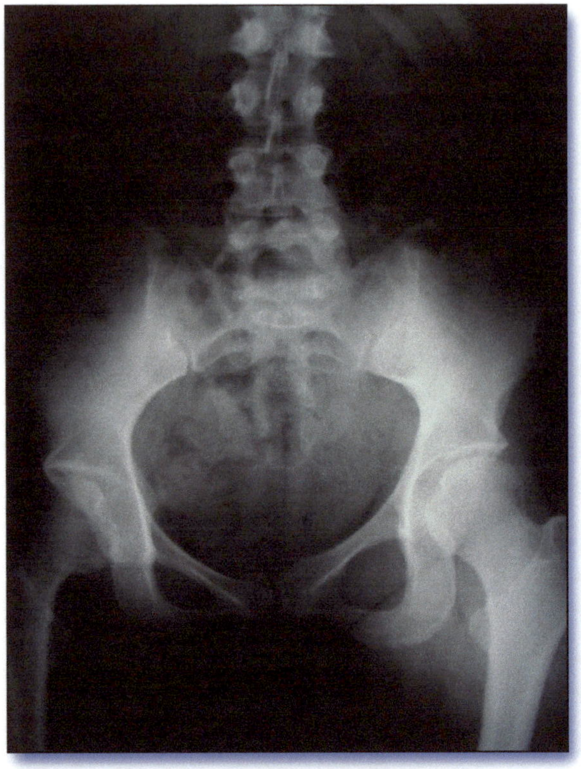

FIGURE 11-1 AP X-RAY LUMBOPELVIC VIEW

Patient had "foot-drop", bladder dysfunction, and was diagnosed with TBI. Resolved with chiropractic care.

Case 2: Marilyn

One case history in particular characterizes the group. Marilyn was in the front passenger seat of a car that got hit by a truck that lost its brakes. The windshield came in contact with her head and her knees contacted the dashboard as the car was crushed. Her inability to walk properly and straighten her knees was blamed on her head injury. No one evaluated her knee injuries and her complaints of difficulty walking, especially up and down stairs. The second floor of her house, where her bedroom is, was completely unused by her since the accident. Chiropractic care got her upstairs again and she was able to reduce her medications enough to regain her mental focus and energy, and went back to work.

Case 3: Female Stroke Victim

This patient came to me as a patient six months after the stroke. Her right hand and forearm were swollen, blue and rigid, causing her significant pain. The pain meds were keeping her dull and listless, but they were not affecting the pain. I found her rib cage subluxated on the right side, her clavicular joints were both out of place, her humerus was at a grade two dislocation and her ulna was also significantly subluxated. The muscles of her whole right pectoral girdle were rock hard. She couldn't move anything, so it was called paralysis. I think this is a mistake. When the muscles are rock hard, there is motor firing, thus it cannot be true paralysis. The subluxation patterns were causing the muscles to be guarding and therefore rigid.

It took 45 minutes to adjust everything and restore the circulation and motion to her hand and arm. The swelling, blueness and rigidity were gone within moments of restoring the multiple joint displacement patterns to normal. She could flex her fingers and shake my hand when we were done. The problem is managing such cases: between the medications and the stroke itself, a patient might have little ability to be a full participant in her recovery and rehabilitation. Since this is not always the case, each patient has to be evaluated.

Case 4: John

A few years ago a long time patient's son had a stroke. He was 48 years old, over weight-- not in good shape. He was diagnosed with an irregular heart beat and given a "blood thinner" that has a nasty side affect of causing clotting. She called me because he was in so much pain on his left side. We did a home visit to assess him and see if he could tolerate care. His left rib cage, clavicle (both proximal and distal) were out of alignment. His humerus was mildly dislocated, his ulna was also misaligned causing part of his hand pain. He had pain down the whole left arm and shoulder. He had been given stretching exercises that were contraindicated for this type of injury, making him worse.

We started with midline subluxations first, *see Figure 11-2*. The patient was on his side, affected side up, while his rib cage was adjusted. When the ribs are in place, the arm and shoulder are easier to move. This allows for less pain in the arm so that care of the arm and shoulder is more comfortable. Note that adjustments of the shoulder and elbow are done with very specific, isolated gentle maneuvers (*See Figure 11-3*). When working on the shoulder you must be mindful that it is connected to an unstable shoulder. A rib belt was applied to his chest when all the adjusting was done (*See Figure 11-4*). He was at that time "out of pain". He had follow up care with 90% recovery. He has been back to work, but not at the pace he had before, which he says was "nuts."

This chapter will be somewhat repetitive and like the previous chapters. I feel it is important for you, the doctor, not to be intimidated by the terms "traumatic brain injury" or "stroke." These patients deserve a full evaluation of all the adverse effects of traumatic brain injury and stroke. When taking the case history of the

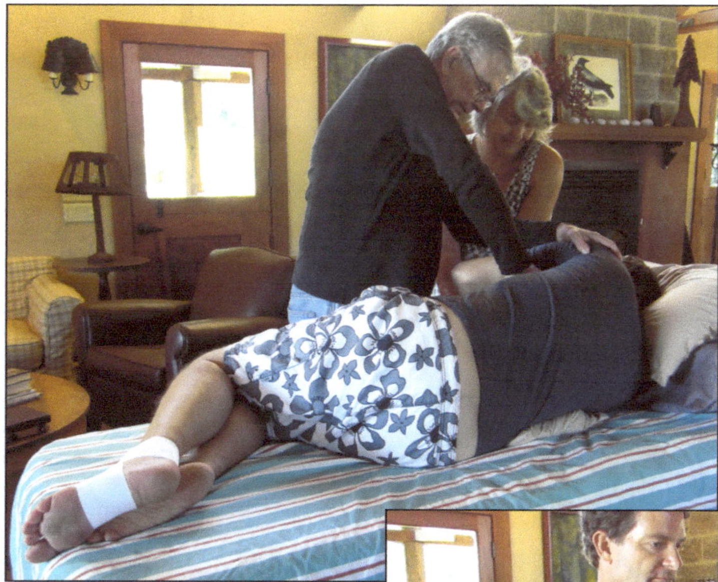

FIGURE 11-2 RIB ADJUSTMENT OF STROKE VICTIM

Stroke victim with affected side up having ribs adjusted with the SLI.

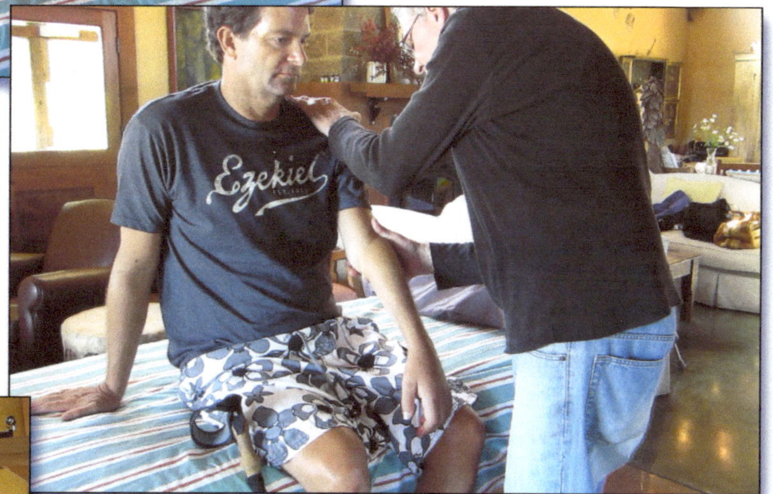

FIGURE 11-3 SHOULDER ADJUSTMENT OF STROKE VICTIM

Patient having left shoulder adjusted

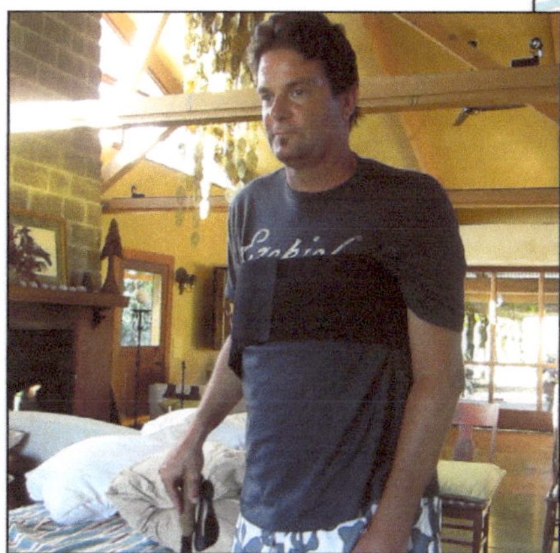

FIGURE 11-4 POST ADJUSTING

Patient has been adjusted and has 6" rib belt on holding the ribs in place. At this point he said "I am out of pain". This brace is no longer needed because of recovery.

TBI patient, it is usually apparent that most of them had multiple injuries occur at the time their head was traumatized. Please evaluate fully all of their complaints and injuries.

A stroke is a discrete event in the brain that affects the motor function of usually one side of the body. In my opinion, the event not only affects the muscles, but also affects the ligaments. I believe that ligaments have a tone that is a neurological phenomenon. When the wave of the neurological event sweeps through the brain, it will affect the muscles as well as the ligaments. So joints can and usually do fall apart, involving mostly the upper body, including the rib cage, clavicles, shoulders, elbows and wrists. The spine can also be affected, especially if there is a history of previous spinal trauma and arthritic changes. If there is a recovery from the stroke, the muscles will start to function again and become more toned. In this awakening process, the displaced or subluxated joints will be perceived by the nervous system, and the neuromuscular guarding reflex initiated by the spinal cord will go into effect and lock everything up to try to preserve stability. That's why stroke victims will frequently have twisted limbs and dysfunctional conditions.

One of the reasons I've put stroke and traumatic brain injury together is that there is a wide variation in how a stroke affects a person and how a traumatic brain injury affects a person. Both conditions are primarily events adversely affecting the brain and the effects are unique to that individual. But what is common to both conditions are the peripheral injuries and distress patterns that I find in a full examination. No matter how extensive or mild a stroke or traumatic brain injury might be, trying to recover with dislocated shoulders, subluxated knees and the associated muscle contractions makes full recovery very difficult and challenging, if not impossible.

Another feature of strokes and brain injuries is reduced blood flow to and from the brain. So the chiropractic care should be focused on realigning the occiput and the upper cervical vertebrae, and addressing all of the injuries that are affecting the patient. If we assume that the condition we find the patient in is totally related to the brain, then the patient is being underserved. Full recovery would include proper proprioceptive input from the periphery into the aligned spine that has optimum blood flow to and from the cranium. This can only happen with a full assessment of all the patient's injuries.

TBI AND STROKE VICTIMS SHARE COMMON FEATURES: NEGLECT OF THE ADDITIONAL INJURIES.

- *Traumatic Brain Injury (TBI) victims have, almost certainly, mechanisms of injury that include other parts of their bodies. These additional injuries are assumed to be manifestations of the brain injury. Usually no one evaluates the additional complaints.*
- *Stroke victims can be suffering from a multiple joint dysfunction that is related to the stroke. The therapy for these patients focuses on the NON-stroke side. So the joint dysfunction that results from the stroke is neglected.*
- *A stroke will affect the muscular tone and function, but will also affect the ligaments. Ligaments have tone and this will be lost in a vascular event.*
- *Upper cervical care is needed to optimize the blood flow to and from the brain*

TBI patients all have unique experiences and adverse responses to the events they have suffered. I've had patients that have made a full recovery. Cognitive function and executive function were not affected in these individuals, thankfully. Their entire complaints were actually spinal subluxation and peripheral subluxation, including the rib cage and pelvis. A resolution of these injuries resulted in full recovery, leaving the patient and myself wondering how much actual brain injury occurred with the trauma. Any loss of consciousness including memory can preclude you from having a full examination of your injuries. This sounds fairly ridiculous, but I'm just reporting what I've found with more than three dozen TBI patients over the years. So if anyone comes into your chiropractic office reporting a traumatic brain injury, please do them the courtesy of examining all of their complaints and their entire body. As I jokingly say, they didn't leave anything home on the day of their traumatic brain injury.

Stroke victims can be suffering from multiple joint dysfunctions related to the stroke. The therapy for these patients focuses on the non-stroke affected side. Medicare will not approve therapy for the stroke-affected side, and most insurance companies follow suit. So the therapy that is used is focused on strengthening the good side and training in becoming one-handed or one-legged in their activities of daily living.

A stroke will affect the muscular tone of the affected tissues but will also affect ligaments. I observe that ligaments have tone and this tone will be lost, at least temporarily, with a stroke. This will allow parts of the body to subluxate. These patients can present with a flaccid paralysis of various parts of their body. This might change over time as the brain recovers. If neurological function returns to the periphery and the joints are out of place, the muscles will respond with a neuromuscular guarding reflex from the spinal cord. It is very likely the musculature involved will be rigid and there will be minimal to no motion. There is commonly a severe pain pattern usually not relieved by the medications. This can be agony for the patient. My finding is that rock-hard muscles have motor firing, which is good in the context of paralysis. My job is to find what structures are causing the neuromuscular guarding reflex of the spinal cord and to relieve the joint distress. If the rigid muscles are the result of peripheral joint dysfunction, they will frequently respond quickly to the relief of the joint dysfunction.

Almost every victim of these conditions has upper cervical needs. I can go into the adverse affects of subluxations of the upper cervical spine, but I covered that subject already in Chapter 4. The brain's full recovery, or as much recovery as possible, can be limited by reduced blood flow to and from the brain. I keep saying "from the brain" because I think that 'venous stasis' is common in post-TBI and stroke. I also think it is common in motor vehicle accidents and other injuries to the upper body. This can lead to confusion, inability to focus, "brain fog," insomnia and irritability. Care to the whole upper body is critical, including the rib cage and clavicles. I am of the opinion that you could have the best upper cervical care and if the ribs and clavicles are subluxated, then the sternocleidomastoid and levator scapulae will pull everything back out of place with weight bearing and daily activities. This opinion is part of the reason for examining and assessing every part of the body.

EVALUATION

> *Evaluate everything. Focus on the rib cage, sternoclavicular joints and costosternal joints to optimize blood flow to and from the head, especially if swallowing and vocalization are issues.*

> *Upper extremity function will be impaired by a rib cage injury. Brachial plexus, subclavian artery (and their rami) entrapment is common with both conditions.*

> *Lower extremity problems are common with both conditions. All joints should be inspected for ligament integrity and alignment.*

> *Rigid paralysis common in stroke should be considered a neuromuscular response to joint subluxation. There is motor firing, so make use of it!*

ADJUSTING THE TBI PATIENT

> *At a first examination, the patient can be very frail. If there is a rib cage injury and instability is found, avoid prone positions.*

> *Initially, the Spring Loaded Instrument (SLI) should be used.*

> *The previous chapters in this book will provide the various adjusting protocols.*

ADJUSTING THE STROKE VICTIM

> *Adjusting the ridged patient: start with the rib cage, get the stretching off the neurovascular bundles in the axilla and clavicular region. Get the humerus and ulna back in place. The same protocols are used for the lower body.*

> *The other adjusting protocols are covered in the previous chapters in this book.*

MANAGING THE TBI AND STROKE PATIENT

> *Assessing cognitive function is paramount*

> *The length of time from the event plays a big factor in recovery. The sooner the chiropractic intervention, the better the chances for recovery.*

> *It might be impossible, initially, to tell which of the injuries will recover and which*

might be permanent impairments.

- *With TBI, some joint injuries might completely recover. Remember that some injuries were concomitant injuries with the brain injury, but not affected by the brain injury.*
- *Mobility, mobility, mobility. The therapeutic goal is to get everything moving again, as that will positively affect the brain, as well as the injured joints.*
- *Hydrotherapy can be very helpful to some of these patients. Restoring normal motion in the water can be the beginning of normal motion without the support of the water.*
- *Beware of previous providers' (especially MDs & PTs) exercises and stretches, attitudes and notions.*

In managing the traumatic brain injury and stroke patient, cognitive function is critical for a full recovery. Basic assessment techniques should be used to evaluate the condition of the patient. Sometimes, it's really clear that they are not totally present. If that's the case, then the providers and family members have to be brought in to assist with the case and therapy. Sometimes, the patient has full cognitive function present but there is no drive to improve. I have had some patients that are like this, and from talking to family members, the opinion is that there never was any drive to stay fit or conditioned. If that's the pre-event personality, then full participation in rehabilitation is unlikely. It is really nice to work with fully cognitive patients that have a great desire to recover and will do everything and more to improve themselves.

The length of time from the date of the event to your contact is critical. If decades have passed, then contracture and permanent peripheral nerve damage will have developed. An ulna that's been out of place for a long time can be impossible to realign because of the contracture of the tendons of the biceps and triceps. Anatomical studies show that chronic deformation of nerves causes the nerves to become fibrotic. Persistent mechanical tension can change the histology of the tissue, including the nerves. This would stop nerve conduction. Your goal is to keep that from happening by having an early intervention.

I've had some TBI patients make full recoveries. This again reinforces my view that every part of the body must be assessed. I have found most injuries were concomitant to the brain injury, but were not caused by the brain injury. I feel this is one of the common mistakes with these types of patients: the assumption that the brain is the main and only injury.

Mobility is so important that it's hard to overstate. A study at Duke University years ago showed that depression, when measured by brain scans, can change with regular physical activity. In fact, it beat the pharmacology that is generally used to treat depression. So the assessment of TBI and stroke patients is to be thorough, and our goal in that effort is to restore normal alignment and motion. Sometimes, the easiest part is restoring the alignment and it's harder to manage its recovery because you have a person involved! People can be unpredictable and tell you one thing, yet do something different. So I recommend multiple daily exercise sessions. These would be very short sessions initially with gradual incremental increases and after three to six months, a fair amount of time should be spent in activity.

Hydrotherapy can be very helpful for some of these patients. Restoring normal motion in the water can be the beginning of normal motion without the support of the water. This is especially true when there are lower extremity injuries, pelvic girdle instability, balance problems and some kinds of pain that will benefit from warm water. Easily half my patients will not do hydrotherapy. They don't like the chlorine, they don't want to get a bathing suit or many other problems, like expense and transportation. But those that have gotten into the pool have gotten positive results from it and it greatly adds to their conditioning. Usually, there are other people in the pool in similar conditions and sometimes, there are classes they can get involved with. The buddy system can really be helpful. The studies on this show that buddies keep each other motivated and sticking to the regimen.

Previous providers, most commonly MDs and physical therapists, will have given the patient exercises and stretches that need to be reviewed, modified or eliminated from the routine. Unstable joints with ligament damage don't seem to be one of the diagnostic observations that are made by these providers. Pain is viewed as caused by a lack of exercise, yet there is little evidence to support this since few people exercise on a regular basis and this doesn't seem to lead people to terrible pain patterns. Again, all exercises and stretches should be reviewed to make sure that your work to align the subluxated joints is not hindered by the therapeutic attempts to stretch things further out of place. For example: tight pectoralis muscles will be stretched with the arm behind the door frame and the patient moving forward pulling on their chest. If the tight pectoralis muscle is from costosternal joint subluxation, then the stretching is adding to the cycle of tightness and inflammation of the chest wall, affecting the shoulder, head and upper cervical spine adversely.

Additionally, previous providers, including family members, can have attitudes and assumptions that, because the brain has been affected, there is no recovery possible. So the chiropractor needs to be a source of positive input and the best prognosis has to include a good attitude in the recovery process.

BRACING AND TAPING

> *I am in favor of the use of braces to restore normal alignment and to promote activity.*

> *I have used taping for these patients, but this can be less effective because of bathing and hydrotherapy.*

> *The weight of the arm and shoulder (12 -24 lbs.) can pull the injured, unstable rib cage apart. Use a brace to keep this from occurring.*

> *Rib belts can be very useful.*

I've been surprised at how much recovery some patients can make and they have been a joy to work with. I always go back to a basic chiropractic principle: ***the body wants to heal.*** But it must be acknowledged that there are some injuries that will be permanent. We have to come up with ways to modify the effects of the injury and manage the injury for activities of daily living and work of our patients. So I use rib belts, low back braces, knee braces, shoulder braces, etc.

This notion is in conflict with a lot of my colleagues. When my patients have traveled and need care away from home, other practitioners take the braces away, saying they are concerned that the patient would become dependent on the brace. Yes, let me repeat that some of them might be dependent on the brace. But if the brace keeps them moving, out of pain and gives stability so that the ligaments have a chance to heal, then the brace is efficacious. I wear braces daily to work in my office. I have permanent injuries that I have to manage while I perform manual medical techniques.

I am not going to let my injuries interfere with my capacities as a doctor, or a householder. So I am dependent on my braces, due to the severity of my injuries, and I don't think that's anything to be ashamed of. That is the attitude that I try to convey to my patients.

Most people want to remain independent for as long as possible. Some patients cannot handle the braces for various reasons, and modifying them or using them in specific situations becomes necessary. I term it "prophylactic use," when the braces are used to prevent further joint injury during a specific activity – for instance, while driving a car – and then it is removed at the end of the activity. Some people get swelling and other adverse responses, including rashes, from a brace. This can complicate the managing of the injuries.

Taping can be very helpful, and is usually more temporary. Adverse dermal responses have to be expected at some point in patients with long-term problems. Most patients can handle five to eight tapings before the skin starts to become inflamed and irritated. We have to stop the taping at that point; a rash from the taping can be as painful as the joint dysfunction. The tape I use can be used in a brief hot shower and kept on for three or four days at a time. If the person is doing hydrotherapy or needs long bath time, then the tape will come off. So for some people, taping is a godsend and for others, it is not very helpful. It is one of those techniques that you have to try before you know if it's effective.

Bracing and supporting injured shoulders can be necessary for similar patients whose injuries have left the upper extremity joints unstable. Again, a patient's arm and shoulder can weigh between 12 and 24 or more pounds. If the rib cage joints are injured and unstable, if the AC joint is injured and unstable and the glenohumeral joint is injured and unstable, the weight of the arm and shoulder can be too heavy and cause pain.

There are many approaches to aid in the initial phases of recovery from these injuries. The braces I use are applied after all the adjusting has been performed.

Then I direct the patient to walk around the office for five minutes for a ligament stability test. Ligament stability is evaluated after the adjusting by having the patient perform normal walking motions and swinging his arms. If the joints fail after a brief period of normal weight bearing activity, then operating a motor vehicle and other activities of daily living will be a problem for the integrity of the joints. I use this approach to determine the need for the braces and possibly taping.

Bracing and taping of the shoulder and arm can be particularly challenging. The weight of the arm and shoulder varies among individuals and its gravitational pull on the clavicle, rib cage and spine can be excruciating for some patients. So using tape and braces to support the weight of the arm and shoulder can be very helpful, at least temporarily, for some patients. I find the "AC Splint" to be helpful when the distal clavicle joint is unstable. This brace has a component that comes across the top of the clavicle and can be cinched down to the patient's comfort. The shoulder sling is useful when there is glenohumeral joint instability. The Sully Brace is a sports device meant for keeping an athlete on the field. I have used this brace to keep myself in the office adjusting patients after I've had a car accident.

If a patient has positive signs of relief from the rib cage compression test, then using the rib belt should be considered. I apply the rib belt when the patient has taken a full deep breath, and then it is put on snugly, so it is snappily tight. I have a patient keep the brace on for five minutes or more. I direct them to walk around and then we take the brace off. And then they spend a few minutes without it, and are asked if they want the brace again. Ninety percent of the time they want the rib belt. If rib cage pain is keeping them awake at night, I recommend the use of the rib belt at night to facilitate sleep. The rib belt can be helpful for any of the neck or shoulder problems related to the modern injuries that I have been describing.

There are some innovative taping procedures for the upper body with new types of tape, and these can be very helpful. Please remember that taping for some people can only be temporary because of their dermal responses, so the taping must be monitored. Job descriptions and personal activities are part of the factors in prescribing these devices. Keeping somebody at work is of paramount importance and these devices can be helpful with this goal. The rib belt and the Sully Brace can be worn under the clothing and be completely inconspicuous.

In conclusion, I must advise that for a full recovery from any of these types of injuries, being clever, persistent and committed to recovery is necessary for both the patient and the doctor.

CHAPTER TWELVE

Evaluating, Adjusting and Managing the Spinal Cord-Injured Patient

This chapter describes the chiropractic care for patients with spinal cord injury. The focus is on evaluating, adjusting and managing the spinal cord injured patient. It is necessary to do a bit of a review of the anatomy and physiology of the spinal cord, including the biomechanics of the spinal cord. By biomechanics I mean the movement of the spinal cord.

My experience with the chiropractic college curriculum is that the biomechanics of the spinal cord are not covered. This is truly a shame because in my dealing with injured patients and their neurologists and neurosurgeons, the biomechanics of the spinal cord are not one of their concerns. Leaving the injured spinal cord stretched and immobile is not going to benefit anyone's neurological recovery. What I have discovered is that the care of the spinal cord injured person is dictated by their insurance reimbursement. After stabilizing the patient's injuries and vital signs, the patient is then put in a wheelchair. Mastering the wheelchair obstacle course becomes the prime therapeutic goal. This is not rehabilitation of the injured spinal cord. Also, there will be some of the same issues I've discussed in the previous chapter: the additional, concomitant neglected injuries that occurred at the time the spinal column was damaged and the spinal cord injured.

Impairment of any part of the body will be written off as manifestations of the spinal cord injury – without any inspection of those additional injuries. Patients will be trying to move their wheelchairs with dislocated shoulders or elbows, which adds to their pain and discomfort. Over years, the limited motion and contractures of these additional injuries will confirm in the minds of other providers that this is all part of the spinal cord injury.

I'm assuming that the chiropractor's first contact with the spinal cord injured patient is after they have been released from the hospital. They have been through the wheelchair obstacle course and have gained some proficiency in its use. Unless, of course, they are a total quadriplegic and need all the necessary assistance to travel about and get to the chiropractor's office. I make this assumption because the introduction to the hospitals to provide chiropractic care in the hospital setting has not been accomplished by the time this book went to publication. A lot of the techniques we have discussed and will discuss can be done in a hospital bed or rehabilitation center and also at the patient's home.

As with the stroke and TBI patient, family and staff support and understanding of the patient's needs are really critical. As with these other injuries, the person with a spinal cord injury must have some executive function left after the injury for chiropractic care to be of any more value than temporary palliative care. Which is not to say that's not necessary, since reducing someone's pain can be very important. But if the chiropractic care can increase function, then the patient's alertness and motivation to recover is essential for progress.

A SPINAL CORD INJURY CAN BE DEVASTATING

> *It is necessary to evaluate the patient body and emotions.*

> *Many additional injuries that occur simultaneously with the injury to the spine are neglected.*

> *Caring for the injured spinal cord is usually not appropriate.*

First, it should be said that a spinal cord injury is a serious and devastating injury. The chiropractor has to be able to handle the fallout of a patient's normal life being over and helping them through the various levels of recovery. This would include the psychological and emotional aspects of such a devastating injury. As chiropractors, we all have had to say things to patients to motivate them to co-manage their injuries for their optimum recovery. There has to be some personal responsibility and a willingness to work very hard to make even small improvements. I've had patients that can't do that, as they are too emotionally and psychologically devastated to be of much help to themselves, though they can participate in self-destructive behavior. I feel that these psychological problems are out of the scope of chiropractic practice. However, motivating your patient and helping them have a positive attitude can be a very important part of recovery.

Giving a patient hope that things will get better can appear from the outside to be an unrealistic or even suspicious impression. Yet, there have been many remarkable recoveries, and most of these cases involve someone with high spirits and hope, which can be essential components for any recovery.

So in assessing these patients, it must be thought that everything was injured in the event that damaged the vertebral column and spinal cord. Don't make any assumptions, except that everything is possibly injured with ligament instability throughout the body. One the main things to search for are peripheral entrapment syndromes that can mimic the central canal injury. An example of this is a patient I treated, a quadriplegic in a halo brace. Her rib cage was so subluxated that it tractioned or stretched the axial and brachial plexus to the point of no motor conduction to the upper extremity. This was assumed to be a manifestation of the spinal cord injury. The only assumption that should be made in evaluating a spinal cord injury patient is that there were many additional injuries that occurred at the time the spinal cord was injured. Next, we should know the spinal cord injury itself is not being treated properly. Care of the spinal cord injury is usually characterized by immobilization and a persistent stretching of the spinal tissue.

SPINAL REHABILITATION

> *"Spinal Rehabilitation" occurs after the patient is stable.*

> *This therapy is devoted to mastering the "Wheelchair Obstacle Course."*

> *The long-term studies on these patients usually show gradual neurological decline over the years.*

> *This is the expected outcome if the injured spinal tissue is persistently stretched and immobilized.*

What is spinal rehabilitation? I found that the actual injured spinal tissue is not of any therapeutic interest. There will be in all likelihood some kind of spinal surgery that the patient will have after the injury. These surgical wounds will usually need to be healed before the rehabilitation starts. There might be physical therapy for the patient's additional injuries, but a physical therapist does not evaluate joint dysfunction, restore normal joint function or stabilize injured ligaments. These have been my findings in my encounters with physical therapists, and I have reviewed their educational curriculum. They have no training in their program about diagnosis. For the most part, they feel exercise is the source of all pain relief, and if you can't move it, then they don't know what to do. Possibly, there will be some massage and compressive squeezing on the limbs to promote circulation. From my point of view, these strategies verge on neglecting the actual injuries.

Fixing the vertebral column in an unnatural position while making no attempt to reestablish the normal architectural features of the vertebral column is also common. In the case I will describe in the next section, the patient's neck was fused into kyphosis with two procedures, one anterior and one posterior. This has contributed to her long-term problems. In reviewing the spinal surgery procedures, a main focus was putting the spine into a position to give the surgeons the greatest space to get their tools, screws and plates into position. There was no thought about aligning the facets or general architecture of the normal curves of the spine. If the surgeons had been carpenters when I was a superintendent of construction, I would've had to fire them.

Once a patient is stable after these surgical interventions, the therapy starts. Again the main therapy is mastering the wheelchair obstacle course. Once this is accomplished, then an occupational therapist goes to the residence and orders necessary ramps and bars to make the home wheelchair accessible and functional for a handicapped person.

Long-term studies on these patients reported in the Archives of Rehabilitative Medicine shows that they decline over the years, post-injury. The example I use to show my objection to leaving the injured spinal tissue stretched and immobile is this: I'm going to strike your biceps muscle with a baton to contuse it. Then we're going to extend your shoulder and your elbow, stretching the biceps to its maximum length and then we are going to leave it immobile. Does anyone honestly feel that this would be an appropriate way for damaged muscle tissue to recover? I think that no matter how you've been trained, or what specialty you have, that form of treatment for a contused and bruised muscle would be inappropriate and full recovery would not be the expected outcome. This is what is done to the injured spinal cord, and providers and researchers wonder why the patient degrades neurologically over time. So I suggest a different and more appropriate method of treating injured spinal tissue. But first, the normal spinal cord and its physiology must be discussed.

THE BIOMECHANICS PHYSIOLOGY OF THE CENTRAL NERVOUS SYSTEM

- *A capillary blood flow in the spinal cord is dependent on motion.*
- *The spinal canal and cord increase in length with forward flexion.*
- *The persistent stretching of neurological tissue causes a decline in conductivity.*
- *The extension of the vertebral column shortens the canal and therefore the spinal cord.*

The spinal cord moves around in the spinal canal when the vertebral column is moving. It is not static, it has flexibility and deforms in shape and position. This is normal. The motion of the vertebral column is translated to the spinal tissue. The spinal tissue has no contractile fibers like muscle tissue does. Contractile fibers of muscle tissue are responsible for capillary blood flow, and this is accomplished even in static positions because of the tone of the muscle tissue. The tone at rest is responsible for capillary blood flow. Spinal tissue needs to be moved via the vertebral column for optimum capillary blood flow. Fixed prolonged immobility impairs the microcirculation of the capillaries of the spinal cord. So normal blood flow to the lower parts of the central nervous system are motion-dependent for optimum circulation. That means that constant sitting at computers and in motor vehicles is bad for our central nervous systems.

The spinal cord and spinal canal get longer with flexion. The spinal canal is longer than the spinal cord. The spinal cord in the adult ends around T12- L1 in the spinal canal. The canal goes from the base of the occiput to the coccyx. When a person goes into flexion, the spinal canal increases in length five to seven centimeters. There is a variation because of the difference in height among individuals. When someone goes into extension the spinal canal shortens, and so does the spinal cord. When the spinal canal is stretched into flexion, the dura mater or thecal sac will also be stretched. When we over-stretch spinal tissue, conductivity is reduced. When the spinal canal is flexed, the anterior surface changes less than the posterior surface. This makes the front of the canal shorter than the back of the canal causing the spinal cord to translate or move to the front of the canal. This causes the spinal cord to have direct contact with any bulging discs or bone spurs possibly causing increased neurological deficit. When a person bends, the side of the spinal cord also displaces to the convex side of the canal moving away from the concave side. This is accomplished by the dentate ligaments, that are on either side of the spinal cord, stretching or relaxing.

The following illustrations show the mechanics of increased canal length with flexion (*see Figure 12-1*). Also demonstrated are the length of the canal differences from the front to the back of the canal. In extension, there is a closing of the space between lamina and spinous processes, and the overall change decreases the length of the canal. In flexion, the opposite is happening, the lamina and spinous processes move away from each other and this, over the length of the vertebral column, increases the length of the canal. The anterior surface does not have as much motion with the discs in vertebral bodies, having less than the more movable laminar and spinous processes.

Fig. 12-2 A & B is a dissection where we have sequentially removed, on the left side, the lamina and spinous processes. On the right, we have additionally removed part of the occiput to reveal the cerebellum. We have left at this point C1 contact. You can see how close the upper cervical structures are to the cranium.

In the next picture, the dissection has progressed. We have removed more of the occiput, we've removed the cerebellum exposing the pons and the brain stem and we have removed part of the thecal sac. We have exposed the spinal cord and brain stem with all its fine hair-like rootlets which go off to form cranial and spinal nerve roots. You can see on the inside left of the spinal cord the beginnings of the dentate ligament.

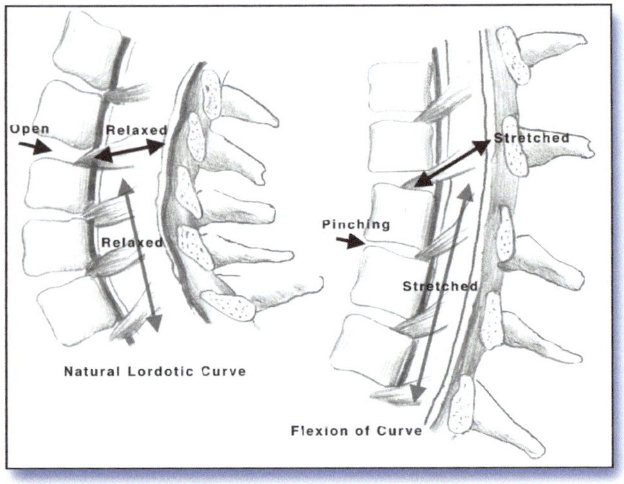

FIGURE 12-1 NORMAL ROM OF THE CERVICAL SPINE

The extension of a lordotic curve in comparison to flexion. The closeness of the lamina and spinous processes in extension shortens the posterior aspect of the canal. Compare the flexion position with the large space between each lamina and spinous process. The spinal cord and thecal sac go from being on the inside of a concavity to the outside of a convexity.

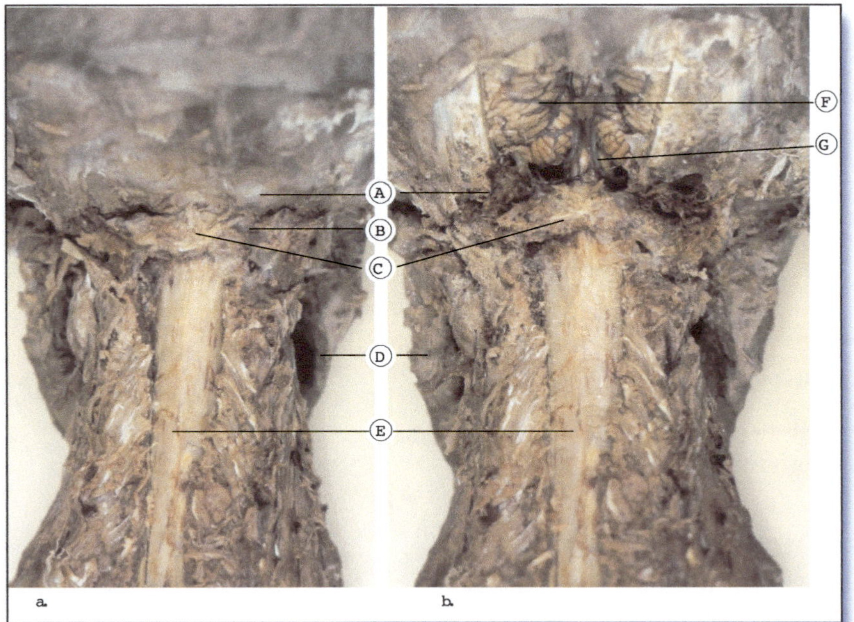

(A) Base of Skull (Occiput)

(B) Vertebral artery

(C) Atlas

(D) Mandible

(E) Thecal Sac

(F) Cerebellum

(G) Posterior Inferior Cerebellar Artery

FIGURE 12-2 A & B THE NORMAL ANATOMICAL RELATIONSHIPS OF THE SKULL AND VERTEBRAL COLUMN

Photo (a). Laminectomized specimen with skin removed from back of skull, to show relationships of structures. (Posterior view.)

Photo (b). Same specimen with occiput partially removed to show the cerebellum.

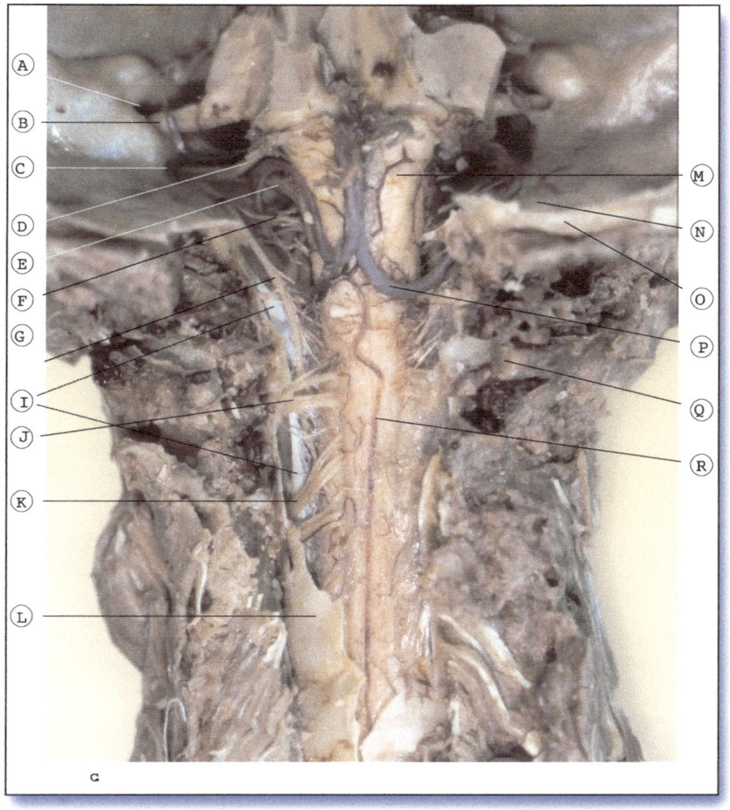

FIGURE 12-3 THE NORMAL ANATOMICAL RELATIONSHIPS, CONTINUED

Same specimen with occiput opened and cerebellum removed, with the skull in the neutral position relative to the neck.

(A) Internal Auditory Meatus

(B) Acoustic Nerve(VIII)

(C) Jugular Foramen

(D) Glossopharyngeal Nerve(IX)

(E) Vagus Nerve(X)

(F) Hypoglossal Nerve (XII)

(G) C1 nerve rootlets

(H) Spinal Accessory Nerve (XI)

(I) Dentate Ligament

(J) C2 Nerve rootlets

(K) C3 Nerve rootlets

(L) Thecal sac (dural side)

(M) Brainstem

(N) Cerebellar Fossa

(O) Occiput (cut edge)

(P) Posterior Inferior Cerebellar Artery

(Q) Arch of Atlas

(R) Dorsal Spinal Vein

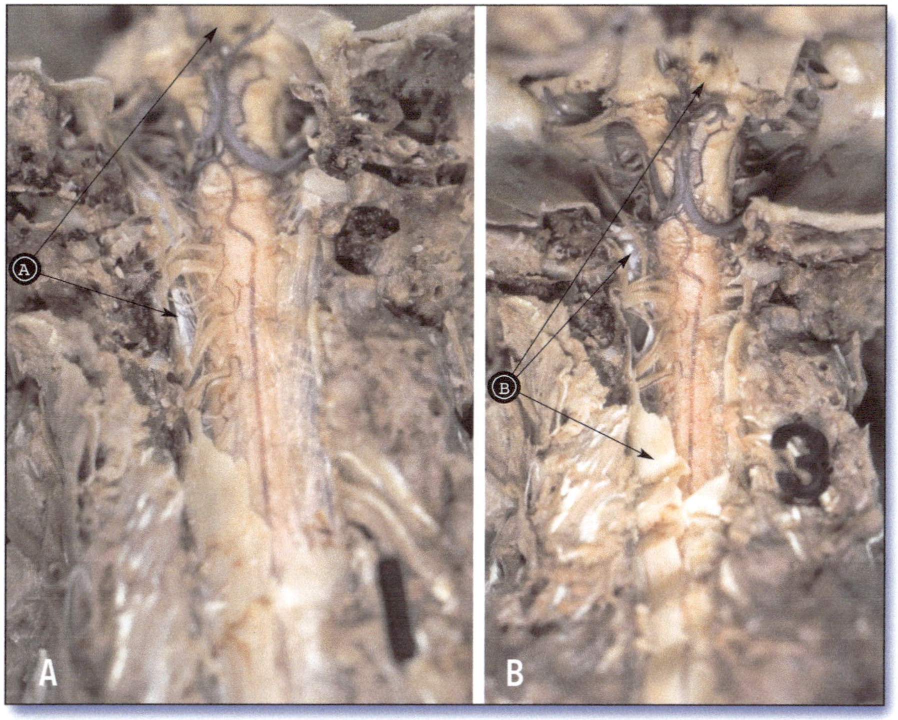

FIGURE 12-4 A & B

EFFECTS OF HEAD FLEXION AND EXTENSION ON THE CENTRAL NERVOUS SYSTEM

12-4A: Flexion(head tipped forward) increases the distance between the occiput and the coccyx, therefore lengthening the neural canal and the stretching the cord and brainstem.

A) Note the stretching of the dentate ligament and the movement of the brainstem down toward the occiput. Note positions of Dentate Ligament, Brainstem, Base of Occiput, Arch of Atlas

12-4B: Extension (head tipped backward) decreases the distance between the occiput and the coccyx, shortening and relaxing the cord and brainstem.

B) Note the relaxed left dentate ligament, the folded, relaxed dura mater (thecal sac), and the distance of the brainstem from the occiput. Note positions of Dentate Ligament, Brainstem, Base of Occiput, Arch of Atlas, Thecal sac.

Refer to Figure 12-03 for keys to anatomical structures

Fig. 12-3 A & B shows an experiment illustrating the difference between flexion and extension of the cervical spine. One study reveals that on measuring the length of the spinal canal from the base of the occiput to the bottom of C7 in flexion, and comparing it to extension, there is a difference of three centimeters in length between the two positions. The picture on the left is flexion and the one on the right is extension. Note that the picture of flexion shows the brainstem being pulled down into the upper cervical region.

With the specimen, we were also able to show that the caudae equinae in the lumbar spine stretched in flexion of the cervical spine and relaxed with the extension of the cervical spine. Most of this is detailed to a much greater extent by Dr. Alf Breig in his book *Adverse Mechanical Tension on the Central Nervous System*. He was a neurosurgeon and he would put the patient's cervical spine into extension when he was doing surgery on the lumbar spine. This would allow the caudae equinae to be relaxed and easily moved aside to avoid harm during the surgery. The subtitle to his book is *Relief by Functional Neurosurgery*. So I would think we would want to take note of these relationships that the bony canal has with the spinal tissue when we are helping someone recover from a spinal cord injury.

Fig. 12-5 is a picture of a normal spinal cord on cross-section. Note the nearly round appearance of the spinal cord and that it is laying on the back or posterior aspect of the canal. Gravity should have the cord in the back of a canal when seen on advanced

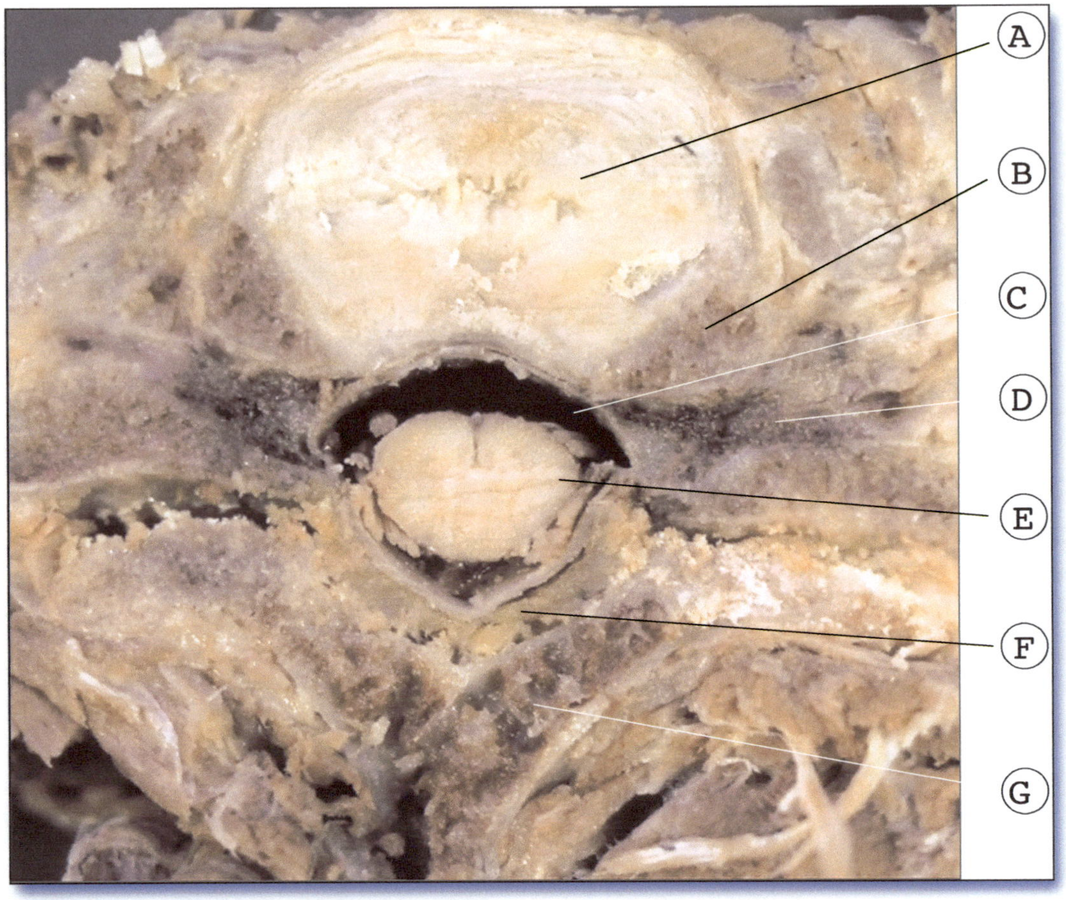

FIGURE 12-5
A CROSS SECTION OF NORMAL VERTEBRAL COLUMN

Note the spinal cord has a nearly round appearance or 1:1 ratio between the sagittal and coronal diameters. Also it is in the posterior aspect of the spinal canal indicating a relaxed lower central nervous system in the supine position, which is normal.

A. Disc
B. Uncinate process
C. Spinal canal
D. Dorsal root ganglion
E .Lateral columns of spinal cord
F. Ligamentum flavum
G. Lamina

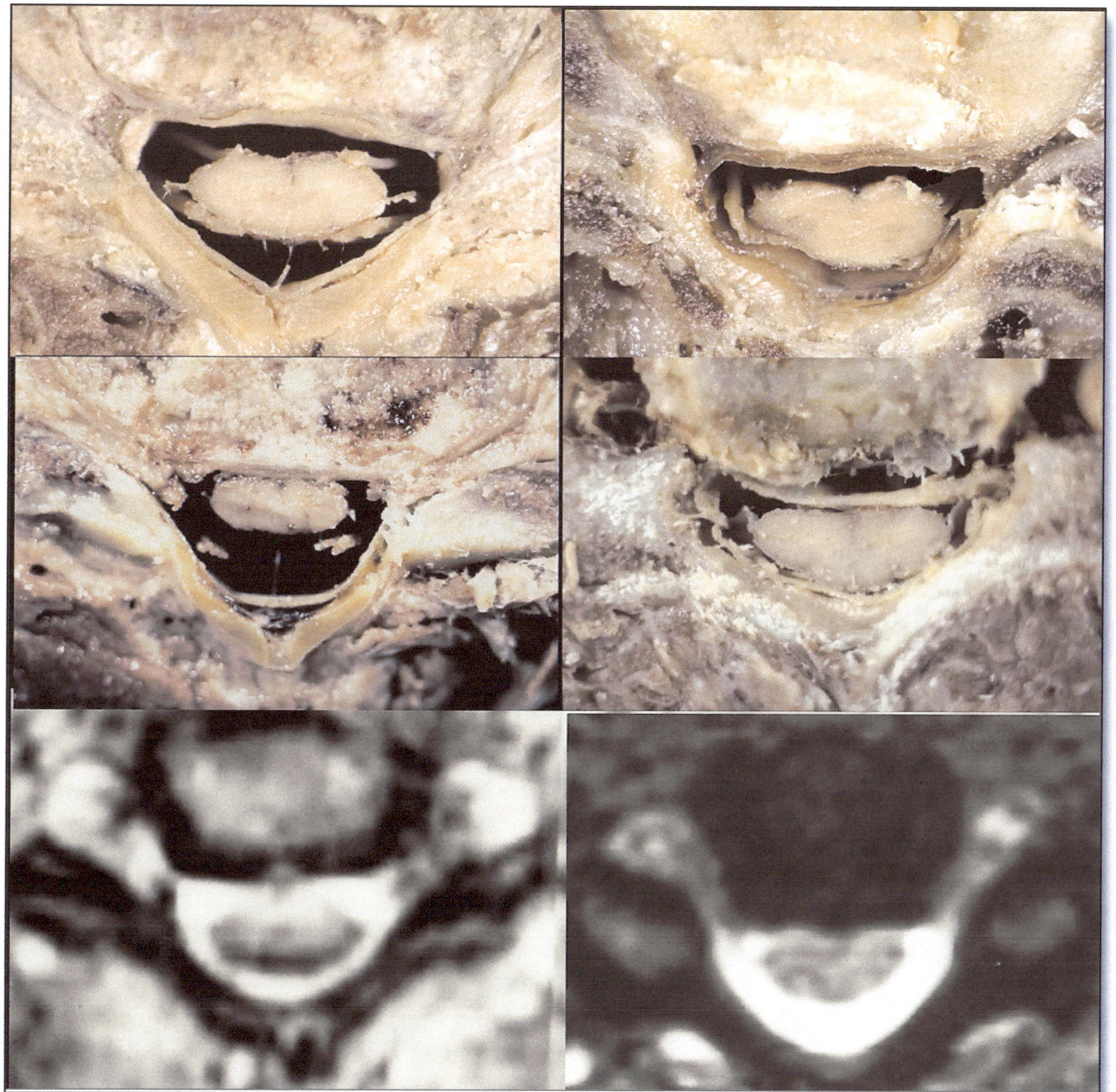

FIGURE 12-6 A SERIES OF VERTEBRAL COLUMN CROSS SECTIONS OF 6 INDIVIDUALS.

The top 4 are cadavers and the bottom 2 are patients' MRIs. All are in the supine position. Note the lack of 1:1 ratio of the saggital and coronal diameters; the oval appearance is due to an increase in length of the spinal canal and therefore the spinal cord. Both of the patients would lie down to get relief, which is the position in which the MRI was taken.

imaging. If the cord is not round and it is elevated or raised off the back canal, defying gravity, then there is adverse mechanical tension on the spinal cord. This could impair conductivity and blood flow and should be avoided.

In Fig. 12-6 top four pictures show our more typical findings. The top four are cadaver specimens and the bottom two are MRIs of living patients. They all demonstrate an increase in width from right to left, indicating that the dentate ligaments are being stretched by the increase in canal length. This tension is also raising two of them on the upper right off the back of the canal. The other two on the upper right have canal stenosis, which is an additional issue in cord compression. The bottom two pictures also demonstrate mechanical distress.

The individual on the lower left was referred to my office as a second opinion. She was suffering from left shoulder and arm pain following a motor vehicle accident. A cervical spine injury was suspected and an MRI was ordered. It was found to be relatively normal from the radiographic point of view, no herniating discs or other positive findings. I did an evaluation of her and found her left acromioclavicular joint was separated and her upper rib cage was subluxated. This could not be seen on an MRI of the cervical spine. This is another case of a mistaken assumption that radiating arm pain had to be caused by the cervical spine.

The individual in the lower right is a professor who was editing books. He realized his hands and arms were going numb as he sat at his desk with his head and neck bent. When the symptoms got to be too much, he would get up and go to his bedroom and lay down flat on his back until the symptoms went away. Then he would get up, go back and deform himself in that position at his desk until the symptoms returned. Please note that the MRI of his cervical spine was taken in the supine position – the position he would assume to get relief. We have no picture of what his spinal cord looks like when he was seated with his chin to his chest. In radiology land, the position the patient gets relief in and the position that the symptoms are produced in are not considered important. If he looks this bad in his position of relief, what does he look like when he's really irritating everything? I gave him my opinion about what we needed to do: chiropractic care with an ergonomic change to his workstation. He took his MRIs back to the neurologist that ordered the study. He returned that evening with a rigid cervical collar on his neck and reported to me that the neurologist had never looked at MRIs like that before, that I was right and he should never bend his neck again. Fortunately, he chose my less extreme (than surgery) form of intervention, and in less than three weeks, we had him working with no symptoms.

CASE HISTORY OF A QUADRIPLEGIC

Molly is a personal friend, a former co-worker from my construction days. In 1995, she fell asleep at the wheel while driving. The car cartwheeled six times. She had a fracture of C5 and C6 lamina and was told she would be a "talking vegetable" for the rest of her life. I began treating her five weeks after her surgery.

Molly had multiple injuries. In reviewing her x-ray imaging I noticed the rib cage was separated from spine. Her arms were suffering a placid paralysis. I took her left arm in my hand and put the other one up underneath her halo brace and pressed from lateral to medial. Her arm immediately toned up and she lifted it up away from my hand. She left the hospital and we started care. One of the first things we did was adjust her ribs and put her in a rib belt (*See Figure 12-8*). Her shoulders were dislocated posteriorly and her ulnas were also dislocated. Her hands were stuck in extension due to the deformation of the forearms, subluxation of her carpal bones and the beginning of contractures to the tendons and muscles from having to use a wheelchair. These upper body injuries were not examined, treated or taken into account during her "spinal rehabilitation". Adjusting and taping of her elbows and wrists gave her back some of her fine motor skills (*See Figure 12-9*).

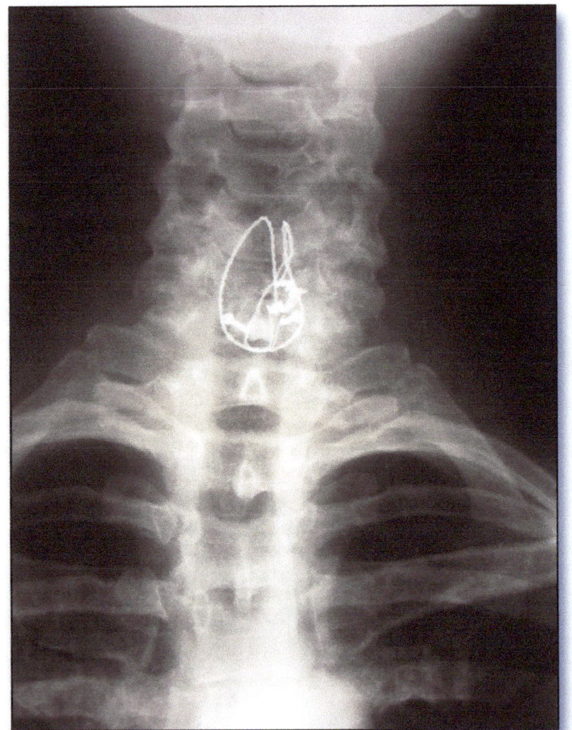

FIGURE 12-7. AP CERVICAL X-RAY POST SURGERY

The loss of the cervical curve is surgically fixed with wire posteriorly and bone anteriorly. Note the subluxated ribs that turned out to be the main cause of her upper extremity paralysis.

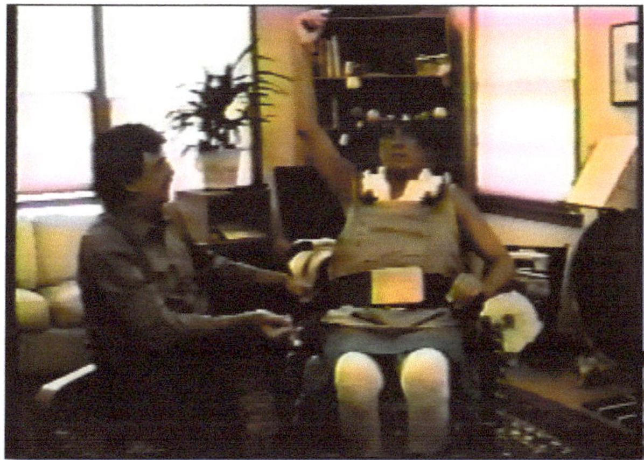

FIGURE 12-8. A "TALKING VEGETABLE" RAISES HER ARM

Adjusting ribs relieves nerves stretched by rib subluxation

FIGURE 12-9 PATIENT WITH TAPED ELBOW AND WRISTS WITH RIB BELT

Note halo brace.

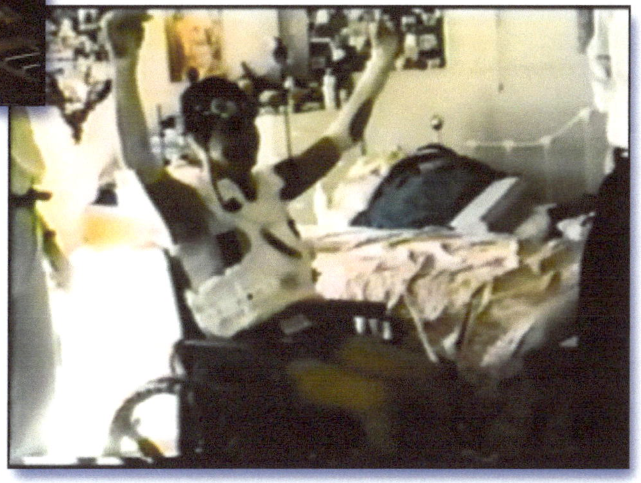

Upon her first treatment outside the hospital we unfastened the lower part of the halo brace and inserted a four-inch foam roll to induce lordosis of the lumbar spine, then bolted the halo brace back together. She started moving her legs. We have a video of this. She is far from a talking vegetable. She is quite ambulatory in the pool and is an active equestrian. Now 22 years later, she has degeneration of the spine *(see Figures 12-10 and 12-11).* She has some atrophy of her forearms and hands. Her spinal cord injury has degenerated. In her MRI view of her mid cervical spine, it is flattened and therefore stretched *(see Figure 12 – 10).* She has continued problems on all counts. I have wondered what my forearms and wrists would be like if I had luxated (dislocated) both elbows and wrists. Would there be any residuals despite not having a spinal injury?

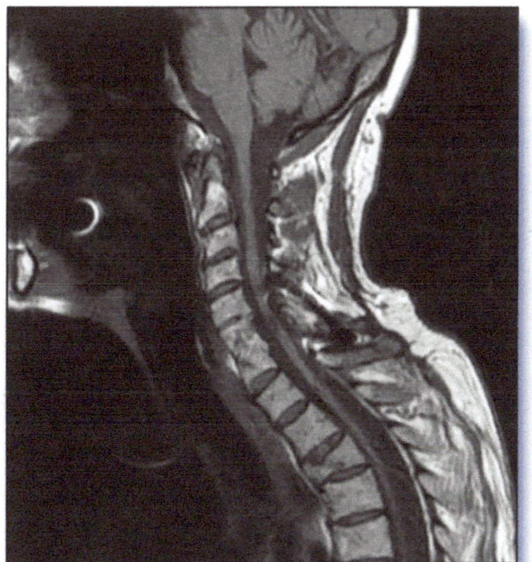

FIGURE 12-10 LATERAL MRI OF QUADRIPLEGIC

Note the mid Cervical Spine is flattened and therefore stretched.

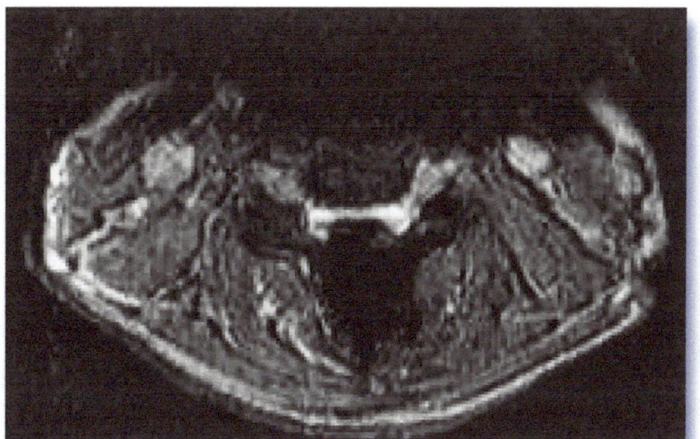

FIGURE 12-11. AXIAL MRI OF THE CERVICAL SPINE 20 YEARS LATER

Note the spinal cord is oval instead of round and therefore in a state of tension from an elongated canal

ALL INJURIES SHOULD BE IDENTIFIED AND TREATED

> *The previous chapters in this book should be used to evaluate and treat all the injuries.*

> *I have found "luxations" (complete dislocations) of peripheral joints that were affecting quality of life and functionality.*

> *The sooner these injuries are treated, the less likely that they will turn into permanent impairments.*

> *Chiropractors should be on site in hospitals so these patients will have the best chance to recover.*

OPTIMAL TREATMENT FOR THE INJURED SPINAL CORD.

> *The Vertebral Column, if possible, should have the normal curves supported to establish the relaxed Spinal Cord. (Avoid surgeries that lengthen the canal, i.e. putting a Kyphosis in the Cervical Spine.)*

> *A motion machine should be used to establish CFS and capillary blood flow. (CHI Machine) This allows passive motion to be used to increase circulation in the injured spinal tissue. (See Figure 12-14)*

> *Avoid stretching and flexing the spinal canal until recovery is under way.*

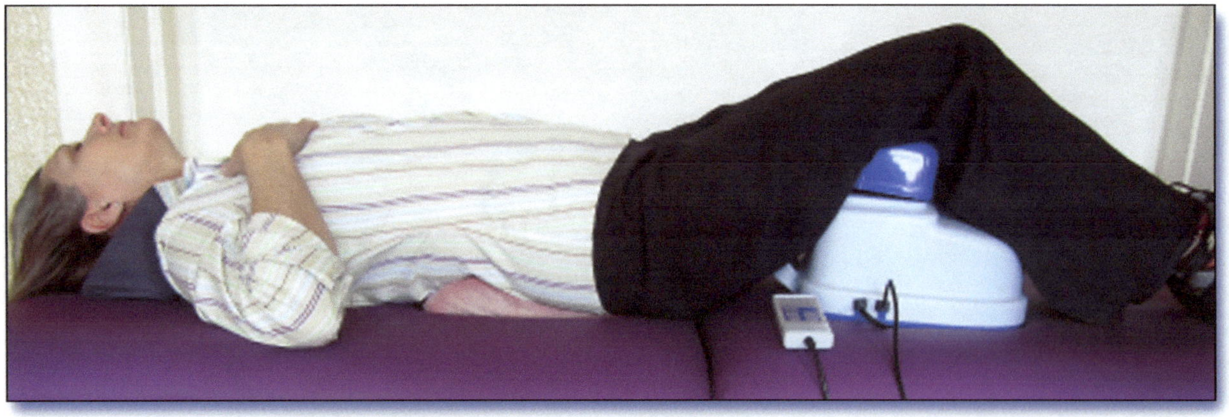

FIGURE 12-14. PATIENT WITH SPINAL CURVES SUPPORTED WITH A CHI MACHINE

Note the cervical fulcrum supporting the cervical curve and lumbar support for the lumbar curve. The CHI Machine is not under the ankles as directed by the instructions, but under the thighs. This reduces the motion into the spine.

GLOSSARY · INDEX

abdominal oblique muscles (internal and external) • 23

The external obliques originate at the lower eight ribs and insert at the iliac crest and linea alba (midline aponeurosis). Contraction of both compresses the abdomen. Contraction of one side alone bends the vertebral column laterally. Also rotates vertebral column. A disruption in the pelvic girdle will cause these muscles to partially or fully contract causing a disruption in the spinal curve and muscle guarding.

AC Compression Test • 70

An Orthopedic test that involves the sustained (30 Seconds) compression or depression of the distal clavicle with the doctorís hand and noting changes in the symptoms. A positive finding is relief from the complaints and results in a diagnosis of a subluxated distal clavicle or a ìseparated shoulderî or AC joint separation

AC Joint • 71

The joint between the acromion (part of the scapula) and the clavicle.

acromion 69

A bony projection of the scapula that articulates with the clavical. Commonly called the "AC Joint."

adhesions • 71

A joining of parts normally free to move independently to each other with fascia. This occurs as a response to injury, edema, or irritation due to subluxation and resulting altered motion.

Adjustment, adjusting

A specific manual procedure that realigns joints.

A.L.L. • 90

Anterior longitudinal ligament

allopathic • 11

The name given to "Western Medicine", which emphasizes pharmaceutical and surgery interventions.

anterior longitudinal ligament • 90

A broad ligament that extends from the occipital bone to the sacrum. It supports the vertebral column and unites the vertebrae anteriorly.

antero/posterior

Directed from the front toward the back.

apex • 26

1. The outermost point of a convexity.
2. The apex of the sacrum is at the bottom where it joins with the coccyx.

arthritis • 7

Inflammation of a joint. The most common arthritic inflammatory condition of the spine is caused by subluxation.

atlas • 59

The first cervical vertebra, C1, having a two point weight bearing system, lacking a body, and articulating superiorly with the occipital condyles of the occipital bone, which permits nodding of the head. The atlas articulates differently with C2, the axis, at the inferior articular facets.

avascular • 22

Lacking a direct supply of blood; oxygen, carbon dioxide, nutrients, and waste, all diffuse through connective tissue via motion.

axial • 58

1. Pertaining to the axis, C2.
2. Pertaining to the axial plane of the Cartesian coordinate system, the Y plane. 3. Pertaining to the axial skeleton, consisting of the bones of the skull, hyoid, ribs, sternum, and vertebral column.

Axilla • 43

The area under the arm that is the lateral part of the chest

axis • 10

The second cervical vertebra, C2, is the first three-point weight bearing system in the vertebral column. The dens of the axis projects through the atlas, C1, and makes a pivot on which the head and atlas rotate, permitting side-to-side rotation of the head. The axis articulates superiorly with the atlas at the two superior articular facets and inferiorly with C3 at the two inferior articular facets and the body of the vertebra via the intervertebral disc.

Babinski's Reflex

Stroking the bottom of the great toe causing it to extended and flinch. If it occurs is a "positive Babinski" and indicates Upper Motor Neuron lesion, i.e. brain damage.

Backwards push • 36

The maneuver that pushes or moves the anterior innominate posteriorly or backwards

brain stem • 151

The portion of the brain immediately superior to the spinal cord, made up of the medulla oblongata, pons, and midbrain. The brain stem is contiguous with the spinal cord and subject to forces initiated in the vertebral column. The blood supply to the brain stem is dependent on the integrity of the vertebral artery.

Calcaneal Draw Test • 130

An orthopedic test that involves the doctor gripping the foot and with the heel contacting a firm surface pushing the heel towards the toes. It can be done with the hands; the doctor grips the lower leg and with the other hand grips the heel and draws it towards the toes. A positive test is relief of plantar fascia pain, medial arch pain and or big toe pain.

canal stenosis • 15

The narrowing of the spinal canal.
1. A congenital condition, a narrower canal than normal, can be a silent condition until injury occurs.
2. A developed or acquired spinal canal stenosis is a result of subluxation of vertebrae and the subsequent widening endplates.

Cartesian Coordinate System • 20

A three-dimensional coordinate system in which the coordinates of a point are its distances from three intersecting perpendicular straight lines or planes. These are described as the X, Y and Z axes or planes. It is used to describe position in human anatomy.

central nervous system • 11

The part of the nervous system that is condensed and centrally located; the brain and spinal cord.

cerebellum • 150

The portion of the brain lying posterior to the medulla and pons, concerned with coordination of movement. Damage can cause ataxia (lack of muscle coordination), disturbance of gait, and severe dizziness. The position of the cerebellum in the occiput can be changed with vertebral column changes. The blood supply is vertebral artery dependent.

cervical • 8

Of or pertaining to the neck.

cervical curve 62

An essential architectural feature of the human spine. Changes in the shape of the cervical spine result in central nervous system deformation and joint pathology. The cervical curve is lordotic or the convex side of the curve is ventral.

chronic • 9

Long-term or frequently recurring.

chronic inflammation

A long-term, localized protective response to tissue injury designed to destroy, dilute, or wall off an infecting agent or injured tissue. Characterized by redness, pain, heat, swelling, and sometimes loss of function. Loss of joint integrity generates inflammation.

clavicle • 44

The collarbone. The medial end of the clavicle, the sternal end, is rounded and articulates with the sternum. The broad, flat, lateral end, the acromial extremity, articulates with the acromion of the scapula. These articulations are primarily ligaments and capsules and form the only bony articulation of the pectoral girdle to the chest.

coccyx • 149

The lowermost element in the backbone. It is the fusion of the three or four coccygeal vertebrae and is triangular in shape. Articulates superiorly with the sacrum. The sacrococcygeal ligament is contiguous with the sacrotuberous ligaments.

conductivity • 82

The capacity of a tissue to conduct current.

contracture • 101

1. A permanent shortening of a soft tissue, such as a muscle or tendon, so that it cannot passively attain its normal length.
2. A state of diminished or loss of compliance of a normally pliant tissue. A shortening with a decrease range of motion, a common feature of chronic subluxation.

coronal • 71

1.The frontal plane. It divides the body into anterior (front) and posterior (back) portions.
2.The X plane in the Cartesian Coordinate System.

cortex • 113

1. The dense bone that forms the external surface of a bone called cortical bone.
2 The outer part of an organ.

cortical bone

The dense outer wall of a bone.

costotransverse • 16

Pertaining to the ribs and transverse processes of the vertebrae. The transverse process is posterior to the rib and articulates with the neck of the rib.

costo-vertebral • 16

Of or pertaining to a rib and a vertebrae. The typical costo-vertebral joint (T2-T10) is a three joint complex made up of the head of the rib, superior and inferior demifacets and the intervertebral disc.

cross section • 152

1. A section formed by a plane cutting through an object, usually at right angles to an axis.
2. The Z plane of the Cartesian coordinate system.

cranium/cranial

The cranium can be defined as the bones of the skull that protects the brain and the organs of sight, hearing, and balance, including the frontal, parietal, temporal, occipital, sphenoid, and ethmoid bones. Cranial can be defined as a subdivision of the superior body cavity formed by the cranial bones and containing the brain.

decompression • 9

In physical medicine the act of stretching or pulling apart segments of the body. To increase space or open an area.

Deconditioning • 18

The state of becoming less capable of doing Activities of Daily Living

degeneration • 32

The deterioration of the cells of a tissue by alteration of the tissue. A pathological process of a progressive nature.

degenerative joint disease • 19

A chronic joint disease characterized by a degeneration of articular cartilage, hypertrophy of bone, and formation of new bone in the subchondral areas and margins of the joint, particularly the weight-bearing joints. The most common pathological feature of this condition is subluxation and resulting loss of joint space.

dehydration • 113

The removal or reduction of water from the body or from a substance.

dermatomal • 111

The distribution of sensation by specific nerve structures, identifiable nerve roots that go to certain areas.

deviation • 26

1. A variation from normal.
2. Displacement of one of the bodyís masses relative to the others. When at rest, it is no longer aligned with one or more coordinate system planes.

disc • 9

The intervertebral disc.

Distal • 68

The end of the structure further away from the center or top of the body.

DJD, D.J.D.

Degenerative joint disease.

dorsal • 9

Relative to or situated on the posterior or back surface; opposite of ventral. Synonym: thoracic.

erector spinae • 20

This is the largest muscular mass of the back and consists of three groupings: iliocostalis, longissimus, and spinalis. These groups, in turn, consist of a series of interlapping muscles. The iliocostalis group is laterally placed, the longissimus group is intermediate in placement, and the spinalis group is medially placed. The proprioceptive links are to the sacroiliac joints and the position of the ilium relative to the ribs and vertebrae.

extension • 55

The straightening of a joint so that the two adjacent segments are moved apart, thereby decreasing the joint angle. Relating to the vertebral canal, when the head and or spine is tipped backward the canal length is shortened.

extremity • 14

1. A distal or terminal portion.
2. An arm or leg.

facet

The posterior zygopophyseal joints of the spine. They are endowed with articular cartilage and synovial capsules, with a shape and planar geometry specific to the area of the spine in which they occur. These capsules are imbedded with proprioceptors.

fascia • 112

A sheet or band of connective tissue that envelops muscles and muscle groups, usually of similar function. Fascia is pervasive and interconnects with the body tissues. It can proliferate with injury and chronic inflammation, causing adhesions.

FIB-TIB Squeeze Test • 117

An Orthopedic test involving the doctor squeezing the lower leg bones together near the top of the lower leg for 20-30 seconds to see if there is any relief of symptoms

fibrocartilage • 22

Cartilage that contains dense, parallel bundles of collagenous fibers in the matrix. The bundles are separated by narrow clefts containing chondrocytes. This type of cartilage is found in the intervertebral discs, the pubis symphysis, and at the attachments of tendons and ligaments to bone.

Fibromyalgia • 12, 13

A chronic condition involving multiple subluxations that are not corrected, resulting in persistent guarding of the injuries. The symptoms are pain, trigger points, contractures, lymphatic and vascular changes.

Fibrous • 21

Containing or composed of fibers.

flexion • 84

The act of bending or condition of being bent. In the spine, it can refer to forward bending, head moving towards knees, elongating the spinal canal and spinal cord.

foramen • 58

An opening, orifice, perforation, or passage through which nerves or blood vessels pass. Usually found in bones.

fusion • 7

1. The normal process for bone formation.
2. The end stage of the degenerative process of joint pathology, i.e. the end stage of degenerative joint disease.

guarding • 11

A description of a functional aspect of muscle tissue, a muscle spasm i.e. to protect a distressed joint complex. this is a neurological reflex.

Hallicus tendon (Big Toe)

The big toe muscle (hallicus) has a tendon that passes uder the medial arch of the foot, calcaneal subluxation can inflame this tendon

herniation • 15

A rupture of an intervertebral disc so that the nucleus pulposus protrudes outside the annulus fibrosus. Trauma and other excessive forces on the disc can result in a loss of annulus fibrosus integrity.

hyperkyphosis • 93

A kyphosis of the thoracic spine greater than normal range.

iliacus • 23

The iliacus originates at the iliac fossa and inserts at the tendon of the psoas major. Action is to flex and rotate the thigh laterally and also flexes the vertebral column. Innervation is at the femoral nerve. Proprioceptive links are to the sacroiliac joint and the pubis symphysis.

ITB or Iliotibial band • 114

Muscle/fascia structure that arises off the top of the proximal fibula and attaches to the top of Illium, covering the lateral thigh. Fibula subluxation can result in IT Band Syndrome.

ilium • 21

The ilium is the largest of the three original bones of the hip. Its superior border, the iliac crest, ends anteriorly in the anterior superior iliac spine. Posteriorly, the iliac crest ends in the posterior superior iliac spine.

imbibition • 22

The flow of fluid through tissue via motion.

inferior • 23

Lower in place or position.

inflammation • 19

The reaction of living tissues to all forms of injury and irritation. It is a vascular and neurological process characterized by heat, redness, swelling, pain, and loss of function.

innominate • 19

The hip bone. In early life it is three bones, the ilium, ischium and pubis. The three bones fuse as the individual reaches adolescence.

intercostal

Between the ribs.

Interosseous ligament • 78

There is one between the ulna and radius and

another between the tibia and fibula. Both cam become injured and cause pain and other symptoms in the arm and the leg.

intervertebral disc • 19

Composed of a nucleus pulposus (center) and an annulus fibrosus (outer wall). It is largly composed of water and therefore a hydraulic system and it transmits force to the vertebral body. It is, therefore, not a shock absorber but allows a flexible vertebral column (this is essential to spinal cord vascular function).

ischial tuberosity • 24

The blunt, inferior aspect of the ischium on which the body rests in the sitting position.

ischium

The inferior and posterior of the three bones that make up the innominate. It contains a prominent ischial spine, a lesser sciatic notch below the spine, and an ischial tuberosity. The rest of the ischium, the ramus, joins with the pubis and together they surround the obturator foramen.

I.V.D. • 19

Intervertebral disc.

kyphosis • 59

Pertaining to a kyphotic curve.

kyphotic curve • 62

A normal architectural feature of the human vertebral column in the thoracic and sacral regions. It is characterized by the concavity of the curve facing the ventral or anterior surface. Alteration of the kyphotic curve changes the shape of the central nervous system and other associated tissues.

lamina • 61

The flat bone that forms the roof of the posterior vertebral arch. In a typical vertebra, it is a paired structure on either side of the midline that unites posteriorly to form the spinous process.

Laminectomized or laminectomy • 14

The surgical removal of the posterior bony arches of one or more vertebrae in order to expose the neural elements in the spinal cord. A laminectomy allows inspection of the spinal canal as well as identification and removal of pathologic tissues from the cord and roots.

lateral • 14

On the side. Opposite of medial.

ligament • 7

A cord, band, or sheet of fibrous connective tissue linking two or more bones, cartilages, or other structures together. A ligament imparts stability, usually to a joint, preventing excessive motion in certain directions. It is embedded with proprioceptors and other nerve structures.

ligamentum flavum • 152

Any of a series of bands of yellow elastic tissue attached to and extending between the ventral portions of the laminae of two adjacent vertebrae, from the junction of the axis and the third cervical vertebra to the junction of the fifth lumbar vertebra and the sacrum. They assist in maintaining the erect position of the spine and serve to close the spaces between the vertebral arches.

lordosis • 14

Pertaining to a lordotic curve.

lordotic curve • 62

A normal architectural feature of the human vertebral column in the cervical and lumbar regions. It is the angle formed by perpendicular lines drawn from the superior endplate of L1 and the inferior endplate of L5. Alteration of these curves changes the shape of the central nervous system and other tissues.

lumbar • 13

Pertaining to the lower region of the Lumbar spine or pertaining to the lower region of the spine, specifically the lower five vertebrae, L1-L5.

lumbar curve • 157

An essential architectural feature of the human

spine. Changes in the shape of the lumbar region of the spine result in central nervous system deformation and joint pathology. The lumbar curve is lordotic or the convex side of the curve is facing the ventral or anterior surface.

luxation • 11, 12

A complete dislocation of an articulation.

magnetic resonance imaging • 7

An imaging technique that employs radio frequency waves and a strong magnetic field to produce clinically useful images. The resulting image gives excellent soft tissue contrast without bony artifact. There is also excellent imaging of medullary bone.

mandible • 58

The lower jawbone. The bone comprises the tooth-bearing, horseshoe shaped body and two upright plates of bone, the rami, each of which is surmounted by two processes, an anterior process called coronoid and a posterior, or condyloid process and articulates with the temporal bone.

mastoid process • 58

A rounded projection of the temporal bone posterior to the external auditory meatus.

medullary bone

The marrow part of bone, the space within the diaphysis of a bone.

MRI • 7

Magnetic resonance imaging. A form of advanced imaging.

nerve root • 58

One of the two bundles of nerve fibers that emerge from the spinal cord to join together as a spinal nerve. These bundles are the dorsal and ventral nerve roots.

nerve rootlets • 58

Hair-like fibers extending from the spinal cord. They converge laterally and gather into a nerve root.

neuron • 139

A nerve cell consisting of a cell body, dendrites, and an axon.

neutral position • 61

Normal anatomical position; body is erect and facing observer, arms hanging at the sides with palms turned forward.

neurovascular bundle • 128

A grouping of nerves and blood vessels that both innervate and supply blood to a given region.

nucleus pulposus

The central, semielastic, spongy zone of the intervertebral disc. It is a hydrodynamic structure that has a greater fluid content than the rest of the disc and is composed of glycoproteins and interlaced collagen fibers.

ossification • 90

Formation of or conversion into bone.

osteoarthritis • 7

A progressive joint disorder characterized by a deterioration of the articular cartilage and reactive new bone formation in the subchondral regions. Although the name implies an inflammation, this process is not primarily inflammatory, therefore, it can more accurately be called degenerative joint disease. This condition can occur as a result of the pathogenesis of subluxation.

osteophyte • 43

A projection or outgrowth of bone; a bone spur. The tissue attaching or inserting into bone can be under mechanical distress causing its calcification and forming the outgrowth.

osteoporosis • 10

A common bone disorder characterized by decreased density of normally mineralized bone resulting in bone fragility. Causes of osteoporosis are post-menopausal, age-related, disuse, dietary deficiencies, chronic illness, neoplasm, endocrine abnormalities, genetic disorders, and idiopathic problems.

pedicle

A bony process projecting backward from the body of a vertebra, which connects with the lamina on either side.

pelvis/pelvic girdle • 10

The bony, basin-shaped ring that provides the weight-bearing for the trunk and lower extremities while protecting the lower abdominal viscera. It consists of the two innominate bones that articulate posteriorly with the sacrum. Distally, the pelvis articulates with the proximal end of the femurs at the acetabuli. The pelvic ring is joined posteriorly by the sacroiliac joint and anteriorly by the symphysis pubis. More than half of an individuals muscle mass arises from the pelvis.

pelvic shearing • 24

A non-physiologic displacement of the innominates relative to each other in the Y and/ or Z planes. Significant ligament injury occurs in both the sacroiliac joints and the pubis symphysis.

Palpation, palpate • 7

The act of touching a patient to determine information, i.e.: does something hurt

PIIS

posterior inferior iliac spine

P.L.L.

Posterior longitudinal ligament

pons • 150

Part of the CNS that lies directly above the medulla and anterior to the cerebellum. It connects the spinal cord with the brain and parts of the brain with each other. The longitudinal fibers of the pons belong to the motor and sensory tracts that connect the spinal cord or medulla with the upper part of the brain stem.

posterior • 9

Rear, back, or dorsal surfaces of the body.

posterior longitudinal ligament

A ligament that runs on the posterior surfaces of the vertebral bodies, extending from the axis down through the entire length of the vertebral column, and fanning out at the vertebral margins to reinforce the intervertebral discs.

proprioception • 141

The sensation of position and change of position of the body and its parts. Proprioception is transmitted through special organs, most of which are in muscles, tendons and joint tissues.

protrusion

The state of being thrust beyond a boundary forward or laterally.

Proximal • 100

The end of a structure closer to the center or top of the body.

PSIS

The posterior superior iliac spine.

psoas major • 38

The psoas major originates at the transverse processes and bodies of the lumbar vertebrae and inserts at the lesser trochanter of the femur. The action flexes and rotates the thigh laterally and also flexes the vertebral column. Innervated at the lumbar nerves L2-L3. It has a proprioceptive link to the sacroiliac joints and pubis symphsis. The lumbar nerve roots exit the spine into the psoas and the lumbar plexus is in the belly and tendons of the muscle. The psoas attaches to the diaphragm.

pubis symphysis

The pubis symphysis has annular rings and a spongy center, is avascular, and motion is a major component of its physiology. This joint can tear and subluxate and suffer major stability problems. Misalignment of this joint automatically misalign one or both sacroiliac joints. Proprioceptive links are to the psoas, iliacus, all the hip muscles, medial and anterior muscles of the thigh and the abdominal and erector groups.

rectus abdominus

The rectus abdominus originates at the pubic crest and pubis symphysis and inserts at the cartilage of the fifth to seventh ribs and the xiphoid process. Action is to compress the abdomen to aid in defecation, urination, forced expiration, and childbirth. It also flexes the vertebral column. Innervation is from the branches of thoracic nerves T7-T12. Proprioceptive innervation is between pubic bone and lower rib cage. Unilateral rectus abdominus splinting can be a sign of pubis symphysis subluxation.

recumbent position • 53

The body position of lying down on a horizontal surface.

Rib • 4

A curved, slightly twisted strip of bone that forms part of the skeleton of the thorax. There are twelve pairs of ribs. The head of each rib articulates with one of the twelve thoracic vertebrae. The other end is attached to a section of cartilage. The first seven pairs, the true ribs, are connected directly to the sternum by their costal cartilages. The next three pairs, the false ribs, are attached indirectly to the sternum. Each is connected by its cartilage to the rib above it. The last two pairs, the floating ribs, end freely in the muscles of the anterior body wall.

Rib Cage Compression Test

An orthopedic test that is performed with a patient with loss of cervical range of motion and or neck pain complaints. It involves the doctor standing behind the patient and who places their hands in the axilla under each arm, as high or superior as possible. The doctor compresses the ribs towards the center, compressing the ribs. During sustained compression the patient reassess range of motion or other complaints. The test is positive for increased range of motion or reduction of other complaints.

rotation • 25

The turning or moving of a part around its axis of rotation. The unit of measure is degrees or radians.

sacral apex • 26

The inferior aspect of the sacrum, articulating with the superior portion of the coccyx.

sacral base • 28

The superior aspect of the sacrum, articulating with the inferior portion of L5.

sacral disc

The disc between sacral segments. As the sacrum ages, it begins to fuse, becoming for all practical purposes, a single but flexible bone. When these bones, S1-S5, articulate, the intersacral discs remain in place and act just the same as the intervertebral discs of the other vertebrae. The cortex of the sacrum is contiguous but this must be a flexible structure. Physiological function of intrasacral discs necessitates motion as the only mechanism of nutrition and waste elimination. The sacral discs do what the intervertebral discs do: confer flexibility. There is only one mechanism for fluid and nutrient exchange for the intervertebral disc and that is imbibition through motion. This must also be true for sacral disc physiology and function.

sacroiliac joint • 19

The paired articulations between the sacrum and the iliac bone in the pelvis. These two joint complexes are different in each individuals. Some of the factors are the size of the joint, size of each portion, shape of each portion, and orientation of each portion to each other. These factors could explain the different responses to the same treatment with the same diagnosis.

sacroiliac ligament • 32
(anterior and posterior)

Anterior: This ligament is contiguous with periosteum of ilium and sacrum. This is one of the structures involved with S.I. joint injuries, sustaining a sprain with either physiological or non-physiological subluxations.
Posterior: This ligament is contiguous with and attached to the lumbosacral fascia from above and the medial attachment of the gluteus maximus muscle from below. It connects the sacrum and

the ilium behind and forms the chief connection between these bones.

sacrospinous ligament

The ligament from the lateral edge of the sacrum to the spine of the ischium. This ligament along with the sacrotuberous ligament is primarily responsible for conferring motion to the sacrum. As the leg swings forward for heel strike, the innominate nutates with the ilium moving posterior and the ischial tuberosity moving forward and via the sacrotuberous and sacrospinous ligaments, moves the ipsilateral side of the sacrum forward.

sacrotuberous ligament

The ligament from the lateral edge of the sacrum to the ischial tuberosity. Fibers of the sacrotuberous can be contiguous with the tendon of the biceps femoris. Unilateral shortening of the ligament can rotate and or angle the sacrum between the ilium creating a contralateral stretching and irritation to various structures, this could be a factor in a number of syndromes. The sacrotuberous ligament, along with the sacrospinous ligament, confer motion to the sacrum with motion of the leg.

sacrum • 20

The sacrum is a triangular shaped bone formed by the partial fusion of sacral vertebrae. It articulates laterally with the ilium, superiorly with L5, and inferiorly with the coccyx. The sacrum is five separate segments in the child and S1-S5 are fused by age 25 to form, for all practical purposes, a single but flexible bone.

sagittal • 154

A vertical plane that divides the body into left and right portions.

segment • 61

A portion of a larger body or structure.

shearing • 24

A type of deforming force applied in the axial plane to the spine resulting in angular deformation. Involves numerous ligament, joint, muscle and nervous tissue structures besides the vertebrae.

Shoulder Compression Test

An orthopedic test that involves the doctor standing behind the patient and with their hands compresses the shoulders of the patient together for 30 seconds or more. This test is to bring the two sternal clavicular joints together, reducing joint distress found on examination. Sterno-clavicular joint injury can cause headaches, sinus pain, vertigo, loss of hearing and difficulty swallowing among other complaints. The test is positive when relief of symptoms occurs during the test.

SI joint

Sacroiliac joint

soft tissue • 14

The non-osseous tissue of the body, including intervertebral discs, tendons, muscle, the brain, connective tissues, nerves, vascular structures and ligaments.

spasm • 28

Involuntary musculature contraction. It can be due to proprioceptive sensory bombardment, peripheral nerve entrapment or central nervous distress, all of which can be due to subluxation.

spinal canal • 11

A continuous channel running longitudinally through the vertebral column. The anterior wall is formed by the posterior surfaces of the vertebral bodies and intervertebral discs and by the posterior longitudinal ligament. The posterior wall is formed by the vertebral laminae, the ligamentum flava and the intervertebral foramina. Canal length (flexion increases 5-7 cm the length over extension) and shape (side bending and rotation create a concave-convex formation of the lateral surfaces of the canal) are affected by the shape or posture of the spinal column. The anatomic relationship with the spinal cord and caudae equinae determine the shape of the lower central nervous system. A kyphosis of the cervical spine is a flexion deformity that affects the entire length of the canal, spinal cord, brain stem and nerve roots.

spinous process • 60

That part of a vertebra that projects posteriorly from the arch, producing a lever arm for introduction of motion by attaching muscle groups.

stenosis • 151

A narrowing of an opening or passage, such as the spinal canal, can be congenital or acquired. It is a common finding with chronic subluxation with involved segments.

Sterno-clavicular joint • 47

The joint that the clavical has with the manubrium of the sternum. It is a very important joint that can cause headaches, sinus pain, hearing loss, vertigo, difficulty swallowing among other symptoms when injured..

subluxation • 4

Loss of joint alignment and integrity. This describes an injury to the joint structures such as the ligaments, discs, joint capsules, supporting tendons, and fascia. Subluxation is the most common etiology of osteoarthritis and is characterized by immobilization, inflammation, pain and muscle spasms.

superior • 20

Situated above or towards the upper part of the body; opposite of inferior.

supine • 25

Lying on the dorsal surface with the face upward.

sympathetic chain • 46

Long nerve complexes on each side of the vertebral column from the base of the skull to the coccyx. It is the extravertebral portion of the central nervous system containing part of the autonomic nervous system.

sympathetic nervous system

One of the two subdivisions of the autonomic nervous system, having cell bodies of preganglionic neurons in the lateral gray columns of the thoracic segment and first two or three lumbar segments of the spinal cord. It is primarily concerned with processes involving the expenditure of energy. Paravertebral ganglia as well as spinal nerve roots have been observed to be adversely affected by chronic degenerative processes of the vertebral column.

synovial joint • 22

A joint in which there is a space between the articulating bones. A synovial joint is freely movable and is classified as a diarthroses. They are surrounded by a capsule and held together by ligaments. Disruption of normal relationships (subluxation) causes inflammation, muscle guarding and limited range of motion leading to arthritic changes if allowed to become chronic.

Talus • 128

The ankle bone, it articulates with the lower leg bones at itís top and with the heel or calcaneus at itís bottom.

Tempromandibular joint • 59

The mandible is the lower jaw, itís joint with the part of the skull, called the temporal bone, is the Tempromandibular joint or TMJ.

tendon/tendinous

A band of dense fibrous tissue that forms the termination of a muscle and attaches it to a bone. When the muscle contracts, it pulls on the tendon, which moves the bone. The tendons are embedded with proprioceptors and other neurological structures.

tethered cord syndrome

A collection of signs, symptoms and complaints that are the result of central nervous system distress from chronic elongation of the neural canal in the vertebral column. Characterized by translation of the spinal cord into the anterior canal wall obliterating the patency of the anterior spinal artery. Also known as filum terminale syndrome or cord traction syndrome.

www.ingramcontent.com/pod-product-compliance
Lightning Source LLC
LaVergne TN
LVHW070818210926
848482LV00004B/288